Quick Look Nursing:

Oxygenation

Second Edition

LISA KENNEDY SHELDON, PHD(c), ARNP
St. Joseph Hospital
Nashua, NH

JONES AND BARTLETT PUBLISHERS
Sudbury, Massachusetts
BOSTON   TORONTO   LONDON   SINGAPORE

World Headquarters
Jones and Bartlett Publishers
40 Tall Pine Drive
Sudbury, MA 01776
978-443-5000
info@jbpub.com
www.jbpub.com

Jones and Bartlett Publishers Canada
6339 Ormindale Way
Mississauga, Ontario L5V 1J2
CANADA

Jones and Bartlett Publishers
International
Barb House, Barb Mews
London W6 7PA
United Kingdom

Jones and Bartlett's books and products are available through most bookstores and online booksellers. To contact Jones and Bartlett Publishers directly, call 800-832-0034, fax 978-443-8000, or visit our website www.jbpub.com.

The authors, editor, and publisher have made every effort to provide accurate information. However, they are not responsible for errors, omissions, or for any outcomes related to the use of the contents of this book and take no responsibility for the use of the products and procedures described. Treatments and side effects described in this book may not be applicable to all people; likewise, some people may require a dose or experience a side effect that is not described herein. Drugs and medical devices are discussed that may have limited availability or are controlled by the Food and Drug Administration (FDA) for use only in a research study or clinical trial. Research, clinical practice, and government regulations often change the accepted standard in this field. When consideration is being given to use of any drug in the clinical setting, the health care provider or reader is responsible for determining FDA status of the drug, reading the package insert, and reviewing prescribing information for the most up-to-date recommendations on dose, precautions, and contraindications, and determining the appropriate usage for the product. This is especially important in the case of drugs that are new or seldom used.

Production Credits
Executive Editor: Kevin Sullivan
Acquisitions Editor: Emily Ekle
Associate Editor: Amy Sibley
Editorial Assistant: Patricia Donnelly
Production Director: Amy Rose
Production Editor: Carolyn F. Rogers
Senior Marketing Manager: Katrina Gosek
Associate Marketing Manager: Rebecca Wasley
Manufacturing and Inventory Coordinator: Amy Bacus
Composition: Graphic World
Cover Illustrator: Cara Judd
Cover Layout Artist: Timothy Dziewit
Printing and Binding: Malloy, Inc.
Cover Printing: Malloy, Inc.

Library of Congress Cataloging-in-Publication Data
Sheldon, Lisa Kennedy.
    Oxygenation / Lisa Kennedy Sheldon. — 2nd ed.
      p. ; cm. — (Quick look nursing)
    Includes bibliographical references and index.
    ISBN-13: 978-0-7637-4475-5 (pbk. : alk. paper)
    ISBN-10: 0-7637-4475-1 (pbk. : alk. paper)
    1. Nursing. 2. Respiratory organs—Diseases—Nursing. 3. Respiratory therapy. 4. Oxygen therapy.
    I. Title. II. Series.
    [DNLM: 1. Oxygen Inhalation Therapy—nursing—Case Reports. 2. Biological Transport—Case Reports.
    3. Cardiovascular Diseases—nursing—Case Reports. 4. Oxygen Consumption—Case Reports. 5. Respiration
    Disorders—nursing—Case Reports. WY 163 S544o 2007]
    RT51.S54 2007
    610.73'6--dc22
                                    2007005322
6048

Printed in the United States of America
11 10 09 08 07   10 9 8 7 6 5 4 3 2 1

DEDICATION

To my husband, Tom, for his continuing patience and love.

CONTENTS

ACKNOWLEDGMENTS

Like most books, this text is the culmination of the efforts of many people who encourage and support my work. I continue to be grateful to Joanne Farley, PhD, RN, who presented me with an opportunity nine years ago to be an author in a series of books on nursing concepts. I have never looked back since beginning this journey of words to capture the nursing experience and its effect on patients. I would also like to thank Mary M. Sanford, RN, MSN, ANP-C, CCRN, who contributed significantly to the previous edition. To my colleagues at St. Joseph Hospital, I am always amazed by your enthusiasm for my projects and grateful for your friendship. Ultimately, I am driven by experiences with my patients, who humble me with their trust and inspire me with their courage and resilience. Wherever you are, know that I am honored to have been a part of your care. I am blessed by the presence of my children: Bradford, Gregory, Andrea, and Luke. You are the lights of life. Finally, I want to thank my husband, Tom, for his steadfast love.

ABOUT THE AUTHOR

Lisa Kennedy Sheldon, PhD(c), ARNP, is an oncology nurse practitioner at St. Joseph Hospital in Nashua, New Hampshire. She has extensive clinical experience in medical-surgical nursing, intensive care, and oncology as well as teaching at the baccalaureate level. A graduate of Saint Anselm College and Boston College, Ms. Sheldon is currently a doctoral candidate at the University of Utah. Her program of research focuses on nurse–patient communication. Recent publications include a text, *Communication for Nurses: Talking with Patients,* and articles on communication research. Ms. Sheldon is also a founding partner of Barrett & Sheldon, LLC, a nursing services development company in New England. She lives in New Hampshire with her husband and four children.

INTRODUCTION

Does my patient need oxygen just because he is anemic? How does oxygen saturation differ from the oxygen level on the arterial blood gas? Why do I have to be careful about oxygen administration when my patient is hypoxic and has chronic obstructive pulmonary disease?

As I sat with my nursing students at our postclinical conference, I realized how confusing it was to synthesize coursework and apply it to individual patients. With previous classes in anatomy and physiology, chemistry, microbiology and, of course, nursing, I knew the students understood the fundamental principles involved in the process of oxygenation. The difficulty arose in synthesizing and applying the coursework with actual patients in the clinical setting. Perhaps a conceptual approach was more applicable across an array of clinical situations.

The concept of oxygenation can be applied to disorders from the common cold to lung cancer and coronary artery disease. Oxygenation is not just about two lungs and a breathing cycle. It involves complex relationships between the respiratory, cardiovascular, and hematologic systems. Oxygenation requires physiologic processes such as ventilation, perfusion, diffusion, and transport to deliver oxygen to tissues and organs.

This text combines the physiologic principles of oxygenation with interventions for specific disorders in an interdisciplinary format. Physiologic findings, diagnostic procedures, medical interventions, and nursing care are combined to provide a holistic view of health care for the patients with disorders of oxygenation. Medical interventions range from preventive health strategies to pharmacologic treatments and surgical interventions. Many diseases such as asthma, chronic obstructive pulmonary disease, and heart disease require collaborative care from multiple healthcare providers.

Nurses provide a comprehensive approach to patient care, integrating interventions from multiple disciplines to optimize patient outcomes. *Quick Look Nursing: Oxygenation, Second Edition* incorporates an interdisciplinary approach to care, exposing nurses to a variety of disorders and their treatments, each with specific nursing implications. Special facts are highlighted in the text to clarify important aspects of a concept, disease, or treatment. Ultimately, the goal of this text is to integrate the concept of oxygenation into comprehensive care at the bedside of each patient.

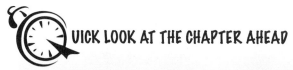

The respiratory system provides several important functions:

- Gas exchange

- Humidification and filtration of air

- Regulation of acid–base balance

- Speech production

- Taste and smell perception

The respiratory system is composed of the upper and lower respiratory tracts.

The upper respiratory tract is composed of the nasal cavities, pharynx, and the larynx.

The lower respiratory tract consists of the trachea, bronchi, bronchioles, alveolar ducts, and alveoli.

The gas is exchanged in the respiratory system through pulmonary and alveolar ventilation, and it is influenced by gas pressures, air flow, perfusion, diffusion, compliance, and control of ventilation.

1

Anatomy and Physiology of the Respiratory System

TERMS
- ☐ pharynx
- ☐ larynx
- ☐ trachea
- ☐ bronchi
- ☐ alveoli
- ☐ mucociliary blanket
- ☐ alveolar membrane
- ☐ ventilation
- ☐ diffusion
- ☐ perfusion

CASE STUDY

Code Blue! Room 622! Code Blue! Room 622!

Hearing those words over the intercom always perks up a nurse's ears and attention. Everyone moves quickly to assure the best outcome for the patient. But much of what goes on during a code involves understanding the anatomy and physiology of the respiratory system. Let's return to the code and watch the interventions of the staff.

Mrs. T is a 68-year-old woman who had a colectomy 2 days ago. The surgery was uncomplicated, but since her oxygen saturation levels were low postoperatively, she was receiving oxygen via nasal cannula at 4 liters (L) per minute. Her vital signs 1 hour ago were: blood pressure (BP)—168/88 mmHg, pulse—92 beats per minute, respiration—24 breaths per minute, and her temperature was 100.8°F orally. Her prior medical history includes hypertension, obesity, and smoking one pack of cigarettes per day for 50 years. Mrs. T had just ambulated in the hall with the nursing assistant and felt short of breath, so she was returned to bed. The nursing assistant came to find the nurse to report Mrs. T's symptoms. The nurse entered the room and found the patient unresponsive and not breathing. She called for help and began cardiopulmonary resuscitation (CPR). As the nurse positioned the patient's head and listened for breathing, she watched the chest and did not observe any movement. She tried to deliver a breath but had difficulty ventilating the patient. She repositioned the head and was then able to deliver a breath and observe the chest rise and fall. As she checked for a carotid pulse, the anesthesiologist arrived and determined that Mrs. T needed to be intubated. The nurse felt for a carotid pulse and noted a faint pulse. Using the laryngoscope, the anesthesiologist visualized the vocal cords and inserted the endotracheal tube. After inflating the cuff on the tube, lungs were ventilated by manual inflation. Listening with the stethoscope, the anesthesiologist noted that there were no breath sounds on the left side of the chest.

Important Questions to Ask

- Why did changing the position of the head allow the nurse to ventilate the patient?
- If rescue breathing involves exhalation, why does it help to oxygenate the patient?

- Why are the vocal cords visualized prior to intubation?
- After intubation, why were breath sounds not heard on the left side of the chest?

The primary function of the respiratory system is gas exchange. In aerobic organisms, such as humans, oxygen is required for the production of energy. This efficient system provides the body with oxygen and removes carbon dioxide, the waste product of metabolism. The lungs provide an extensive area for the exchange of gases between air and circulating blood. The respiratory system also performs several secondary functions, including regulation of acid–base balance, humidification and filtration of air, speech production, and taste and smell perception.

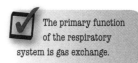
The primary function of the respiratory system is gas exchange.

THE ANATOMY OF THE RESPIRATORY SYSTEM

The respiratory tract is divided into the upper and lower respiratory tracts (see Figure 1-1). The upper respiratory system includes the nasal cavities, the pharynx, and the larynx. The lower respiratory tract includes the trachea, bronchi, bronchioles, lungs, and alveoli. The lungs are encased in the thoracic cage and utilize multiple muscles, including the diaphragm and the intercostal muscles, to facilitate ventilation.

The Upper Respiratory Tract

The Nasal Cavities

The **nasal cavities** or **passages** are the two sides of the nose divided by the **nasal septum** (see Figure 1-2). The upper third of the nose, the bridge, is bony while the lower third of the nose is cartilaginous. The **nostrils** (or **nares**), the two external openings to the nasal cavities, are lined with skin and hair follicles (vibrissae). The **vibrissae** are the first line of defense for filtering foreign objects and preventing them from being inhaled into the respiratory tract. The interior portion of the nasal passages and nasopharynx, which is the posterior aspect of the nasal cavities that connects with the pharynx, are lined with a **mucous membrane** that is well-supplied with blood. The mucous membrane serves to warm, filter, and humidify air. It is composed of **columnar epithelial cells** and **goblet cells** and produces mucus, which forms the **mucociliary blanket**. This blanket

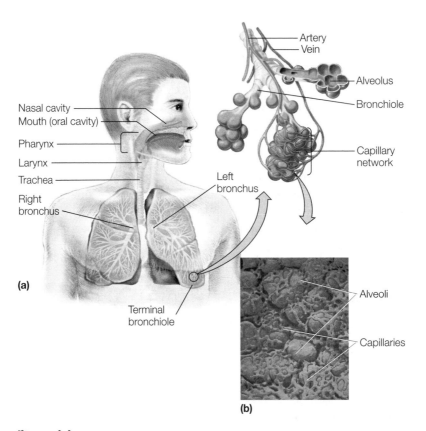

Figure 1-1 Structures of the respiratory tract. (a) This drawing shows the air-conducting portion and the gas-exchange portion of the human respiratory system. The insert shows a higher magnification of the alveoli, where oxygen and carbon dioxide exchange occurs. (b) A scanning electron micrograph of the alveoli, showing the rich capillary network surrounding them.

protects the respiratory system by entrapping foreign particles and pathogens. Cilia are tiny hairlike projections that move the mucociliary blanket and its entrapped particles toward the **oropharynx** where they can either be expelled by coughing or sneezing or swallowed. Anatomically, the nasal passages make a 90° angle down into the oropharynx, allowing additional filtering of particles from inspired air.

The **cribiform plate** is inside the nasal passages, below the ethmoid bone. It is covered with mucous membrane and contributes to the sense of smell. This region is supplied by the first cranial nerve—the olfactory nerve—which passes through holes in the cribiform plate. **Turbinates**

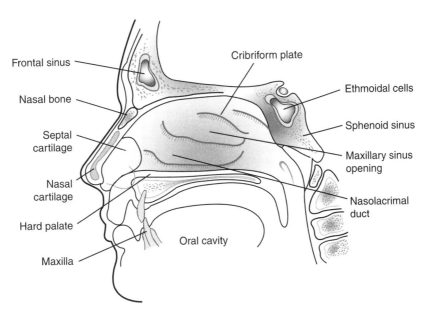

Figure 1-2 Anatomy of the nose.

are bony projections covered with mucous membrane along the sides of the nasal vestibule. The turbinates are highly vascular and serve to cleanse, warm, and humidify inspired air. They also increase the turbulence of inspired air, enhancing capture of particles in the mucociliary blanket.

 The mucous membranes serve to warm, filter, and humidify air. It is composed of columnar epithelial cells and goblet cells and produces mucus, which forms the mucociliary blanket. This blanket protects the respiratory system by entrapping foreign particles and pathogens.

The **paranasal sinuses** are hollow spaces in the facial bones surrounding the nasal passages. The sinuses are named for the bones in which they are located: sphenoid, ethmoid, and maxillary. The paranasal sinuses drain into the nasal cavities, as do the **nasolacrimal ducts** that drain tears from the surface of the eyes.

The Pharynx

The **pharynx** is located on the posterior aspect of the oral and nasal cavities and extends down to the larynx (see Figure 1-3). This tunnel-shaped passageway is shared by the respiratory and digestive systems. It is divided into three parts:

1. The **nasopharynx**, located above the margin of the soft palate

2. The **oropharynx**, located behind the tongue

3. The **laryngopharynx**, located from the base of the tongue to the larynx

The openings for the eustachian tubes are located on either side of the oropharynx. The lingual, palatine, and pharyngeal **tonsils** are nubs of lymphatic tissue in the pharynx. The mouth serves as an alternative air-

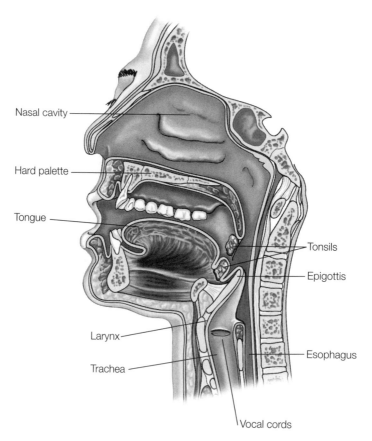

Figure 1-3 Upper respiratory tract.

way when either the nasal passages are obstructed or when high volumes of air are needed, such as during exercise. The mouth is less efficient at humidifying, filtering, and warming air than the nose. The pharynx is the only opening from the nasal passages and the mouth to the lungs, so that any obstruction of the pharynx immediately impairs ventilation.

The **epiglottis** is a thin, leaf-shaped structure of elastic cartilage that helps to protect the larynx during swallowing (see Figure 1-4). The epiglottis covers the larynx during swallowing to prevent food and fluids from entering the lungs. The closed vocal cords are the final lines of defense for the lungs. At the point where the epiglottis covers the larynx, the pharynx divides into the larynx and the esophagus.

> The pharynx is the only opening from the nasal passages and the mouth to the lungs, so that any obstruction of the pharynx immediately impairs ventilation.

The Larynx

The **larynx**, commonly called the voice box, connects the pharynx with the trachea (see Figure 1-5). The larynx has two purposes:

1. Production of sound and speech

2. Protection of lungs from entrance by substances other than air

The larynx lies in the midline of the neck and contains two folds of mucous membrane known as the **vocal cords**. Vibration of the tightened vocal cords allows phonation to occur. The **arytenoid cartilage** is used in vocal cord movement. The epiglottis is attached at the top of the larynx. The esophagus is just posterior to the larynx. Should anything other than air enter the larynx, the cough reflex and laryngeal spasms would reflexively try to expel it. The epiglottis is essential in creating the cough reflex. Nine cartilage rings form the larynx; the largest of which, the **thyroid cartilage**, is sometimes called the Adam's apple. The **cricoid cartilage**, that lies below the thyroid cartilage, contains the vocal cords. The **cricothyroid membrane** connects the cricoid and thyroid cartilage and may be incised for emergency access to the airway.

> The cricothyroid membrane connects the cricoid and thyroid cartilage and may be incised for emergency access to the airway.

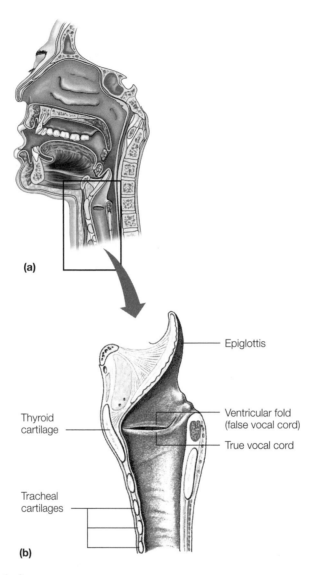

(a)

Epiglottis

Thyroid
cartilage

Ventricular fold
(false vocal cord)

True vocal cord

Tracheal
cartilages

(b)

Figure 1-4 The vocal cords. (a) Uppermost portion of respiratory system showing location of the vocal cords. (b) Longitudinal section of the larynx showing the location of the vocal cords. Note the presence of the false vocal cord, so named because it does not function in phonation.

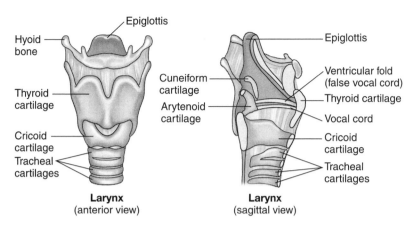

Larynx
(anterior view)

Larynx
(sagittal view)

Figure 1-5 Larynx and trachea.

The Lower Respiratory Tract

The lower respiratory tract consists of the **trachea**, the two mainstem **bronchi**, lobar, segmental and subsegmental bronchi, **bronchioles, alveolar ducts**, and **alveoli**. The tracheobronchial tree can be viewed as a system of branching tubes, each smaller, carrying air to the site of gas exchange: the alveolar membrane. There are about 23 levels of branching from the trachea down to the alveoli. Smooth muscle is wound about all the structures of the lower respiratory tract and constricts airways in disorders such as asthma.

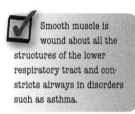 Smooth muscle is wound about all the structures of the lower respiratory tract and constricts airways in disorders such as asthma.

The Trachea
The trachea or windpipe is a flexible tube that connects the larynx with the major bronchi of the lungs. It begins at the lower border of the cricoid cartilage and extends down to the level of the posterior fifth or sixth thoracic vertebrae or the anterior sternal angle, where it branches into the left and right mainstem bronchi. The site of this bifurcation is referred to as the **carina**. The strongest cough reflex is at the carina. Tracheobronchial suctioning may stimulate vigorous coughing if the carina is stimulated. The walls of the trachea contain about 20 horseshoe-shaped cartilages that stiffen the trachea, preventing collapse or expansion of the trachea

when intrathoracic pressures change. The cartilages are open posteriorly to allow stretching of the esophagus when a bolus of food passes. The walls of the trachea are composed of mucus-secreting, ciliated cells (the mucociliary blanket) that carry particles away from the lungs and up to the pharynx. These ciliated cells are destroyed by smoking, resulting in the loss of this valuable function.

 The strongest cough reflex is at the carina. Tracheobronchial suctioning may stimulate vigorous coughing if the carina is stimulated.

The Bronchi and Bronchioles

The right and left mainstem bronchi begin at the carina. These bronchi are similar in structure to the trachea, with cartilage surrounding the airway and maintaining the shape. Smooth muscle, controlled by the parasympathetic nervous system, wraps around the bronchi. The right mainstem bronchus is more like a linear extension of the trachea and is shorter and anatomically more vertically downward than the left. Therefore, aspirated foreign bodies and even accidental intubations are more likely to occur in the right mainstem bronchus.

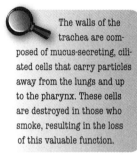
The walls of the trachea are composed of mucus-secreting, ciliated cells that carry particles away from the lungs and up to the pharynx. These cells are destroyed in those who smoke, resulting in the loss of this valuable function.

The bronchioles spread in an inverted treelike formation throughout each lung. The segmental and subsegmental bronchi further branch into smaller and smaller bronchioles until they reach the terminal bronchioles. These bronchioles are only about 1 mm in diameter. They do not have cartilage rings and therefore depend on the elastic recoil of the lungs to maintain patency. They do not have cilia or participate in gas exchange.

The right mainstem bronchus is more like a linear extension of the trachea and is shorter and anatomically more vertically downward than the left. Therefore, aspirated foreign bodies and even accidental intubations are more likely to occur in the right mainstem bronchus.

The Alveoli

The alveoli are cup-shaped structures that are grouped like clusters of grapes at the end of the terminal bronchioles (see Figure 1-6). There are

150 to 300 million alveolar sacs in an adult's lungs. Thin walls separate the alveoli from each other, and within the walls is an extensive network of capillaries that is so dense

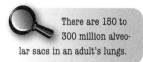
There are 150 to 300 million alveolar sacs in an adult's lungs.

that it has been referred to as a sheet of blood. It is within these walls that the actual gas exchange takes place. Oxygen in the alveoli diffuses across the **alveolar membrane** into the blood, and carbon dioxide in the blood diffuses back into the alveoli (see Figure 1-7). **Surfactant**, a phospholipid protein, is secreted by cells called type II pneumocytes within the alveoli. Surfactant reduces the surface tension in the alveoli, allowing more surface area for gas exchange and preventing collapse of the alveolar sac. Lack of surfactant may cause respiratory failure in premature infants and has also been implicated in adult respiratory distress syndrome (ARDS). As there are no mucus-secreting glands in the alveoli, the majority of particle removal is done by alveolar macrophages and the lymphatic channels of the lungs.

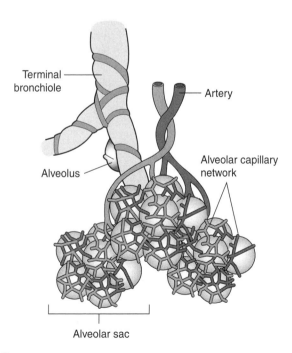

Terminal bronchiole

Artery

Alveolus

Alveolar capillary network

Alveolar sac

Figure 1-6 The alveoli with the network of capillaries.

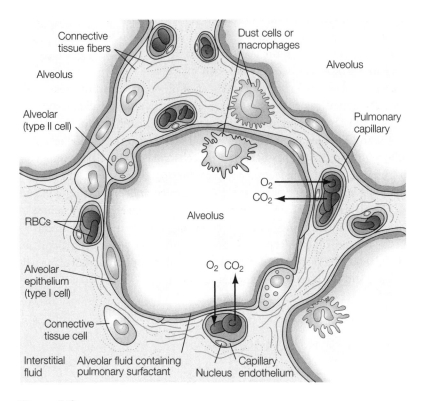

Figure 1-7 Diffusion of gases across the alveolar membrane.

The Lungs

The **lungs** are the functional units of the respiratory system. They are spongy, cone-shaped organs located within the **thoracic cavity** on either side of the heart. Between the two lungs is a space called the **mediastinum**, which contains the heart and great vessels, the esophagus, part of the trachea and bronchi, and the thymus gland (see Figure 1-8). The upper part of the lung is called the **apex**, and the lower part, the **base**, rests upon the diaphragm. Each lung is divided into **lobes**, two lobes in the left lung and three lobes in the right lung. The lungs are further divided into 10 bronchopulmonary segments. The lungs are elastic structures that are capable of inflation from within, as well as external pulling sources. Elastic and collagen fibers

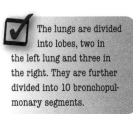

The lungs are divided into lobes, two in the left lung and three in the right. They are further divided into 10 bronchopulmonary segments.

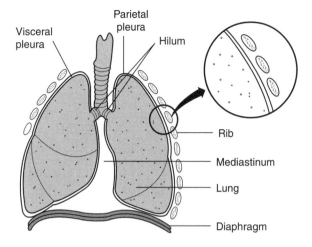

Figure 1-8 The mediastinum, lungs, and pleural cavity.

are contained within the alveolar walls and allow the lungs to stretch in all directions and recoil to return to their normal resting state.

The Thorax, Diaphragm, and Pleura

The **thorax** or **thoracic cavity** contains the lungs, heart, and great vessels. The bony, outer shell of the thorax is comprised of the sternum, thoracic vertebrae, and 12 pairs of ribs that are connected to the thoracic vertebrae of the posterior spine. The first seven pairs of ribs are connected to the sternum by cartilage, the next three pairs are connected to each other by **costochondral cartilage**, and the last two pairs are unattached, the so-called floating ribs, which allow complete expansion of the lungs during inspiration (see Figure 1-9).

Many muscles are used during **inspiration**. The **scalene** and **sternocleidomastoid muscles** elevate the upper thorax. The **intercostal muscles** between the ribs pull the ribs upward and forward, increasing the anteroposterior and transverse diameters.

The **diaphragm** is the principle muscle of respiration. It serves as the lower boundary of the thorax and is attached to the xiphoid process and the lower ribs. When it is relaxed, the diaphragm is dome shaped. Contraction of the diaphragm occurs by stimulation of the **phrenic nerve**, allowing the chest to expand from top to bottom. The phrenic nerve originates from the spinal column at the level of the third cervical vertebrae.

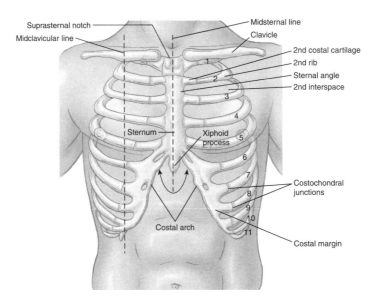

Figure 1-9 Anterior thorax, ribs, and sternum.

Cervical injuries may result in damage to the spinal cord above or at the origination of the phrenic nerve with subsequent paralysis of the diaphragm and an inability to ventilate.

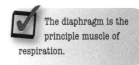 The diaphragm is the principle muscle of respiration.

Cervical injuries may result in damage to the spinal cord above or at the origination of the phrenic nerve with subsequent paralysis of the diaphragm and an inability to ventilate.

The **pleura** are thin, serous membranes that encase the lungs and the thoracic cavity. The **visceral pleura** cover the lungs and the fissures between the lobes. The **parietal pleura** lines the thoracic cavity (see Figure 1-8). The visceral and parietal pleurae allow the lungs to remain against the thoracic wall, creating a pulling force to hold the lungs in the expanded position. A thin film of serous fluid separates the visceral and parietal pleura, acting as a lubricant and allowing the two to glide

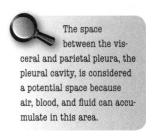 The space between the visceral and parietal pleura, the pleural cavity, is considered a potential space because air, blood, and fluid can accumulate in this area.

over each other without any separation. The space between the visceral and parietal pleura, the **pleural cavity**, is considered a potential space because air, blood, and fluid can accumulate in this area.

 # RESPIRATORY PHYSIOLOGY

The exchange of gases in the respiratory system requires the integration of multiple processes. During respiration, the conducting airways of the upper and lower respiratory tracts deliver air to the alveolar membrane, the site of actual gas exchange. The mechanics of breathing or **ventilation**, the effect of respiratory pressures and airflow, the control of ventilation, the relationship of ventilation to **perfusion** in the exchange of gases, and the system of gas transport will be discussed in the following sections.

Ventilation

The term *ventilation* refers to the entire process of air flow between the human body and the atmosphere. **Pulmonary ventilation** or breathing is the actual flow of gases into and out of the respiratory tract. **Alveolar ventilation** is the exchange of gases across the alveolar membrane between the respiratory and the circulatory systems.

Pulmonary Ventilation

Breathing or pulmonary ventilation is controlled by the movement of the chest cavity, the compliance of the lungs, and the surface tension within the alveoli. A single cycle of ventilation consists of **inhalation** or **inspiration** followed by **exhalation** or **expiration**. During inspiration, the diaphragm and accessory muscles enlarge the thoracic cavity, creating negative pressure within the chest. Air is drawn into the lungs because the **intrathoracic pressure**, pressure of the air within the chest, is less than the **atmospheric pressure**, pressure of the air in the environment. The diaphragm is the principal muscle of inspiration. Normal, quiet breathing is almost entirely performed by the diaphragm. When the diaphragm contracts during inspiration, the abdominal contents are pushed downward and the chest expands. The diaphragm moves down about 1–3 cm on normal inspiration and as much as 10 cm on forced inspiration. The lungs are pulled outward as they are adhered to the pleural lining of the thorax. The scalene muscles and the sternocleidomastoid are the accessory muscles of inspiration. The scalene raises the first two ribs and the sternocleidomastoid pulls the sternum slightly forward, increasing the anteroposterior dia-

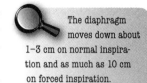

The diaphragm moves down about 1–3 cm on normal inspiration and as much as 10 cm on forced inspiration.

meter. The trapezius and pectoralis muscles also play a minor role by fixing the shoulders in place during inspiration. The accessory muscles contribute little to normal ventilation but are used more intensively during physical exertion or when air exchange is hampered in disease states, such as chronic obstructive pulmonary disease (COPD).

Whereas inhalation requires the active involvement of muscles, exhalation is normally a passive activity. The elastic components of the lungs and chest wall recoil, increasing the pressure in the chest to more than atmospheric pressure, thereby forcing air out of the lungs. The abdominal and intercostal muscles can be used to increase the force of expiration. The use of these accessory muscles may be seen in disorders, such as asthma, which narrow the airways. In asthmatic lungs, the narrowed air passages necessitate greater pressure during exhalation so the accessory muscles are used to force air out of the lungs.

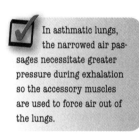

In asthmatic lungs, the narrowed air passages necessitate greater pressure during exhalation so the accessory muscles are used to force air out of the lungs.

Alveolar Ventilation

The rate at which new air reaches the areas for gas exchange in the lungs is referred to as alveolar ventilation. During quiet inhalation, very little new air reaches as far as the alveoli. The air which remains in the nasal passages, pharynx, trachea, bronchi, and bronchioles is not involved in gas exchange and is called dead air space. An inspiration with a tidal volume of 500 mL results is approximately 150 mL of dead space in a 70 kg person. The remaining 350 mL are involved in gas exchange in the alveoli.

Lung Compliance

Lung compliance refers to the ease with which the lungs are inflated. The elastic nature of the lungs causes them to stretch when the lungs are inflated and recoil when the lungs are deflated. The force required to expand the lungs to a particular volume is referred to as compliance. The normal lung compliance for an adult is 200 mL per cm of water pressure. Diseases, such as emphysema, increase compliance, perhaps because the elastic tissues have been over distended or destroyed. Other disorders, such as pulmonary fibrosis, result in a "stiffer" lung with decreased elasticity and decreased compliance.

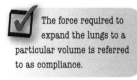

The force required to expand the lungs to a particular volume is referred to as compliance.

Surface Tension

Lung compliance is affected by the surface tension of the alveoli. As previously mentioned, the alveoli are lined with surfactant, which is produced by the type II cells in the alveoli. Surfactant lowers the surface tension of the alveoli, providing stability and even inflation of the alveoli. Without surfactant, lung inflation would be very difficult.

Respiratory Pressures

The pressure difference between the atmosphere and the pulmonary system affects the flow and **diffusion** of gases. The pressure within the respiratory tract is referred to as the **intrapulmonary pressure** (see Figure 1-10). Normal atmospheric pressure is 760 millimeters of mercury (mmHg). When air is not moving into or out of the lungs and the glottis is open, the difference between the intrapulmonary pressure and the atmospheric pressure is 0 mmHg. During quiet breathing, the difference between the atmospheric and intrapulmonary pressures is about 3 mmHg, dropping 3 mmHg below atmospheric pressure during inspiration and increasing 3 mmHg above atmospheric pressure during expiration. Variations in pressure increase from 3 to 5 mmHg during normal activity. During extreme exertion, these pressure differentials may increase dramatically to −80 mmHg during inspiration and +100 mmHg during expiration.

The pressure in the slim space between the visceral and parietal pleura is known as the **intrapleural pressure**. A thin layer of fluid separates the visceral and parietal membranes, providing a powerful force that holds the lung against the chest wall. This force is similar to what happens when a piece of glass is placed on a wet surface. It slides easily back and forth but is very difficult to lift off the surface. Intrapleural pressure falls about 6 mmHg during inspiration and rises as air fills the lungs. It always remains negative relative to the alveolar pressure. This negative pressure holds the lungs against the chest wall.

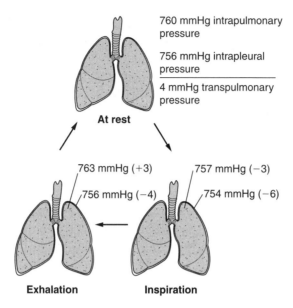

Figure 1-10 Respiratory pressures within the lungs and pleural space during breathing.

Although the intrapleural space is considered a potential space, air can enter the space due to a perforation in the lung or chest wall. When air accumulates in this potential space, causing the lung to collapse, this is called a **pneumothorax**. Blood accumulation in the intrapleural space is known as a **hemothorax**. If serous fluid accumulates in the intrapleural space, it is referred to as a **pleural effusion**. When any accumulation in the pleural space exceeds the atmospheric pressure, the alveoli can collapse causing **atelectasis**. Removal of the air or liquid and the reestablishment of negative pressure in the intrapleural space are required to prevent complete collapse of the lung and shifting of the thoracic contents toward the side of the chest with the collapsed lung. This is called a **mediastinal shift**, a potentially life-threatening condition requiring immediate attention.

The collapse of a lung and shifting of the thoracic contents toward the side of the chest with the collapsed lung, a mediastinal shift, is a potentially life-threatening condition requiring immediate attention.

Gas Pressures

The air in the atmosphere is composed of different gases that move because of changes in pressure. **Atmospheric air** is composed of roughly 20.8% oxygen and 78.6% nitrogen. Each gas comprises a portion of the total atmospheric pressure, which is 760 mmHg. So if nitrogen comprises 78.6% of atmospheric air, then nitrogen makes up 600 mmHg of that total pressure of 760 mmHg. The other gases making up air each contribute their partial pressure to the total pressure. This can be stated in a formula with P representing the partial pressure of each component:

$$P_{O_2} + P_{CO_2} + P_{N_2} + P_{H_2O} = 760 \text{ mmHg}$$

Alveolar air differs in composition from atmospheric air because of humidification, which occurs in the upper airways and by the partial replacement of air with each inspiration (see Table 1-1). Not all alveolar air is replaced during each inspiration. Rather, a portion of the remaining air in the alveoli mixes with the fresh air. Even at the end of expiration, air remains within the pulmonary structures and is referred to as the **residual volume**. Carbon dioxide and oxygen are rapidly and constantly diffusing across the alveolar membrane, making exact measurements of these concentrations difficult.

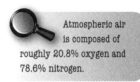

Atmospheric air is composed of roughly 20.8% oxygen and 78.6% nitrogen.

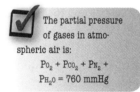

The partial pressure of gases in atmospheric air is:
$P_{O_2} + P_{CO_2} + P_{N_2} + P_{H_2O} = 760 \text{ mmHg}$

Table 1-1 Composition of Atmospheric and Alveolar Air

	Atmospheric Air (%)	Alveolar Air (%)	Expired Air (%)
N_2	78.6	74.5	75
O_2	20.8	15.7	14
CO_2	0.04	3.6	5
H_2O	0.5	6.2	6

Air Flow

The movement of air into and out of the lungs is directly related to the difference between the pressure in the lung, the intrapulmonary pressure, and the atmospheric pressure. It is inversely related to **resistance** in the airways. Airway resistance is normally small, and only 1 mmHg of pressure change is required to move 500 mL of air into and out of the lungs. But in conditions such as asthma, where the airways are narrowed by swelling and bronchospasm, the resistance is markedly increased. Airway resistance is influenced by lung volumes and is less during inspiration and more during expiration. In patients with asthma, the combination of narrowed airways and increased resistance during expiration requires far greater pressure changes to effectively move air.

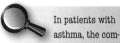

In patients with asthma, the combination of narrowed airways and increased resistance during expiration requires far greater pressure changes to effectively move air.

Control of Ventilation

Higher functions are also involved in maintaining adequate oxygenation in the body. Breathing is controlled by the brain and the **peripheral chemoreceptors**. The respiratory center of the brain is located in the medulla oblongata and the pons. The **central respiratory center** adjusts the respiratory rate and volumes to maintain appropriate oxygen and carbon dioxide levels. Excess carbon dioxide levels (**hypercapnia**) cause a lowering of the blood's pH and stimulate the respiratory center to increase inspiratory and expiratory effort. Carbon dioxide is easily diffused across the blood-brain barrier, and the neurons can sense small changes in carbon dioxide levels and quickly adjust respiratory effort. The central respiratory center is a very effective and rapid control center because of the ease with which carbon dioxide molecules diffuse across the blood-brain barrier. Oxygen levels do not directly affect the central respiratory center. Rather, they affect the peripheral chemoreceptors near the carotid sinus (carotid bodies) and the aortic arch (aortic bodies) (see Figure 1-11). The aortic and carotid bodies are sensitive to levels of dissolved oxygen in the plasma. They do not respond to conditions such as anemia or carbon monoxide poisoning where the hemoglobin is less saturated with oxygen.

Stimulation of the peripheral chemoreceptors, the carotid and aortic bodies, by decreased oxygen levels (**hypoxia**) results in increased inspiratory effort. In certain disease states, such as COPD, the central

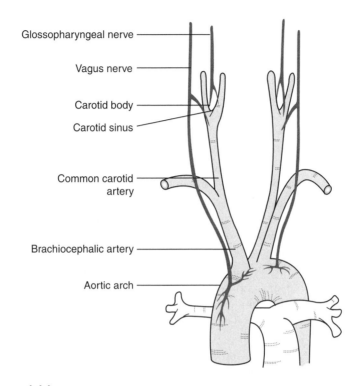

Glossopharyngeal nerve

Vagus nerve

Carotid body

Carotid sinus

Common carotid artery

Brachiocephalic artery

Aortic arch

Figure 1-11 Location of peripheral chemoreceptors.

respiratory center becomes desensitized to high carbon dioxide levels, and the peripheral chemoreceptors use arterial oxygen levels to regulate respiration. Therefore, oxygen should be administered cautiously in patients with COPD and the effect should be assessed frequently. In these patients, the administration of high-flow oxygen may decrease the respiratory drive.

 Oxygen should be administered cautiously in patients with COPD because respiratory drive is regulated by low oxygen levels.

Ventilation and Perfusion

As described previously, alveolar ventilation is crucial for gas exchange to take place. Diffusion is the process by which oxygen and carbon dioxide molecules are exchanged across the alveolar membrane. But diffusion requires not only that the alveoli are ventilated with fresh air but that the ventilated alveoli are perfused by pulmonary capillaries. When there is a discrepancy between ventilation and perfusion optimum gas exchange does not occur. A review of the concepts of diffusion and the pressures of gases will clarify this concept.

Diffusion is the random movement of molecules from areas of high concentration to areas of lower concentration. The source of energy for diffusion is the random movement and collisions of the gas molecules (see Table 1-1). Gases move from areas of high concentration to areas of lower concentration. When air enters the alveoli, it has a higher concentration of oxygen than the blood in the pulmonary capillaries. The oxygen molecules move across the alveolar membrane to the red blood cells in the capillary. Likewise, when venous blood reaches the alveolar membrane, the carbon dioxide levels in the blood are higher than the alveolar air, and the carbon dioxide molecules move into the alveoli. Carbon dioxide diffuses 20 times more rapidly than oxygen. The exchange of gases across the alveolar membrane depends on the perfusion of the pulmonary capillaries, as well as the ventilation of the alveoli. The effect of perfusion of these capillaries ($\dot{Q}$) on alveolar ventilation ($\dot{V}$) is quantifiable as a ratio—the ventilation/perfusion ratio ($\dot{V}/\dot{Q}$). If the alveoli are well ventilated and the capillaries are well perfused, then the ratio is approximately 1. Usually, there is relatively more perfusion than ventilation, yielding a $\dot{V}/\dot{Q}$ ratio of 0.8. But when there is a mismatch between the perfusion and the ventilation, there are serious respiratory consequences.

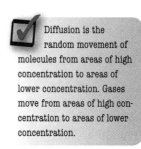

Diffusion is the random movement of molecules from areas of high concentration to areas of lower concentration. Gases move from areas of high concentration to areas of lower concentration.

 When there is a mismatch between the perfusion and the ventilation, there are serious respiratory consequences.

In the case of adequate alveolar ventilation but poor capillary perfusion, there would be no blood flow to carry away the fresh oxygen or remove the carbon dioxide from the portion of the lung, and the $\dot{V}/\dot{Q}$ ratio would be equal to infinity. For example, when a **pulmonary embolus** blocks a pulmonary artery, circulation to lung tissue distal to the blockage is impaired. The ventilation of the alveoli is useless because no gas exchange can take place without perfusion of the affected lung tissue.

When the reverse situation occurs, adequate perfusion without ventilation, then the $\dot{V}/\dot{Q}$ ratio is said to be 0. An example of this would be the obstruction of a bronchiole by a mucus plug. In this case, circulation in the alveoli would be normal, but ventilation of the lung tissue distal to the blockage would be impaired. Therefore, a certain portion of blood returning via the pulmonary veins to the left side of the heart would not be oxygenated. This is known as shunting, and the quantity of unoxygenated blood is described as the **physiologic shunt**. Normally, the physiologic shunt is about 5 mL/dL.

Even in normally perfused and ventilated lungs, the $\dot{V}/\dot{Q}$ ratio differs between the upper and lower portions of the lungs. When the body is upright, gravity affects the amount of blood flow to the upper and lower portions of the lungs. The upper lobes receive less perfusion, resulting in physiologic dead space that is adequately ventilated but has underperfused. During exercise, increased circulation to the upper lobes increases the effectiveness of gas exchange. Conversely, the lower lobes are well perfused but somewhat underventilated. For these reasons, when the lungs are mechanically ventilated, frequent changes of position help to increase ventilation and perfusion to all parts of the lungs.

When the lungs are mechanically ventilated, frequent changes of position are needed to improve ventilation and perfusion in all parts of the lungs.

CASE STUDY RESOLUTION

Let's return to Mrs. T as she is being resuscitated by the nurse and the anesthesiologist. When the anesthesiologist could not hear breath sounds on the left side of the chest, she deflated the cuff of the endotracheal tube and withdrew the tube 1 to 2 cm. Then the cuff was reinflated and breath sounds could be auscultated on both sides of the chest. This maneuver solved the problem because the tube had traveled past the carina and into the right mainstem bronchus. This is a common scenario, as the right mainstem bronchus is straighter and more vertical than the left.

While the nurse manually ventilated Mrs. T, she noticed that the lungs were difficult to inflate. Due to Mrs. T's smoking history, the lung compliance was decreased, making it more difficult to ventilate. Breath sounds were distant in both lower lobes, and the nurse also heard gurgling, coarse sounds (rhonchi) that she assessed as phlegm in the airways, and decided to suction the patient. Suctioning through the endotracheal tube produced large amounts of thick sputum. Smokers frequently have large amounts of sputum because the lung's response to foreign particles from cigarettes causes increased sputum production. Due to the decrease in ciliated cells available to move mucus out of the respiratory tract (another result of smoking), mucus accumulated in the lungs. The surgery and anesthesia further complicated the problem, as the patient had some atelectasis of the alveoli resulting in decreased oxygenation. Nursing interventions, such as assisted coughing and deep breathing, as well as instruction on the use of the incentive spirometer may have prevented this event. Pain from her abdominal incision was probably preventing Mrs. T from deep breathing, so adequate pain medication would have made these interventions more effective.

After suctioning, breath sounds were heard in both bases of both lungs. After 5 minutes of ventilation with oxygen, Mrs. T started to respond and opened her eyes. She was transferred to the intensive care unit for further ventilatory support.

The answers to the questions listed in the introduction are as follows:

- Why did changing the position of the head allow the nurse to ventilate the patient?

Repositioning the head brought the tongue away from the posterior oropharynx and allowed ventilation.

- If rescue breathing involves exhalation, why does it help to oxygenate the patient?

Exhaled air contains 15.7% oxygen (atmospheric air has 20.8% oxygen), so rescue breathing still delivers oxygen to the patient.

- Why are the vocal cords visualized prior to intubation?

The vocal cords are visualized prior to intubation so that the endotracheal tube passes through the vocal cords into the trachea and not into the esophagus.

- After intubation, why were breath sounds not heard on the left side of the chest?

Breath sounds were not heard on the left side after intubation because the endotracheal tube had passed into the right mainstem bronchus, and only the right lung was being ventilated.

CHAPTER 1 MULTIPLE-CHOICE QUESTIONS

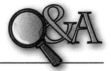

1. What structures prevent foreign bodies from being aspirated into the lungs?
   a. Tongue
   b. Epiglottis, vocal cords, and mucociliary blanket
   c. Carina, bronchioles
   d. Teeth, tonsils, and adenoids

2. In the patient with COPD, why can it be dangerous to give supplemental oxygen?
   a. Supplemental oxygen may decrease respiratory drive.
   b. Oxygen levels in the blood increase the respiratory rate in patients with COPD.
   c. Hyperventilation may occur if supplemental oxygen is given.
   d. Supplemental oxygen may increase sputum production.

3. If a child accidentally inhales a peanut, what lung does it usually lodge in?
   a. Either lung because the force of inspiration is the same in both lungs.
   b. Inhaled objects follow the straightest path, usually the right mainstem bronchus into the right lung.
   c. The left lung, because the left main stem bronchus is wider than the right.
   d. Neither lung because the carina stops the object.

4. Is quiet exhalation active or passive?
   a. Exhalation requires the use of accessory muscles, so it is active.
   b. The diaphragm contracts during exhalation, so it is active.
   c. Exhalation during quiet breathing is usually passive.
   d. The abdominal muscles actively contract during quiet exhalation.

5. When upright, what force of nature makes blood flow greater in the lower portions of the lung?
   a. Pressure from the left ventricle increases blood flow to the lower lungs.
   b. Diffusion of gases is greater in the lower lung fields in the upright position.
   c. Ventilation is better in the lower lungs in the upright position.
   d. Gravity increases the blood flow to the lower lungs when in the upright position.

CHAPTER 1 ANSWERS AND RATIONALES

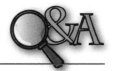

1. **b.**

   Rationale: The epiglottis, vocal cords, and mucociliary blanket all prevent the aspiration of particles into the lungs.

2. **a.**

   Rationale: Patients with COPD use the oxygen levels at the peripheral chemoreceptors to stimulate respiratory drive. Too much supplemental oxygen may actually decrease their respiratory drive. Patients with normal respiratory functioning use carbon dioxide levels to regulate their respiratory rate.

3. **b.**

   Rationale: The right main stem bronchus is straighter than the left and often aspirated particles follow the more direct path into the right lung.

4. **c.**

   Rationale: Exhalation during quiet breathing is usually passive as the muscles, diaphragm, and lungs all recoil.

5. **d.**

   Rationale: Gravity influences blood flow so, when upright, blood flow is increased in the bases of the lungs. But when a patient is supine, blood flow increases in the lung field that is down or lower.

Assessment of the respiratory system combines knowledge of the anatomy and physiology of the respiratory tract with data from the patient's assessment.

- General health history and specific history of respiratory functioning and/or current problem

- Symptoms—Cough, secretions, dyspnea, pain

- Physical assessment—Anatomic landmarks, breath sounds

- Diagnostic testing—Pulmonary volumes, capacities, blood gases, radiologic procedures, laboratory tests

2

Assessment of the Respiratory System

TERMS
- [ ] **dyspnea**
- [ ] **auscultation**
- [ ] **breath sounds**
- [ ] **adventitious lung sounds**
- [ ] **pulmonary function tests**
- [ ] **arterial blood gas**
- [ ] **oxygen saturation level**
- [ ] **hypoxia**
- [ ] **brochoscopy**
- [ ] **thoracentesis**

CASE STUDY

Mr. Z, a 58-year-old man, arrives at the emergency department because his wife states that he "can't catch his breath." Mr. Z is sitting in the chair beside the stretcher with his elbows propped on the arms of the chair. His wife is standing beside him, rubbing his arm. At first glance, he is working hard at breathing, with his shoulders stiff and high, his lips pursed on exhalation. His color is somewhat dusky, especially around the mouth. The nurse takes his vital signs and finds that his temperature is 100.8°F, his heart rate is 94 beats per minute, his respiratory rate is 32 breaths per minute, and his blood pressure is 168/92 mmHg. Using the pulse oximeter, the nurse measures the oxygen saturation (Sao$_2$) at 88%. A round chest circumference and rib retraction are noted on chest examination. Listening with the stethoscope, the nurse notes distant breath sounds with expiratory wheezes throughout his lung fields and rhonchi in his right lung. Breath sounds are absent at the base of the right lung.

Taking a history from his wife, the nurse finds that Mr. Z has smoked two packs of cigarettes a day for 35 years. He has had "trouble catching his breath for several years," but 2 weeks ago he had a cold, and now he can "hardly sleep because he can't breathe." He has no known allergies and takes atenolol, a beta-blocker, for his high blood pressure and pioglitazone for diabetes. A colleague suggests that Mr. Z be put on the stretcher and given oxygen via nasal prongs.

Important Questions to Ask

- Why is Mr. Z sitting in the chair, and should he be lying on a stretcher?
- What should be considered before starting oxygen therapy?
- What changes might be seen on an arterial blood gas, given Mr. Z's smoking history and oxygen saturation?
- What anatomic changes cause wheezes?
- What side effect of beta-blockers is making Mr. Z's breathing more difficult?

To gain an accurate picture of a patient's respiratory functioning, the nurse must combine knowledge of the anatomy and physiology of the respiratory tract with data from the patient's assessment. Every patient has a unique combination of previous medical history, current symptoms, life-style and behavior patterns, and genetic history. The goal is to gather data from the patient's history, physical assessment, and diagnostic testing to compile a complete picture of the patient's respiratory functioning.

THE PATIENT HISTORY

Many aspects of an individual's life impact the functioning of the respiratory system. To gather the necessary information, the nurse must begin by taking a thorough history. Gathering an accurate database provides the nurse with the information that will direct the physical assessment and guide the planning of appropriate interventions. Possible sources of information include the patient, his family or significant others, the patient's appearance and posture, and the medical record(s).

Begin the process of taking a health history with general questions. The nurse might ask the following questions to start the assessment:

- What brings you to seek health care at this visit?
- What is your major problem today?
- How long have you had this problem?
- What makes it better or worse?
- What have you tried to make it better?
- How does it affect your normal daily activities?

The assessment should also include demographic data, such as age, gender, and race. Aging not only affects the functioning of the respiratory tract, but disorders such as emphysema also are more age specific. Gender can influence the incidence of certain diseases of the respiratory tract. For example, oral cancers are more common in men than in women. Race may affect such parameters as normal respiratory volumes. Caucasians have larger lung volumes than Native Americans or Asian Americans. The patient's responses to these general questions will direct the questions in the remainder of the assessment.

Symptoms

Many respiratory problems begin with similar symptoms. Clarifying the nature of these symptoms narrows the possible problems and directs the remainder of the assessment and examination. Some common presentations of respiratory problems include cough, sputum production, nasal secretions, dyspnea (difficult breathing), wheezing, and pain. Each presentation requires further questioning to ascertain the nature of the symptom and how it affects the patient's functioning.

Cough

Coughing is a protective mechanism for clearing the airways. It also can be a reflexive response to irritating stimuli in the tracheobronchial tree or the larynx. The patient may describe the cough as coming in spurts (paroxysmal) or chronic, tickling, hacking, dry, or productive. Some questions might include the following:

- How long has the patient had the cough?
- Is the cough productive?
- How would the patient describe the cough—hacking, dry, or coming in spurts?
- Is the cough worse at certain times of the day or night?

> Coughing is a protective mechanism for clearing the airways.

Sputum

Asking a patient about sputum is an important part of the assessment. When the patient produces **sputum,** inquire about the daily frequency, timing during the day, and amount using a common measurement such as a teaspoon. It is important to note the color and consistency of the sputum. Specifically ask if there is blood in the sputum. If sputum production is a chronic problem, ask about recent changes in the amount and color.

Nasal Secretions

Allergies, rhinitis, infection, and irritants can cause excessive secretions. Allergies may cause thin, watery secretions and pale nasal mucosa. Infection may cause yellow to greenish secretions accompanied by reddened nasal mucosa. Some further questions might include the following:

- Does the patient have problems with excessive nasal secretions?
- What do the secretions look like?
- Do they increase at certain times of the year?

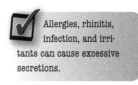

> Allergies, rhinitis, infection, and irritants can cause excessive secretions.

- Do plants or animals affect the amount of secretions?
- Do certain "triggers," such as pollen, dust, or food additives, make the secretions begin or increase?

Dyspnea

Patients do not usually come in complaining of "dyspnea," but they may describe difficulty breathing in a variety of ways. A patient may describe difficulty "catching my breath" or "I can't seem to get enough air." What is significant is not only the patient's perception of the effort but also his or her tolerance for the symptom. The term **dyspnea** is used to describe the symptom of breathlessness and is a common presentation of respiratory problems. Dyspnea is a subjective symptom and varies from person to person. It can be graded as to its impact on the patient's functioning using a dyspnea scale (see Table 2-1). The nurse should ask about fatigue and level of activity to gather information about activity tolerance as it relates to the dyspnea. Also note dyspnea that occurs when lying down (**orthopnea**) and note how many pillows the patient uses at night ("three-pillow orthopnea").

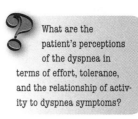

What are the patient's perceptions of the dyspnea in terms of effort, tolerance, and the relationship of activity to dyspnea symptoms?

Some more specific questions might include the following:

- Was the onset abrupt or gradual?
- What relieves the dyspnea—medication, cessation of activity, or change of position?

Table 2-1 Dyspnea Scale

Grade	Degree	Description
0	None	Not troubled with breathlessness except with strenuous exercise
1	Slight	Troubled with shortness of breath when hurrying on level ground or walking up slight hill
2	Moderate	Walks slower than people of same age because of breathlessness or has to stop for breath when walking at pace on level ground
3	Severe	Stops for breath after walking approximately 100 yards after a few minutes on level ground
4	Very severe	Too breathless to leave the house or breathless when dressing

- Is the breathing rapid, labored, or noisy?
- Is the patient assuming certain positions to make the breathing easier, such as sitting upright (orthopnea)?
- In observing the patient, is he using accessory muscles in the shoulders, neck, or abdomen to make the breathing easier?
- Is breathing more difficult at certain times of the day or night?
- Does shortness of breath awaken the patient at night (paroxysmal nocturnal dyspnea)?
- Does the patient appear anxious?
- Is he gasping for breath?
- Are there any signs of **cyanosis** (bluish-gray tinge) or pallor of the lips, mucosal lining of the mouth, inner eyelid, skin, or nail beds?
- How does the dyspnea affect the patient's performance of normal activities?

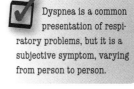

Dyspnea is a common presentation of respiratory problems, but it is a subjective symptom, varying from person to person.

Wheezing

Wheezing is a common symptom described as difficulty breathing or "catching my breath." Wheezing is caused by airways that are constricted by swelling, secretions, or bronchoconstriction, and exhalation requires more effort. Ask the patient about when the wheezing occurs, what makes him or her wheeze, whether others can hear the wheezing, and what makes the wheezing better.

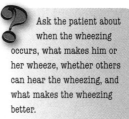

Ask the patient about when the wheezing occurs, what makes him or her wheeze, whether others can hear the wheezing, and what makes the wheezing better.

Pain

Any pain associated with breathing needs to be assessed as to location and timing in the respiratory cycle. Although lung tissue is insensitive to pain, the parietal pleura, the intercostal muscles, the connections between cartilage and bone in the thoracic cage, and the tracheobronchial tree can elicit pain. **Pleuritic pain**, pain caused by inflammation of the pleural membranes, is usually catching in nature and produced by movement of the thoracic cage. It is commonly unilateral and brought on by deep inspiration. **Intercostal pain** is transient in nature and worse during coughing. **Costochondral pain** occurs at the connection of the ribs and cartilage and can be elicited with pressure on the area. When assessing pain, nurses should differentiate between respiratory pain and other pain that may be cardiac or gastrointestinal in origin. Further questions to the patient might include the following:

- How would you rate the pain on a scale of 0 to 10?
- Where is the pain located—beneath the sternum, in the gastric area, or in the shoulder? Does it move to another area?
- What is the nature of the pain—stabbing, burning, or aching?
- When does the pain occur during breathing?
- Does coughing make the pain worse?
- Can you point to the area where you feel the pain?
- Is the pain constant, transient, or catching in nature?
- How long does the pain last?
- Do certain activities or movements bring on the pain, and does stopping the activity relieve the pain?

> When assessing pain, nurses focus questions to differentiate between respiratory pain and other pain that may be cardiac or gastrointestinal in origin.

> Costochondral pain occurs at the connection of the ribs and cartilage and can be elicited with pressure on the area.

Prior Medical History

The patient's prior medical history contains important clues when assessing the respiratory system. A thorough listing of previous illnesses, surgeries, and their respective dates should be recorded. Questions should include the presence of general conditions, such as hypertension, heart disease, and diabetes. Systemic symptoms such as weight loss, night sweats, and fatigue provide valuable information.

Take the time to list all the medications the patient is taking: prescription, nonprescription, herbal remedies, and nutritional supplements. Nurses should obtain a detailed history of all medications for breathing problems including the method of administration and schedule or symptoms that initiate the use of as-needed medications. For example, if a patient with asthma uses an inhaler, it would be important to note if the medication is

> Take the time to list all the medications the patient is taking: prescription, nonprescription, herbal remedies, and nutritional supplements.

used for relief of particular symptoms (as needed) or on a scheduled basis. Also note the frequency of as-needed medications and for what symptoms the patient decides to use these mediations. Nonprescription medications taken for breathing difficulties may include antihistamines, decongestants, nasal sprays, cough and allergy medications, inhalants, herbs, vitamins, and home remedies.

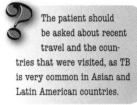

If the patient has a history of asthma, the nurse should inquire about gastroesophageal reflux disease, heartburn, and indigestion.

The patient should be asked about recent travel and the countries that were visited, as TB is very common in Asian and Latin American countries.

Specific patient responses about respiratory symptoms provide details that can direct further questioning and examination. The patient should be asked about any history of asthma, bronchitis, pneumonia, sinusitis, tuberculosis (TB), allergies, or frequent colds during the assessment. Further clarification should be obtained about allergic conditions, such as asthma, eczema, and hay fever, as well as specific allergies to dust, mold, pollen, animal dander, foods, trees, or grass. If the patient has a history of asthma, the nurse should inquire about gastroesophageal reflux disease, heartburn, and indigestion. Allergies also may be associated with asthma. Treatment for allergies, such as desensitization, should be listed with associated dates of treatment.

Any prior surgery to the upper or lower respiratory tract and the dates of surgery should be listed in the assessment. Family history of respiratory and other problems (e.g., emphysema, cystic fibrosis, lung cancer, and asthma) is important because there may be a genetic link in these conditions. The patient should be asked about recent travel and the countries that were visited, as TB is very common in Asian and Latin American countries. TB is also common among household members of an infected person, so it is important to ask about family illnesses. List the dates of the last chest radiograph, TB (Mantoux or PPD) test, vaccinations for influenza, tuberculosis, and pneumococcus, and pulmonary function tests, if appropriate.

One of the most important areas to cover in a respiratory assessment is the smoking history of the patient and his significant others. Questioning should include the use of any tobacco products, such as cigarettes, cigars, pipe tobacco, chewing tobacco, snuff, and marijuana products. Although a patient may state that he or she does not smoke, always ask about smoking in the past. A nonjudgmental attitude about smoking should be maintained to minimize the patient's guilt and encourage honesty. For cigarette smokers, the number of years the patient has been smoking should be ascertained and multiplied by the number of packs per day to obtain the number of "pack-years."

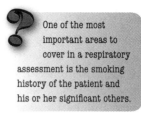

One of the most important areas to cover in a respiratory assessment is the smoking history of the patient and his or her significant others.

$$\text{\# years smoking} \times \text{\# packs per day} = \text{\# pack-years}$$

 A nonjudgmental attitude about smoking should be maintained to minimize the patient's guilt and encourage honesty.

If the patient has already quit using tobacco products, the date(s) should be noted. Also, ask the patient whether anyone in the home has exposed the patient to secondhand or passive smoke. There is increasing

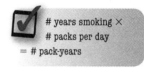

years smoking × # packs per day = # pack-years

evidence that passive smoke exposure increases the risk of asthma in children and lung cancer in nonsmoking adults. Other sources of smoke exposure include wood stoves, kerosene heaters, and fireplaces.

 There is increasing evidence that passive smoke exposure increases the risk of asthma in children and lung cancer in nonsmoking adults.

Reviewing the patient's dietary history provides valuable information about their appetite, nutritional status, eating patterns, and food allergies. Measure and weigh the patient to obtain an accurate height and weight. Review his daily dietary and fluid intake. Patients with dyspnea tend to eat smaller meals because of difficulty catching their breath when eating. Chronic dyspnea may lead to inadequate food intake, increased calorie expenditure, weight loss, and nutritional deficiencies.

Food additives have been linked to allergies and asthma. Beer, wine, restaurant salads, and many processed fruits and vegetables contain sulfites as preservatives. Sulfites may produce allergic responses in sensitive individuals, such as sneezing, urticaria (hives), shortness of breath and wheezing, chest pain or tightness, and **rhinitis** (excessive clear mucus from nose or "runny nose"). Tartrazine, a component of the Food, Drug, and Cosmetic Act (FD&C) Yellow No. 5, is a food additive that has been linked to allergic responses. This is a coloring agent used in many processed foods.

Ask about daily fluid intake. Adequate fluid intake (six 8-oz glasses per day) is necessary for liquefying and mobilizing secretions. The daily fluid requirements of a patient can be calculated by taking his or her weight in pounds, dividing the number in half, and changing the units of measurement to ounces. For example, a woman who weighs 150 pounds should have a daily fluid intake of 75 ounces. Caffeinated and alcoholic beverages have a mild diuretic effect and extra fluids are needed to compensate for this effect. The type, amount, and frequency of alcohol intake should be determined. Excessive alcohol intake has been associated with the increased incidence of head and neck cancers.

Occupational history requires careful questioning during the assessment. The patient's job(s) and date(s) of employment should be listed. Exposure to industrial fumes, chemicals, and dust may damage the respiratory tract. Dust from coal, stone, silicone, and asbestos may cause toxic lung injury. The classic case of occupational dust exposure and resultant disease is coal dust and black lung disease. Other occupations that involve exposure to toxic substances are jobs in dry cleaning, beauty salons, insect control, farming, and painting. Hobbies such as furniture refinishing, model airplane building, and woodworking also may expose the patient to noxious fumes or particles.

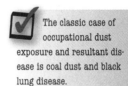

The classic case of occupational dust exposure and resultant disease is coal dust and black lung disease.

Finally, other sources of respiratory problems include pets (e.g., birds, cats), time spent in the armed forces (e.g., Agent Orange exposure, Gulf War syndrome), and exposure to certain farm products (e.g., moldy wheat and hay).

PHYSICAL ASSESSMENT OF THE RESPIRATORY TRACT

After gathering data about the patient's health history and his current symptoms, it is time to perform a physical assessment. Provide the patient with appropriate draping in a warm, well-lit room to make the patient more comfortable during the examination. The room should be private and quiet to facilitate hearing breath sounds. The physical examination of the respiratory tract proceeds in an orderly manner with the following steps: inspection, palpation, percussion, and auscultation.

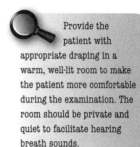

Provide the patient with appropriate draping in a warm, well-lit room to make the patient more comfortable during the examination. The room should be private and quiet to facilitate hearing breath sounds.

The examination begins with a general inspection of the patient. Note the respiratory rate, rhythm, and depth. Assess the breathing pattern without the patient's awareness so as not to make the patient self-conscious, altering the normal pattern. Count the respiratory rate for a full minute to assess the rate. The chest should move symmetrically and evenly during both inspiration and expiration. A normal respiratory rate ranges

A normal respiratory rate ranges from 12 to 20 breaths per minute.

from 12 to 20 breaths per minute. A rate greater than 20 (**tachypnea**) may indicate hypoxemia (low serum oxygen levels), **hypercapnia** (high serum carbon dioxide levels), or anxiety. A low respiratory rate (less than 12 breaths per minute) is called **bradypnea** and may indicate central nervous system (CNS) depression, as seen with head injuries and drug overdoses. Other patterns of respiration are reviewed in Figure 2-1. As the patient breathes, the nurse should watch for the use of accessory muscles in the shoulders, neck, and abdomen or changes in posture that assist the patient in breathing. Normally, the muscles in the neck, shoulders, and abdomen are not needed for respiration, and their use indicates difficulty moving air through the respiratory passages.

> Normally, the muscles in the neck, shoulders, and abdomen are not needed for respiration, and their use indicates difficulty moving air through the respiratory passages.

Check the lips, skin, and nail beds for signs of peripheral cyanosis, such as blue-gray tinge or clubbing of the nails. **Clubbing** of the nails is a sign of long-term, impaired oxygenation. An increase in the angle between the nail bed and the digit is seen in clubbing (see Figure 2-2). Central cyanosis is better assessed by examining the mucous membranes inside the mouth and the inner

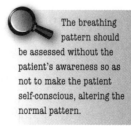

The breathing pattern should be assessed without the patient's awareness so as not to make the patient self-conscious, altering the normal pattern.

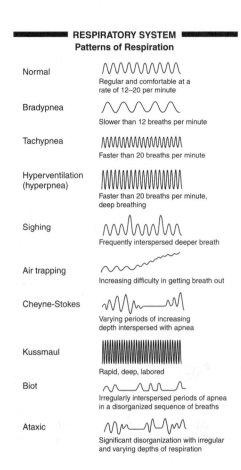

RESPIRATORY SYSTEM
Patterns of Respiration

Normal
Regular and comfortable at a
rate of 12–20 per minute

Bradypnea
Slower than 12 breaths per minute

Tachypnea
Faster than 20 breaths per minute

Hyperventilation
(hyperpnea)
Faster than 20 breaths per minute,
deep breathing

Sighing
Frequently interspersed deeper breath

Air trapping
Increasing difficulty in getting breath out

Cheyne-Stokes
Varying periods of increasing
depth interspersed with apnea

Kussmaul
Rapid, deep, labored

Biot
Irregularly interspersed periods of apnea
in a disorganized sequence of breaths

Ataxic
Significant disorganization with irregular
and varying depths of respiration

Figure 2-1 Patterns of respiration.

eyelid for pallor. Observe the face for nasal flaring and open-mouthed or **pursed-lip breathing**, which may indicate respiratory distress.

 Clubbing of the nails may be a sign of long-term, impaired oxygenation.

Nose and Sinuses

The nose and nostrils should be inspected, keeping in mind the underlying structures. The symmetry of the bony part of the nose (upper

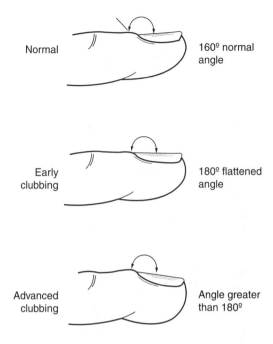

Normal	160º normal angle
Early clubbing	180º flattened angle
Advanced clubbing	Angle greater than 180º

Figure 2-2 Clubbing of the nails.

third) and the cartilaginous part (lower two thirds) should be noted. The patient's head should be tilted back 15° to 30°, and the position should be stabilized by putting a hand on the patient's forehead to prevent sudden changes of position. Using a penlight and a **nasal speculum**, the interior of the nose, or nasal vestibule, should be inspected while not touching the septum, as it is very sensitive. The outermost portion should be skin with fine hairs followed by mucous membranes, which are normally pink and moist. The mucosa may be reddened during infection or pale during allergic reactions. The nasal septum should be inspected for deviation or perforation. The middle and lower turbinates should be visible as well. The third turbinate will not be visible because of its anatomic location. The patency of each side of the nose should be assessed by pressing on one nares to block airflow, asking the patient to inhale through the other nares, and repeating on the other side. An alcohol wipe or essence of peppermint is used to assess whether the sense of smell is intact while the patient closes his eyes and is asked to identify the smell. This determines whether the first cranial nerve, the **olfactory nerve**, is intact.

The nasal septum is very sensitive—be careful not to touch it during the exam of the nasal vestibule.

Two of the four pairs of sinuses in the head, the frontal and the maxillary, are accessible for examination (see Figure 2-3). Swelling and tenderness over these sinuses is checked by palpating the area. Using the thumbs, the nurse should press firmly but gently up on the cheekbones to assess the maxillary sinuses and up on the brow bone to assess the frontal sinuses. Pain or tenderness in these areas may indicate infection (**sinusitis**).

Transillumination is another technique that may be used to assess the sinuses. It is an assessment technique used to evaluate the translucency of the sinuses using an outside light source. In a darkened room, a penlight is placed under the brow bone to assess the frontal sinus. A dim, red glow on the forehead indicates a normally air-filled frontal sinus. Lack of this glow may indicate a fluid or mucous-filled sinus. The same technique can be used to assess the maxillary sinuses. With the patient's mouth opened and head tilted back, the light should be placed downward just under the inner aspect of the eye. A dim glow should be visible in the mouth on the hard palate. Although transillumination is not a definitive test, it may be

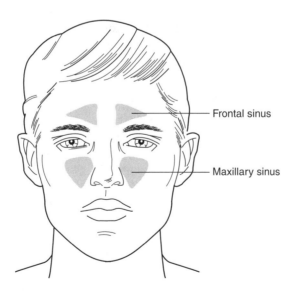

Frontal sinus

Maxillary sinus

Figure 2-3 Frontal and maxillary sinuses.

helpful in conjunction with other findings in the physical examination and history for deciding whether radiographs or computed tomography (CT scan) are needed.

Mouth, Pharynx, Trachea, and Larynx

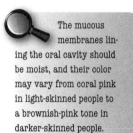

The mucous membranes lining the oral cavity should be moist, and their color may vary from coral pink in light-skinned people to a brownish-pink tone in darker-skinned people.

The examination begins by assessing the lips for cyanosis or pallor, sores, ulcers, cracks, or nodules. Look for signs of peripheral cyanosis on the lips that may indicate poor oxygenation. Sores or ulcers may be present with a herpes infection. Cracks in the corners of the mouth (**cheilitis**) may indicate nutritional deficiencies. The teeth, the quality of the dental hygiene, and the presence of dentures and other dental appliances should be noted. The patient should remove the dentures, if they are present. A penlight and tongue blade should be used to check the gums for soreness or redness that may indicate poorly fitting dentures, **gingivitis**, or **aphthous ulcers** (canker sores). Check the mucous membranes of the mouth for pallor. Because the tongue may interfere with a thorough examination, a dry 4 x 4 gauze should be used to hold the tongue and gently move it side to side to examine the mouth. The mucous membranes lining the oral cavity should be moist, and their color may vary from coral pink in light-skinned people to a brownish-pink tone in darker-skinned people. Any redness, especially along the gum line, white patches (**leukoplakia**), ulcerations, sores, or growths should be noted.

The tongue should have pinkish **papillae** and be without redness or white patches. A shiny surface also is an abnormal finding on the tongue and may indicate nutritional deficiencies. With the tongue wrapped in gauze, the tongue should be moved side to side in order to examine the base of the tongue and the floor of the mouth. This is especially important for people at high risk for oral cancers, such as patients who smoke, have a history of high alcohol intake, and chew tobacco. Any redness, leukoplakia, or ulcerations should be noted.

The posterior oropharynx is visualized with a tongue blade and a penlight. While gently pressing on the middle of the tongue (not too far back, as this may cause gagging), the palate, uvula, tonsils, and posterior oropharynx should be inspected. The color and symmetry from one side to the other should be noted. Abnormal findings include swelling, exudate, and ulceration. Enlargement of the tonsils is an abnormal finding in the adult, because tonsils should be small to nonexistent in adults. Push gently down on the tongue and have the patient say "ahhhh" or yawn to elevate the soft palate and allow visualization of the posterior oropharynx. Asymmetric elevation of the soft palate and the uvula indicates a problem with the 10th cranial nerve.

 Asymmetric elevation of the soft palate and the uvula indicates a problem with the 10th cranial nerve.

Inspect the neck for alignment, symmetry, nodules, or masses. Palpate the lymph nodes in the neck, assessing their size and mobility and whether they are tender (see Figure 2-4). Tender, enlarged lymph nodes usually indicate inflammation, whereas hard, fixed nodes may indicate malignancy. Palpate the trachea gently so as not to stimulate coughing or gagging. The thyroid cartilage (Adam's apple) and the cricoid cartilage beneath it should be identified. The trachea should be uniform and midline, elevating smoothly during swallowing.

 Palpate the trachea gently to prevent coughing or gagging.

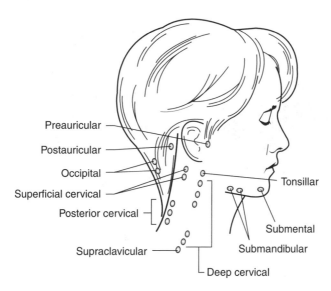

Figure 2-4 Cervical lymph node chains.

Thorax and Lungs

Anatomic landmarks on the thoracic cavity are useful for identifying organs within the thoracic cavity and for labeling abnormal findings (see Figures 2-5 through 2-8). The **midsternal line** is an imaginary line that runs vertically through the sternum. The **midclavicular line** runs vertically down the anterior chest wall beginning at the center of each clavicle. The **anterior axillary line** is another landmark that runs vertically along the anterior aspect of the chest at the anterior fold of the axilla. The **posterior axillary line**, which also starts at the axilla, extends vertically down the posterior chest. Also remember that each **intercostal space** is numbered by the rib just above it. Finally, the bases of the lungs are the lowest portions of the lungs. Anteriorly, the **base of the lung** refers to the lower portion of the lung beginning at the sixth intercostal space at the midclavicular line anteriorly, the eighth space laterally, and the 10th to 12th intercostal spaces posteriorly. The **apex of the lung** refers to the uppermost portion of the lung located above the clavicle anteriorly.

> Anatomic landmarks on the thorax are useful for identifying organs within the thoracic cavity and for labeling abnormal findings.

> Each intercostal space is numbered by the rib just above it.

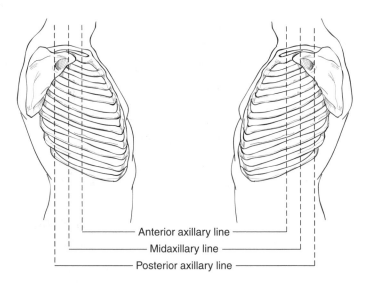

Anterior axillary line
Midaxillary line
Posterior axillary line

Figure 2-5 Lateral landmarks of the thorax.

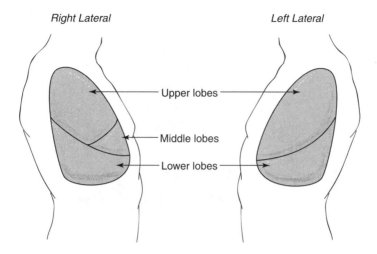

Figure 2-6 Lateral lung structures.

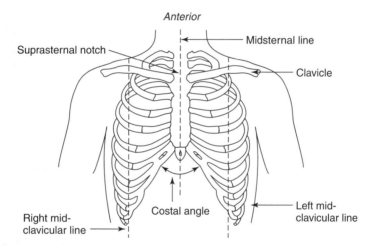

Figure 2-7 Anterior landmarks of the thorax.

The chest is examined by following the same stepwise examination: inspection, palpation, percussion, and auscultation. One side of the patient should be compared with the other side to assess physical symmetry and similarity of breath sounds.

The examination begins with the posterior chest, with the patient sitting with his arms folded across his chest. As the chest is uncovered,

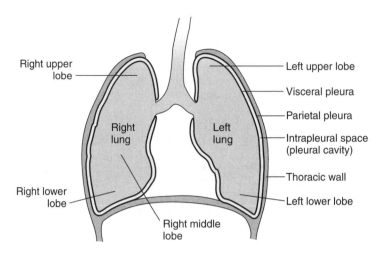

Figure 2-8 Anterior lung structures.

take care to cover the unexamined areas, particularly on female patients. If the patient has difficulty sitting up, ask for assistance or roll the patient from side to side for the examination.

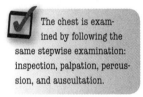

The chest is examined by following the same stepwise examination: inspection, palpation, percussion, and auscultation.

Inspection

Inspection of the chest begins with observing the patient's breathing, watching for chest expansion, and the use of accessory muscles. The rate, rhythm, and regularity

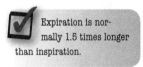

Expiration is normally 1.5 times longer than inspiration.

of the ventilations and the length of inspiration and expiration should be noted. Expiration is normally 1.5 times longer than inspiration. Prolonged expiration indicates narrowed airways or difficulty moving air out of the lungs (air trapping), as seen in emphysema. Slight retraction of the intercostal spaces is normal in thin people during quiet breathing, but any more than slight retraction indicates difficulty moving air, which may occur with chronic obstructive pulmonary disease (COPD) or an obstructed airway. Accessory muscles in the neck and shoulders normally are not used during breathing. The use of accessory muscles may indicate respiratory distress.

The use of accessory muscles in the neck and shoulders during breathing may indicate respiratory distress.

A normal chest has a lateral (side-to-side) diameter, which is twice as large as the anteroposterior (front-to-back) diameter. The ratio of the lateral to **anteroposterior (A-P) diameter** may be increased in patients with emphysema or in infants. Some common abnormalities of the chest are seen in Figure 2-9.

> A normal chest has a lateral (side-to-side) diameter, which is twice as large as the anteroposterior (front-to-back) diameter.

- **Barrel chest**—Increased A-P diameter, giving the chest a rounded appearance with the sternum pulled out. The A-P diameter is normally increased with aging or in diseases such as emphysema.
- **Funnel chest** (pectus excavatum)—Congenital depression of the sternum that decreases the A-P diameter
- **Kyphosis** and **scoliosis**—Abnormal curvature of the spine with vertebral rotation that distorts the thorax

Palpation

Palpation of the thorax provides information about **respiratory excursion**, tender areas or masses on the chest, and the presence of tactile fremitus. Keeping the patient warm and draped, examine the posterior chest beginning with any areas that the patient reports as problematic. Palpate the chest wall gently with the palm of the hand. Note any painful areas and their anatomic location. Gentle palpation should not normally cause any pain. Note any **crepitus**, crackling feelings under the skin that indicate subcutaneous pockets of air. This is an abnormal condition but may occur around chest tube insertion sites.

Respiratory excursion is assessed by placing the thumbs and stretching the hands around the rib cage at the level of the 10th rib at the vertebra with the thumbs touching at the vertebra after exhalation (see Figure 2-10). The patient is asked to inhale deeply

> During deep inhalation, thumbs placed on the chest should separate 5 to 8 cm (respiratory excursion).

while the nurse watches the thumbs separate and feels the symmetry of the chest expansion. The nurse's thumbs should separate approximately

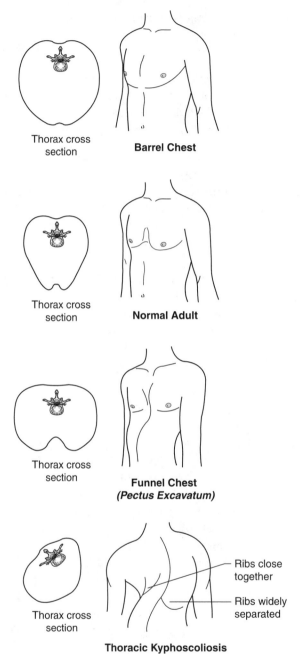

Thorax cross section
Barrel Chest

Thorax cross section
Normal Adult

Thorax cross section
Funnel Chest
(Pectus Excavatum)

Thorax cross section

Ribs close together

Ribs widely separated

Thoracic Kyphoscoliosis

Figure 2-9 Abnormalities of the chest.

5 to 8 cm during inspiration. Any asymmetry or diminished excursion should be noted in the assessment and direct further examination.

Tactile fremitus is the palpable vibrations of the voice transmitted down the tracheobronchial tree and through the chest wall. Tactile fremitus is assessed by placing the palm of the hand on the chest wall and having the patient repeat a phrase or word such as "ninety-nine." Palpate one side of the chest and compare it with the other side at several locations (see Figure 2-11) to assess the symmetry of the vibrations. The transmission of voice sounds is decreased when the tracheo-bronchial tree is obstructed by pleural effusion, tumors, or even a thick chest wall. Tactile fremitus may be increased when part of the lung is consolidated, as seen in pneumonia.

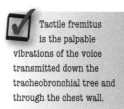

Tactile fremitus is the palpable vibrations of the voice transmitted down the tracheobronchial tree and through the chest wall.

Percussion

Percussion is used to assess lung size and position, to determine whether the lungs are filled with fluid or air, and to evaluate diaphragmatic

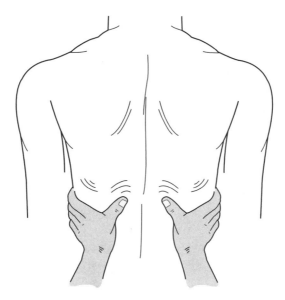

Figure 2-10 Assessing respiratory excursion.

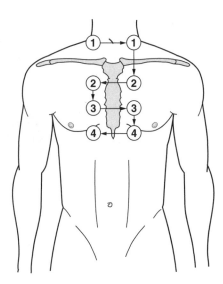

Figure 2-11 Assessing for tactile fremitus.

excursion. It is a technique that requires some practice to differentiate between vibrations. Using the distal joint of the middle finger of the left hand, the joint is placed on the intercostal space to be percussed and the middle finger of the right hand is used to strike the left with a quick, short stroke. The chest is percussed from the apices down to the bases

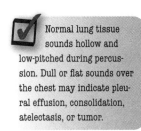

Normal lung tissue sounds hollow and low-pitched during percussion. Dull or flat sounds over the chest may indicate pleural effusion, consolidation, atelectasis, or tumor.

moving from side to side. With time, the different vibrations of air, liquid, and solid can be detected by noting the intensity, pitch, duration, and quality of the sound. Using one side of the chest as a comparison to the other, note the symmetry of the sounds (see Figure 2-12). Normal air-filled lung tissue is resonant, sounding hollow and low-pitched during percussion. The sound is dull and flat over solid tissue such as liver, muscle, and bone. A fluid-filled area, such as a pleural effusion, may also produce a flat sound. Tympanic sounds are loud and hollow sounding, and are found over air-filled spaces such as the stomach. Also, note the anatomic location of areas that do not have the expected percussion sound.

Percussion may be used to assess **diaphragmatic excursion**, the downward movement of the diaphragm as it contracts during inspira-

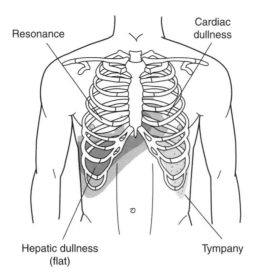

Resonance

Cardiac
dullness

Hepatic dullness
(flat)

Tympany

Figure 2-12 Different vibrations with percussion of the thorax.

tion. The distance between the relaxed dia-phragm (after expiration) and the contracted diaphragm (after inspiration) is a measure of diaphragmatic excursion. The patient is asked to take a deep breath, and the nurse percusses downward on the posterior chest until resonance (lung tissue) is replaced by dullness (diaphragm). This spot is marked with a tiny dot. Then, the patient is asked to exhale force-fully and hold it. The nurse then percusses upward until resonance is detected again. This spot is marked, and the distance between the two spots is measured. Normal diaphragmatic excursion is 5 to 6 cm but may increase to as much as 10 cm with maximal inspiration. Diaphragmatic excursion may be decreased when thoracic expansion is limited by pain or difficulty moving air.

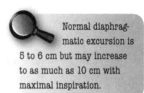

Normal diaphrag-matic excursion is 5 to 6 cm but may increase to as much as 10 cm with maximal inspiration.

Auscultation

Auscultation provides valuable clues to the functioning of the lungs and is one of the most frequently performed assessment techniques. Air moving through the tracheobronchial pathways creates sound waves that can be heard through the chest wall. These sounds change if they pass

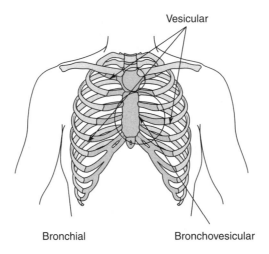

Vesicular

Bronchial   Bronchovesicular

Figure 2-13 Anatomic locations of different breath sounds.

through fluid or constricted airways. Auscultation is an assessment technique using a stethoscope at the same sites as percussion. The diaphragm of the stethoscope is used in auscultation to detect air flow through the

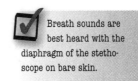

Breath sounds are best heard with the diaphragm of the stethoscope on bare skin.

respiratory passages as well as the sounds of inspiration and expiration. Normal **breath sounds** vary over different parts of the lungs. A systematic approach helps to identify the appropriate breath sound in each anatomic area (see Figure 2-13). Begin with the patient in a sitting position, breathing slowly and deeply through an open mouth. Breath sounds are best heard with the diaphragm of the stethoscope on bare skin. Drape the patient as necessary for warmth and privacy. If the patient is unable to sit up, seek assistance or roll the patient from side to side, listening to the side that is upward.

Normal breath sounds are classified by their pitch, intensity, and duration in the respiratory cycle (see Figure 2-14).

The breath sounds normally heard are tracheal, vesicular, bronchial, and bronchovesicular.

- **Tracheal breath sounds** are heard over the trachea and are harsh and discontinuous. Expiration may be heard slightly longer than inspiration.

Tracheal

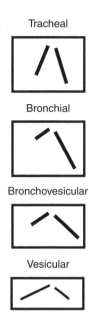

Bronchial

Bronchovesicular

Vesicular

Figure 2-14 Normal breath sounds—location, pitch, intensity, and timing.

- **Vesicular breath sounds** are heard over the majority of the lung fields. They are soft, low-pitched sounds that are heard longer during inspiration than expiration. Vesicular breath sounds are produced by air moving through the bronchioles and filling the alveoli. They are not heard over the sternum or between the scapulae. They are longer during inhalation than exhalation.
- **Bronchial breath sounds**, which normally are heard next to the trachea and mainstem bronchi, are loud, high-pitched, and discontinuous, produced by air moving through the trachea and mainstem bronchi. Bronchial breath sounds are heard over the manubrium of the sternum and between the scapulae. They have a short inspiratory phase followed by a brief pause and then are longer and louder during the expiratory phase. Expiration usually is twice as long as inspiration. Bronchial breath sounds heard over any other part of the lungs may indicate respiratory dysfunction and should be noted by their anatomic location.
- **Bronchovesicular breath sounds** are medium-pitched and continuous with muted characteristics of both bronchial and

vesicular breath sounds. They are produced by air moving through larger airways and are heard over the first and second intercostal spaces along the sternal border and between the scapulae, if they are heard at all. The presence of bronchovesicular breath sounds in any other portion of the lungs is abnormal and indicates consolidation of the lung tissue, as in pneumonia, or the replacement of air-filled lung tissue by solid tissue, such as a tumor. Sometimes they are described as windy.

Note the breath sounds, their pitch, intensity, and characteristic as well as their anatomic location in the assessment. Be specific about any asymmetry such as bronchial breath sounds in the base of the left lung, an area that should only have vesicular breath sounds.

The presence of bronchovesicular breath sounds in any other portion of the lungs is abnormal.

Transmitted voice sounds can be used to further assess portions of the lungs that have abnormal breath sounds. Bronchial or bronchovesicular breath sounds heard over parts of the lungs where vesicular breath sounds should be heard are considered abnormal. Increased transmission of voice sounds in the areas of abnormal breath sounds indicates consolidated lung tissue or the replacement of air-filled lung tissue with solid tissue. The patient is asked to produce sounds while the nurse listens with a stethoscope at the same sites used during percussion and auscultation. Comparing areas of abnormal breath sounds with areas of normal transmission identifies the anatomic location of abnormal transmitted sounds. The following are the three types of transmitted voice sounds:

- **Whispered petriloquy**—The patient is asked to repeatedly whisper a phrase such as "ninety-nine." The transmission is normally almost indistinguishable but may be louder over the area of consolidated lung tissue.
- **Bronchophony**—The patient is asked to repeat a phrase like "one-two-three" or "blue moon." The transmission would normally be quiet and muffled, but in bronchophony, the words are louder and clearer and may indicate consolidation.
- **Egophony** (E-to-A change)—The patient is asked to say "eee." Normally this would be transmitted as a muffled "eee," but in areas of consolidated lung tissue it sounds like "ay."

Adventitious Lung Sounds

Adventitious lung sounds (see Figure 2-15) are heard in addition to normal breath sounds and direct further assessment and testing. They may be identified by their pitch, intensity, and duration during the respira-

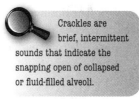

Crackles are brief, intermittent sounds that indicate the snapping open of collapsed or fluid-filled alveoli.

tory cycle. There have been many terms for these sounds, but there are now two classifications: crackles and wheezes. **Crackles** are brief, intermittent sounds that indicate the snapping open of collapsed or fluid-filled alveoli. They may be classified as **fine crackles**, sounding like hair rolled between the fingers close to the ear, or **coarse crackles**, sounding louder with more intermittent popping sounds. Crackles may occur in patients with respiratory disorders such as pneumonia, congestive heart failure, or bronchitis. Their presence should be noted and described by their anatomic location (e.g., fine crackles, base of left lower lung, one-third of the

Crackles (fine)

Crackles (coarse)

Sibilant wheezes

Sonorous wheezes

Pleural friction rub

Figure 2-15 Adventitious breath sounds—location, pitch, intensity, and timing.

way up). The timing of crackles in the respiratory cycle and whether they clear with coughing or changing of position should be noted. Crackles do not normally clear with coughing.

Wheezes are high-pitched, shrill, whistling sounds with a musical quality. They are caused by air moving through narrowed tracheobronchial airways. Wheezes may be heard in patients with asthma or bronchospasm and may be more predominant on expiration but may be heard throughout the respiratory cycle. They do not clear with coughing.

Rhonchi are low-pitched, snoring sounds heard on exhalation that change or disappear with coughing. Rhonchi occur when fluid blocks large airways.

Sonorous wheezes are low-pitched snoring sounds. They are usually produced by secretions in large airways and may clear with coughing.

Stridor is a loud-pitched sound, almost crowing in nature, caused by obstruction of the upper airway. It requires immediate attention.

Pleural friction rub is a harsh, loud, grating sound heard over an area of pleural inflammation. The roughened pleural surfaces grate over each other as the thorax expands in conditions like pleurisy or pneumonia. They are usually heard loudest at the end of inspiration.

The anterior chest is examined using the same steps as for the posterior chest. There are several anatomic differences of note. Inspection of the chest wall during normal breathing may reveal the use of abdominal muscles or retraction of the intercostal spaces. Palpation of the anterior chest is useful for noting tender areas, particularly in **costochondritis**, which is inflammation at the juncture of the ribs and cartilage. Percussion of the anterior chest reveals dullness over the heart and liver, as well as a hollow note over the gastric bubble. Auscultation over the anterior chest proceeds in the same manner as for the posterior chest, progressing from the apices to the bases and moving from one side of the chest to the other while trying to envision the underlying anatomy. Tracheal breath sounds should be heard over the manubrium of the sternum. Bronchovesicular breath sounds may be heard over the first and second intercostal spaces at the sternal border. Vesicular breath sounds should be heard over the remaining lung fields. In women, the breasts may need to be displaced to hear the lower lung fields. In men, chest hair may produce sounds against the diaphragm of the stethoscope that need to be differentiated from adventitious breath sounds such as crackles.

DIAGNOSTIC TESTS OF THE RESPIRATORY SYSTEM

If the patient's assessment detects some changes in respiratory functioning, diagnostic tests may be ordered to evaluate the respiratory system and identify the respiratory dysfunction. The functional ability of the lungs may be measured by a variety of **pulmonary function tests (PFT)** that measure air flow rates and calculate lung volumes and lung capacities.

PFTs are performed to accomplish the following:

* Evaluate the function of the lungs.
* Confirm the presence of respiratory disorders.
* Differentiate between obstructive and restrictive disorders.
* Evaluate disease exacerbation or progression.
* Evaluate lung function prior to surgery.
* Evaluate response to bronchodilators.
* Evaluate the need for mechanical ventilation.

Some different types of PFTs include **spirometry** (which measures lung volumes and calculates lung capacities), measurement of airflow rates, estimation of diffusion capacities, bronchial provocation or inhalation tests, and exercise pulmonary stress testing. **Arterial blood gases** are another important measure of pulmonary functioning that will be discussed later in this chapter.

Lung Capacities and Volumes

Measurement of **lung capacities** and **lung volumes** is performed with spirometry. These are usually the first PFTs performed when a patient needs evaluation. PFTs are ordered to accomplish the following:

* Evaluate ventilatory function.
* Determine the causes of dyspnea.
* Assess the effectiveness of medications.
* Determine the cause of respiratory dysfunction.
* Assess the extent of the dysfunction.

Using a machine called a spirometer, the patient performs various breathing maneuvers. To get accurate measurements, a clip is placed on the nose, and the patient is asked to seal his mouth over the mouthpiece.

The volume of air inspired or expired can be measured during breathing with a recording device called a **kymograph**. If the volumes are measured over time, then air flow rates can be calculated. Measurements of air flow rates are important when there is a question of obstruction or restriction. Normal values for volumes and air flow rates are predicted based on age, gender, height, weight, and race.

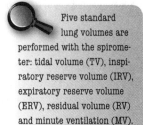

Five standard lung volumes are performed with the spirometer: tidal volume (TV), inspiratory reserve volume (IRV), expiratory reserve volume (ERV), residual volume (RV) and minute ventilation (MV).

Patient values greater than 80% of the predicted values are considered normal. Withholding bronchodilating or sedating medications for 4 hours prior to testing may be necessary to gain an accurate picture of the patient's respiratory functioning. These medications can be resumed immediately after the PFTs.

Five standard lung volumes are performed with the spirometer:

1. **Tidal volume (TV)**—The TV is the amount of air inspired or exhaled during normal, quiet breathing. The amount is approximately 500 mL in a 70 kg person. It can range from 400 to 700 mL and reach 4,500 mL during maximal exercise. Volume capacities are 20–25% lower in women. A decrease in TV without a decrease in respiratory rate indicates a restrictive disorder such as pulmonary fibrosis. A decrease in TV with a decrease in respiratory rate indicates a neurological problem.

2. **Inspiratory reserve volume (IRV)**—The IRV is the amount of air that can be inhaled after a normal or tidal inspiration (approximately 3,300 mL).

3. **Expiratory reserve volume (ERV)**—The ERV is the amount of air that can be forcibly exhaled after normal or tidal expiration (approximately 1,100 mL).

4. **Residual volume (RV)**—The RV is the amount of air remaining in the lungs after forced, maximal expiration (approximately 1,000 mL).

5. **Minute ventilation (MV)**—The MV is the volume of air inspired and expired during 1 minute of normal breathing.

Lung capacities also can be calculated during pulmonary function testing. They are determined by combining two (or more) lung volumes. Figure 2-16 shows the relationship of lung volumes and capacities.

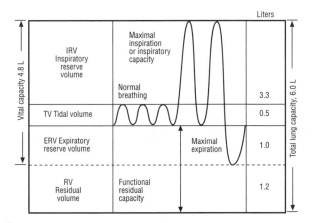

Figure 2-16 Relationship of lung volumes and capacities.

The following is a list of the different types of lung capacities:

- **Vital capacity (VC)**—The VC is the maximal amount of air that can be exhaled after maximal inspiration (approximately 5,000 mL). The VC is the total of the tidal volume, inspiratory reserve volume, and expiratory reserve volume.
- **Inspiratory capacity (IC)**—The IC is the amount of air that can be inhaled with maximal effort after a normal exhalation (approximately 3,000 mL).
- **Functional residual capacity (FRC)**—The FRC is the amount of air remaining in the lungs at the end of normal exhalation (approximately 1,200 mL).
- **Total lung capacity (TLC)**—The TLC is the amount of air in the lungs with maximal inspiration (approximately 6,000 mL). It is also the total of the four lung volumes (TV + IRV + ERV + RV = TLC).
- **Forced vital capacity (FVC)**—The FVC is the amount of air expelled with maximally forced exhalation.

> There is always some air remaining in the lungs even after maximal expiration. This remaining air allows the alveoli to stay partially inflated and minimizes rapid fluctuations of the oxygen and carbon dioxide levels in the blood between breaths.

Lung volumes and capacities also can be determined in specially equipped laboratories. Tests using tracer gases, such as helium or nitrogen, can be performed to determine the FRC. The FRC was previously defined as the amount of air remaining in the lungs at the end of normal expiration.

There is always some air remaining in the lungs even after maximal expiration. This remaining air allows the alveoli to stay partially inflated and minimizes rapid fluctuations of the oxygen and carbon dioxide levels in the blood between breaths. Increased RV indicates that there is an abnormally large amount of air remaining in the lungs at the end of exhalation, seen in conditions that cause air-trapping (e.g., emphysema). The RV and FRC usually decrease together in restrictive conditions like pulmonary fibrosis.

Pulmonary mechanics, the measurements of airflow in the respiratory tract, are calculated by examining air flow versus volume. They can be graphically produced by specific machines or visibly produced by small devices that patients can use at home. Three measurements that are frequently used include the following:

- **Peak expiratory flow (PEF)**—The PEF is the amount of air that can be forcibly exhaled after maximal inhalation. Small PEF devices for home use make this a quick and useful measure of disease exacerbation or response to medications such as bronchodilators.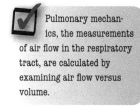

  Pulmonary mechanics, the measurements of air flow in the respiratory tract, are calculated by examining air flow versus volume.

- **Forced expiratory flow (FEF)**—The FEF measures the rate of air flow during forced expiration on a flow-volume graph.
- **Forced expiratory volume (FEV)**—The FEV measures the amount of air exhaled after full inhalation at various times during the exhalation (i.e., 1 second, 2 seconds, 3 seconds). The FEV1 (volume expired at 1 second) is a good measure of airway resistance in disease exacerbations.

> Increased residual volume (RV) indicates that there is an abnormally large amount of air remaining in the lungs at the end of exhalation, seen in conditions that cause air-trapping (e.g., emphysema).

Another measurement of air flow in the lungs is the **airway resistance (R_{aw})**, This test determines whether restrictive or obstructive disease is present. R_{aw} is the difference between the pressure in the mouth (atmospheric pressure) and the pressure in the alveoli. It is calculated from the airflow and changes in pressure in the respiratory tract (i.e., the pressure gradient) during breathing. R_{aw} increases in obstructive diseases (e.g., asthma) due to narrowing of the airways by secretions and edema.

Other PFTs include exercise pulmonary stress testing, diffusion capacities, and bronchial provocation tests. Exercise-induced changes in respiratory functioning can be monitored using spirometry and exercise machinery (e.g., treadmill to help in the diagnosis of exercise-induced asthma).

Diffusion Capacities

Diffusion capacities measure the ability of gases to diffuse across the alveolar membrane. A given amount of carbon monoxide is inhaled by the patient and then exhaled. The exhaled amount is measured and compared to the amount in the blood. The difference represents the amount of gas that diffused across the alveolar membrane and into the blood. A decreased diffusion capacity occurs when defects in the alveoli, such as thickening of the alveolar wall (pulmonary fibrosis), inhibit gas diffusion.

Bronchial provocation tests are used to determine a cause-and-effect relationship between certain inhaled irritants and the reactivity of the patient's airways. Histamine or methacholine are inhaled by the patient. PFTs are then performed to assess for bronchial constriction. These tests are used to establish a diagnosis of hyperactive airway disease.

Arterial Blood Gases

Arterial blood gas (ABG) analysis is performed to evaluate respiratory functioning and determine the level of carbon dioxide ($Paco_2$), oxygen (Pao_2), bicarbonate level (HCO_3^-), and the hydrogen ion concentration (pH). These provide information about the ventilation and diffusion of gases in the lungs and the acid-base balance of the blood, as explained in the following:

- The partial pressure of arterial oxygen (Pao_2) is useful for determining whether a patient is hypoxemic (i.e., low levels of oxygen in the arterial blood) or to determine the effectiveness of interventions such as supplemental oxygen.
- The partial pressure of arterial carbon dioxide ($Paco_2$) reflects the lungs ability to eliminate carbon dioxide and the adequacy of the lungs' ventilation.

- The pH indicates the blood's acidity or alkalinity.
- The bicarbonate level (HCO_3^-) is an indication of the kidney's ability to retain and/or excrete (HCO_3^-).

An important concept used in measuring the levels of gas in the blood is **Dalton's Law.** It states that each gas in the atmosphere contributes to the total pressure of all the gases in the atmosphere. Oxygen, carbon dioxide, nitrogen, and hydrogen each contribute a portion to the total pressure of the atmosphere, which is 760 mmHg. Room air is 20.8% oxygen, 78.6% nitrogen, and less than 1% other gases. The partial pressure of atmospheric oxygen is 160 mmHg and falls to about 100 mmHg in the alveoli after mixing with residual air in the lungs. The average arterial oxygen levels (Pao_2) at sea level is 95 to 100 mmHg (Table 2-2).

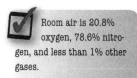
Room air is 20.8% oxygen, 78.6% nitrogen, and less than 1% other gases.

An arterial blood gas sample is taken from the radial, brachial, or femoral arteries. Puncture of the radial artery requires that the patient has adequate arterial perfusion to the hand via the ulnar artery (Figure 2-17). The adequacy of the circulation can be evaluated by **Allen's test**, a simple compression of the radial artery to assess circulation to the hand by the ulnar artery. An arterial blood sample is obtained in a heparinized syringe, which is immediately placed on ice and taken to the laboratory for analysis. Care must be taken not to allow air bubbles in the syringe, as they might alter the gas analysis. The puncture site must be compressed for a full 5 minutes after an arterial blood sample is drawn to prevent bleeding and longer if the patient is on anticoagulant therapy. The sample must be labeled with the time it was drawn, the patient's temperature, and the amount and method of supplemental oxygen (including mechanical ventilation) or room air if the patient is not receiving supplemental oxygen.

Table 2-2 Arterial Blood Gas Ranges

Value	Normal
pH	7.35 to 7.45
Pao_2	95 to 100 mmHg
$Paco_2$	35 to 45 mmHg
HCO_3^-	22 to 24 mEq/L

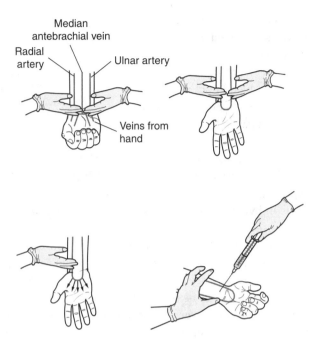

Figure 2-17 Arterial blood gas sampling.

 An arterial puncture site must be compressed for a full 5 minutes after the sample is drawn to prevent bleeding.

The oxygen levels in the blood are an indicator of the ability of the lungs to match capillary blood flow to the ventilated alveoli. Oxygen levels in the blood are also dependent on the cardiac output, the amount of blood the heart is pumping, and the ability of the red blood cells to carry oxygen. **Hypoxemia** (low oxygen levels in the blood), exists when arterial oxygen levels fall below 75 mmHg. **Hypoxia** refers to inadequate oxygenation of the tissues. Of the oxygen carried in the blood, 98% is bound to hemoglobin as oxyhemoglobin. Only 2% of oxygen is actually carried as dissolved gas, which is what is measured as a PaO_2. When hypoxemia exists, the patient may develop signs of cyanosis. The role of the cardiovascular

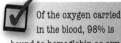 Of the oxygen carried in the blood, 98% is bound to hemoglobin as oxyhemoglobin. Only 2% is actually carried as dissolved gas, measured as the PaO_2.

and the hematologic systems in the process of oxygenation is discussed in more detail in later chapters.

The **partial pressure of carbon dioxide** (**Paco₂**) in arterial blood fluctuates with the respiratory cycle. It is automatically calculated by the blood gas analyzer. The average Paco₂ is 35 to 45 mmHg. The respiratory rate regulates the amount of carbon dioxide in the blood. During hyperventilation, more carbon dioxide is exhaled, decreasing the Paco₂. The reverse is true in hypoventilation, although this is a less efficient system because a decreased respiratory rate also can cause hypoxemia, stimulating the medulla to increase the respiratory rate. An exception to this effect occurs in patients with COPD. The chronically elevated Paco₂ levels no longer stimulate the respiratory centers in the medulla to increase the respiratory rate. The peripheral chemoreceptors take on the role of regulator of respiration based on the oxygen levels in the arterial blood. Blood gas analysis in patients with COPD allows supplemental oxygen levels to be adjusted to not only the Pao₂ but the Paco₂ and pH.

Oxygen levels in the blood are also dependent on the cardiac output, the amount of blood the heart is pumping, and the ability of the red blood cells to carry oxygen.

The average Paco₂ is 35 to 45 mmHg.

Acid-Base Balance

The respiratory system participates in the acid-base balance by altering the respiratory rate. The pH determines the alkalinity or acidity of the blood. A pH of 7.4 is considered neutral in blood, with a normal range being 7.35 to 7.45. When the pH is greater than 7.45, then the blood is considered alkalotic (**alkalosis**). Likewise, if the pH is lower than 7.35, then the blood is considered acidotic (**acidosis**).

Alkalosis or acidosis may originate in the respiratory or metabolic systems or both. By examining the carbon dioxide levels and the bicarbonate levels, the origin(s) of an imbalance may be determined. Carbon dioxide levels reflect the role of the respiratory sys-

The respiratory system participates in the acid-base balance by altering the respiratory rate.

The pH determines the alkalinity or acidity of the blood. A pH of 7.4 is considered neutral in blood, with a normal range being 7.35 to 7.45. When the pH is greater than 7.45, then the blood is considered alkalotic (alkalosis). Likewise, if the pH is lower than 7.35, then the blood is considered acidotic (acidosis).

tem in maintaining the acid-base balance (see Table 2-3). Carbon dioxide is carried in the blood as carbonic acid. Changing the respiratory rate can alter the amount of carbonic acid and the pH of the blood in minutes. When the respiratory rate increases, more carbon dioxide is exhaled, making the blood more alkaline (higher pH). Likewise, a decreased respiratory rate allows the levels of carbon dioxide to increase, making the blood more acidic (lower pH).

Metabolic changes to the acid-base balance are done by the kidneys. The levels of **bicarbonate (HCO_3^-)** in the blood are changed by the kidneys to normalize the blood's pH. This slower system requires 24 to 48 hours to alter the pH of the blood. Bicarbonate functions as a buffer in the blood to keep the pH within the normal range. The bicarbonate level is usually maintained in a 20:1 ratio with carbonic acid to keep the blood pH between 7.35 and 7.45. The normal values for serum bicarbonate are 24 to 30 mEq/L and are calculated by the blood gas analyzer. When the HCO_3^- level increases, the pH increases and the blood becomes more alkaline. Likewise, when the HCO_3^- level decreases, the blood becomes more acidic and the pH of the blood decreases. Generally, bicarbonate levels greater than 30 mEq/L indicate a metabolic alkalosis, and levels lower than 24 mEq/L indicate a metabolic acidosis. All components of arterial blood gas analysis must be examined in reference to each other

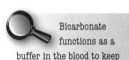 Bicarbonate functions as a buffer in the blood to keep the pH within the normal range. The bicarbonate level is usually maintained in a 20:1 ratio with carbonic acid to keep the blood pH between 7.35 and 7.45.

Table 2-3 Changes in Acid-Base Imbalances

	pH	PaCO₂	HCO₃⁻	Compensation
Respiratory alkalosis	↑	↓	Normal until compensation	Kidneys increase HCO_3^-; 24 to 48 hrs
Metabolic alkalosis	↑	Normal unless lungs compensate	↑	Lungs increase PaCO₂ by decrease in respiratory rate; takes minutes
Respiratory acidosis	↓	↑	Normal until kidneys compensate	Kidneys keep more HCO_3^-; takes days
Metabolic acidosis	↓	Normal until lungs compensate	↓	Lungs decrease PaCO₂ by increase in respiratory rate; takes minutes

and the patient's overall status to determine the nature of the acid-base disturbance.

Metabolic alkalosis (an increase in serum bicarbonate level) is most commonly caused by the loss of gastric contents, such as prolonged nasogastric suction or excessive vomiting. It is also seen in patients with long-standing COPD because the increased bicarbonate levels buffer the chronically high Pco_2 levels. **Metabolic acidosis** (decreased serum bicarbonate level) is seen in patients with lower gastrointestinal losses (e.g., prolonged diarrhea), and in diabetic acidosis, shock, dehydration, and after cardiopulmonary arrest.

There are also cases of acid-base imbalances that are mixed in origin when one system may compensate for the other, resulting in a compensated acidosis or alkalosis. For example, patients with COPD who have chronically elevated carbon dioxide levels and low pH may have increased bicarbonate levels because the kidneys have compensated for the long-term respiratory acidosis by retaining bicarbonate. Because of the complex nature of acid-base balance, the patient's condition must be evaluated with the blood values.

 Because of the complex nature of acid-base balance, the patient's condition must be evaluated in conjunction with the blood values.

Oxygen Saturation

Whereas the Pao_2 measures the amount of oxygen dissolved in the arterial blood, the **oxygen saturation level (Sao_2)** measures the amount of oxygen bound to hemoglobin as oxyhemoglobin. **Pulse oximetry** uses a spectrophotometer to determine the amount of light absorbed by hemoglobin in arterial blood. A clip placed on a finger or ear allows the oximeter to calculate the percentage of oxygenated hemoglobin as compared to the total capacity of hemoglobin available for binding. Painted fingernails and dark pigmentation may overstate the oxygen saturation but acrylic nails do not interfere with readings. Because the clip relies on adequate perfusion of the tissue, conditions that decrease perfusion alter the reading. Pulse oximetry may not be useful during times of rapid desaturation like a "code" because it measures the previous minutes' oxygenation. Hypothermia, hypotension, and drugs that cause vasoconstriction may result in decreased perfusion and a low reading. In cases of reduced blood flow, the finger will provide a more accurate reading than the ear or forehead.

> Painted fingernails, acrylic nails, lipid emulsions, and dark pigmentation may interfere with the measurement of oxygen saturation.

A normal oxygenation saturation level (Sao_2, O_2 Sat, or Spo_2) is 96% to 100% but varies depending on the Po_2, the pH of the blood, the body temperature, and the structure of the hemoglobin. Oxygen saturation levels do not follow the Pao_2 proportionately. For example, an Sao_2 of 89% is equivalent to a Pao_2 of 60 mmHg, far below the level defined as hypoxemia. The **oxyhemoglobin dissociation curve** is a graphic depiction of the relationship between oxyhemoglobin saturation and oxygen tension in the blood. The oxyhemoglobin dissociation curve describes the changes in the oxygen binding and release from hemoglobin with the pH of the blood. The pH of the blood affects the affinity of oxygen for hemoglobin (see Figure 2-18). If the blood is acidotic (pH less than 7.35), then the curve is said to shift to the left with decreased Sao_2, increased oxygen release, and decreased oxygen binding. Conversely, if the blood is alkalotic (pH greater than 7.45), then the oxyhemoglobin dissociation curve

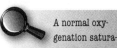

> A normal oxygenation saturation level (Sao_2) is 96% to 100% but varies depending on the Po_2, the pH of the blood, the body temperature, and the structure of the hemoglobin.

shifts to the right with an increased Sao_2 but increased O_2 binding and decreased O_2 release. In either case, the Sao_2 needs to be assessed in relation to the patient's appearance, the vital signs, and, if necessary, arterial blood gases. Temperature increases allow more oxygen to be released from hemoglobin but also increase oxygen consumption by the tissues.

> An Sao_2 of 89% is equivalent to a Pao_2 of 60 mmHg, far below the level defined as hypoxemia.

Hemoglobin is structured to combine with and release oxygen as oxyhemoglobin. Hemoglobin also may combine with **2,3-diphosphoglycerol (2,3-DPG),** an intermediate product of **glycolysis** (the conversion of glycogen in liver stores to glucose). 2,3-DPG causes oxyhemoglobin to more readily release oxygen. The levels of 2,3-DPG in the blood increase when

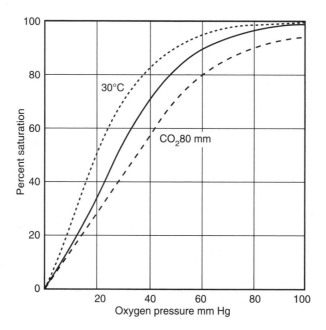

Figure 2-18 Oxygen–hemoglobin dissociation curve.

there is decreased oxygen delivery to the tissues, increased altitude, or when glycolysis is occurring. Blood obtained from blood banks is lower in 2,3-DPG and has reduced ability to release oxygen to the tissues.

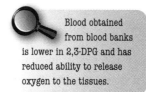

Blood obtained from blood banks is lower in 2,3-DPG and has reduced ability to release oxygen to the tissues.

Other Tests of Respiratory Function and Structure

There are a variety of tests that examine different aspects of respiratory functioning and anatomy. Some of the tests performed in the radiology department include chest radiographs (X-rays), fluoroscopy, computerized axial tomography (CAT) scans, magnetic resonance imaging (MRI), lung scans, bronchography, and pulmonary angiography.

Chest Radiographs

Radiologic examination or X-rays provide information about internal structures. Normal lung tissue is radiolucent, so foreign bodies, infiltrates, tumors, and fluids appear as white areas or densities. The **chest** radiograph (X-ray) is performed from the posterior-anterior and lateral views, where X-rays pass from one side through the other. They are useful for assessing pathophysiologic changes in the thorax, such as tumors, inflammation, fluid and air accumulation, integrity of bony structures, and diaphragmatic hernia. They are most useful when compared to the patient's previous films, allowing the detection of changes. Although chest X-rays may not diagnose every condition, they are useful in visualizing pneumothorax, fibrosis, infiltrates, and atelectasis. Radiographs are useful in evaluating the nose and sinuses, assessing the integrity of the bony and cartilaginous structures, and detecting fluid accumulation in the sinuses or lung tissues.

Chest X-rays are performed in the radiology department or at the bedside with a portable unit. They are completed in a few minutes and are painless. Patients must wear a gown without snaps and remove all metal objects like jewelry. Patients of childbearing age will be given a lead apron to protect their pelvis, particularly the ovaries and testes.

Fluoroscopy

Fluoroscopy uses a continuous stream of X-rays to assess the motion of thoracic contents. Because it exposes the patient to high levels of radiation it is only used to visualize the motion of thoracic structures, like the diaphragm. Decreased or asymmetric movement of the diaphragm may occur after open-heart surgery.

CAT Scans

Computerized axial tomography (CAT) scans provide different views with more detail of internal structures than does traditional radiography. Using X-rays and a computer, a cross section of the body through a horizontal plane can be constructed. This picture provides greater definition of internal structures and organs. Sometimes a contrast agent is injected in a vein to allow greater visualization. Mediastinal tumors are best viewed by CAT scan. Needle biopsies can be performed with CAT scan guidance. The procedure takes 30 to 60 minutes and requires the patient to remain still in a horizontal position. The nurse should explain to the patient that they will lie in a noisy, tunnel-shaped machine. Encourage the patient to lie still as movement may make the test less accurate. If they feel claustrophobic, they should try to relax and breathe normally and visualize a pleasant place or activity. Sedation may be required.

MRI

Magnetic resonance imaging (MRI) uses a powerful magnetic field, radio waves, and computer enhancement to create detailed, cross-sectional pictures of the human anatomy. A noninvasive procedure, MRI is useful for assessing normal internal structure, such as the pulmonary vasculature, lung tissue, and lymph nodes as well as abnormalities

Magnetic resonance imaging (MRI) uses a powerful magnetic field, radio waves, and computer enhancement to create detailed, cross-sectional pictures of the human anatomy.

such as tumors, cysts, and pulmonary edema. MRI is a painless procedure that requires the patient to lie within a tunnel for 30 to 60 minutes. Tell the patient to lie quietly and not talk to avoid distorting the results. Warn the patient that the machine itself is loud and noisy, with repeated banging or pinging.

 Warn the patient that the machine itself is loud and noisy, with repeated banging or pinging.

Lung Scans

Lung scans are performed to assess the perfusion of the lungs by the pulmonary arteries. They are used in diagnosing pulmonary embolism, lung malignancies, COPD, and pulmonary edema. **Ventilation-perfusion scans ($\dot{V}/\dot{Q}$)** are used to assess lung perfusion and ventilation, particularly to detect pulmonary emboli. A $\dot{V}/\dot{Q}$ scan can also be used to detect atelectasis, obstructing tumors, and chronic obstructive pulmonary disease. Albumin tagged with radioactive technetium is used in the perfusion portion of the study. It is injected into the patient's bloodstream. Then, radiographic images are taken of the lungs in the nuclear medicine department. The scintillation camera shows decreased blood flow to part of the lung is blocked by an embolus. Simultaneous ventilation scans, with the patient breathing a tagged gas, can be done to detect defects in ventilation as well as perfusion. Diminished or absent blood flow (i.e., pulmonary embolism) is seen as a defect in perfusion on the scan. Defects in ventilation alone can be the result of an airway obstruction.

Bronchography

Bronchography is used to evaluate the structure of the trachea and bronchi. It is useful for identifying obstruction of the tracheobronchial tree caused by a tumor or foreign bodies, as well as for making the diagnosis of hyaline membrane disease in infants. A dye with radioactive iodine is injected through a catheter in the trachea. Radiographic films are taken with the patient in a variety of positions to move the dye around the structures and to improve visualization. Patients need to be encouraged to cough after the procedure to expel the dye.

Pulmonary Angiography

Pulmonary angiography, also called pulmonary arteriography, assesses the perfusion of the lungs by the pulmonary circulation. A radioactive contrast dye is injected into a vein or artery, a series of X-rays are taken of the chest to detect blood flow abnormalities. These films provide a picture of the vasculature that can detect pulmonary embolism or infarction. Defects in filling of the vasculature indicate blockage of the blood vessel by an embolus or other obstruction such as a tumor. Tell the patient that he must fast for 6 hours prior to the procedure. The test will be done in the radiology or nuclear medicine department. The doctor will place a needle in a vein (antecubital, subclavian, femoral, or jugular vein) and advance a catheter to release the dye in the correct location. Some patients have hypersensitivity reactions to the contrast dye. Watch for dyspnea, itchiness, hives, or changes in blood pressure. The nurse needs to carefully assess for allergic reactions as well as perfusion distal to the catheter insertion.

Some patients have hypersensitivity reactions to the contrast dye. Watch for dyspnea, itchiness, hives, or changes in blood pressure.

Other tests to examine respiratory anatomy are performed by an endoscopic approach. These include **laryngoscopy, bronchoscopy,** and **mediastinoscopy.** Fiber-optic or rigid scopes allow direct visualization of the structures and may detect changes in anatomy and the presence of foreign bodies or tumors. The endoscope also can be used to cauterize bleeding vessels, biopsy tissue, or remove a foreign body. Patients are at least locally anesthetized and sedated during laryngoscopy and bronchoscopy. The endoscope is passed through the nose or mouth and into the larynx and trachea for visualization of the anatomy. Biopsies may be taken during the procedure. Patients should be instructed to refrain from coughing after bronchoscopy with biopsy to prevent dislodging of the clot at the biopsy site.

Patients should be instructed to refrain from coughing after bronchoscopy with biopsy to prevent dislodging of the clot at the biopsy site.

Mediastinoscopy requires general anesthesia because an incision is made at the **suprasternal notch**, at the anterior base of the neck. A mirrored lens instrument is passed into the mediastinum to visualize the anatomy of the mediastinum, identify possible growths, and take tissue samples for pathological examination. Because the lymph nodes in the mediastinum drain the lungs, specimens can be used to diagnose and stage lung cancer, lymphomas, sarcoidosis, granulomatous infections, and histoplasmosis.

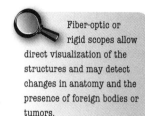

Fiber-optic or rigid scopes allow direct visualization of the structures and may detect changes in anatomy and the presence of foreign bodies or tumors.

Cultures

Laboratory cultures provide valuable information about diseases of the respiratory tract. **Throat culture,** or nasopharyngeal culture, is one of the most commonly performed diagnostic tests. It is performed to detect and identify bacteria in the oropharynx. A swab is brushed along the back of the oropharynx and then sent to the laboratory to culture the growth and identify antibiotic sensitivity if indicated. The most common reason to perform a throat culture is to rule out a streptococcal infection.

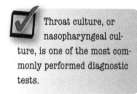

Throat culture, or nasopharyngeal culture, is one of the most commonly performed diagnostic tests.

Tell the patient where the culture will be obtained and warn him that he may feel like coughing or gagging when the swab is on his throat. After putting on gloves, visualize the posterior oropharynx with a light. Swab from side to side but do not touch the cheeks, tongue, or teeth with the swab. If a commercial sterile collection kit is used, break the ampule at the base after reinserting the swab. Label the sample with the date and time as well as recent antimicrobial therapy.

Tell the patient where the culture will be obtained and warn him that he may feel like coughing or gagging when the swab is on his throat.

Sputum cultures are obtained to detect and identify infectious bacteria in sputum, to check for malignancy, and to detect the tubercle bacillus, the organism that causes tuberculosis. Sputum cultures are best obtained early in the morning with deep coughing but may also be obtained through tracheobronchial suctioning, tracheal suctioning, or bronchoscopy. If infecting organisms are identified in the culture, then a sensitivity is done to determine which antibiotics will be effective. Malignant cells from the respiratory tract also may be shed into the sputum, in which case the sputum sample is sent to pathology for microscopic examination.

The sputum test for tuberculosis is called an acid-fast bacillus smear. It requires three consecutive early-morning sputum samples. Another test for tuberculosis is the tuberculin or **Mantoux skin test.** A small amount of purified protein (0.1 mL) is injected intradermally on the forearm. The area is then examined 48 to 72 hours later to note any swelling and erythema. If the indurated or swollen area is greater than 10 mm wide, the test is considered positive for tuberculosis. Follow-up testing is required.

Malignant cells from tumors in the respiratory tract also may be shed into the sputum.

 With the Mantoux skin test, a small amount of purified protein (0.1 mL) is injected intradermally on the forearm. The area is then examined 48 to 72 hours later to note any swelling and erythema. If the indurated or swollen area is greater than 10 mm wide, the test is considered positive for tuberculosis. Follow-up testing is required.

Other pathological tests that may be performed to assess the respiratory tract include **pleural fluid analysis** and **blood cultures**. Pleural fluid is obtained for analysis by inserting a needle into an area where fluid has accumulated in the pleural space. Pleural fluid analysis is performed to detect malignancy. Blood cultures are obtained by venipuncture at three successive times to identify blood infection caused by organisms in the respiratory tract.

Thoracentesis

Thoracentesis, or pleural fluid analysis, is performed to obtain fluid samples from the pleural space, relieve pressure from accumulated fluid, and obtain tissue for biopsy. Usually, the pleural cavity contains less than 20 mL of fluid. Pleural effusions develop from either abnormal fluid production or reabsorption. Thoracentesis is usually performed with a local anesthetic. Chest X-rays are indicated before and after the procedure. The patient can usually feel

Thoracentesis, or pleural fluid analysis, is performed to obtain fluid samples from the pleural space, relieve pressure from accumulated fluid, and obtain tissue for biopsy.

pressure from the needle even after the use of local anesthetic. The nurse should help the patient stay still and in position during the thoracentesis. Careful observation of the patient following the procedure is necessary to assess for pneumothorax, tension pneumothorax, mediastinal shift, and subcutaneous emphysema (crepitus).

> Careful observation of the patient following the procedure is necessary to assess for pneumothorax, tension pneumothorax, mediastinal shift, and subcutaneous emphysema (crepitus).

Biopsies

Biopsies are performed to obtain tissue samples for microscopic examination. Although biopsies may be obtained from most any location in the respiratory tract, two of the most common are lung biopsies and pleural biopsies. Lung biopsies are used to diagnose small and nonsmall lung carcinomas. In lung biopsies, a sample of lung tissue is obtained through either open or closed techniques. Open techniques require general anesthesia in the operating room through either limited or standard thoracotomies. Closed techniques may be done with local anesthesia and include both needle biopsies and transbronchial biopsies during bronchoscopy. Needle biopsies are appropriate for lesions that are easily accessible. Chest X-rays are indicated after lung biopsies to rule out pneumothorax.

Pleural biopsies are used to obtain tissue for pathological analysis. They are usually performed under local anesthesia and may follow thoracentesis (obtaining pleural fluid from an effusion for pathologic analysis). Open pleural biopsies may be required when there is not a pleural effusion.

There are many ways to evaluate the functioning of the respiratory tract. History taking, physical assessment, preparation of the patient for diagnostic testing, and education of the patient and family all are components of the nurse's role. But before the assessment forms are filled out and the numbers are analyzed, there is a person—a patient—who has the most important information. He can tell the nurse how he is feeling, what hurts, what he coughs up, and what makes him feel better. It is the nurse's role to listen to all the cues that the patient provides and let these guide the assessment of the patient's respiratory system.

CASE STUDY RESOLUTION

The emergency department physician examines Mr. Z and orders a portable chest X-ray, complete blood counts, arterial blood gases, sputum for culture and sensitivity, routine PFTs, and serum electrolyte tests. The nurse reassures Mr. Z and his wife because they seem quite anxious. She tells them that the tests will help the medical team decide how best to treat the problem. The arterial blood gas is as follows: PaO_2—65, $PaCO_2$—58, pH—7.29, HCO_3^-—34. Mr. Z is in a respiratory acidosis, but given his PO_2 and SaO_2, the physician orders oxygen at 4 L per minute via nasal prongs. The nurse watches for a decreased respiratory rate and signs of carbon dioxide narcosis. The FEV_1 is markedly decreased, as is the tidal volume. Bronchodilators are ordered to help Mr. Z's breathing. The chest X-ray shows lobar consolidation in the right middle lobe. The tentative diagnosis is COPD and pneumonia. Mr. Z states that he can breathe much better after the bronchodilator treatment, and he is admitted for intravenous antibiotic treatment and respiratory therapy, as well as for reevaluation of his antihypertensive medication.

The answers to the questions in the introduction are as follows:

- Why is Mr. Z sitting in the chair?

Mr. Z. is sitting in the chair with his elbows propped up because this position allows his rib cage to expand more easily, allowing more air in with each inhalation. Laying Mr. Z down on the stretcher would make his breathing more difficult, unless he sat upright and propped his arms on an over-the-bed table.

- What should be considered before starting oxygen therapy?

If Mr. Z has been smoking for a long time (2 packs per day × 35 years), COPD should be considered a tentative diagnosis. His respiratory process may be driven by low oxygen levels in his blood because his central chemoreceptors no longer sense high carbon dioxide levels. Oxygen therapy should be initiated cautiously at 1 to 2 L per min so as not to increase his blood oxygen levels too dramatically and diminish his respiratory drive. His respiratory rate and ABGs should be frequently checked to evaluate his response to therapy.

- Given Mr. Z's smoking history and tentative diagnosis, what changes might be seen on an arterial blood gas?

The arterial blood gas analysis will probably show a low oxygen level (Pao_2), a high carbon dioxide level ($Paco_2$), and either a low pH with a normal bicarbonate or a normal pH with a high bicarbonate level depending upon how his body has compensated for acidosis.

- What anatomic changes cause wheezes?

Wheezes are caused by narrowing of the bronchi and bronchioles due to swelling, secretions, or bronchospasm of the smooth muscle around the bronchi.

- What side effect of beta-blockers is making Mr. Z's breathing more difficult?

Beta-blockers not only vasodilate the peripheral vasculature, a desired therapeutic response in patients with hypertension, but they also block the beta-2 sites in the lungs, causing constriction of the smooth muscle around the bronchioles in susceptible patients (e.g., those with asthma or COPD).

CHAPTER 2 MULTIPLE-CHOICE QUESTIONS

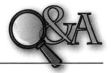

1. Normal breath sounds heard over the mainstem bronchi are:
   a. Vesicular breath sounds
   b. Tracheal breath sounds
   c. Crackles
   d. Bronchovesicular breath sounds

2. The primary abnormality in respiratory acidosis is:
   a. Increased $Paco_2$
   b. Decreased Pao_2
   c. Increased Pao_2
   d. Decreased HCO_3^-

3. The renal system responds to a respiratory acidosis by:
   a. Reabsorbing HCO_3^-
   b. Decreasing hydrogen secretion
   c. Increasing CO_2
   d. Increasing urine output

4. Vesicular breath sounds are best heard:
   a. Over the trachea
   b. At the first and second interspaces beside the sternum
   c. Over most of the lungs
   d. During expiration

5. Pulse oximetry measures:
   a. Carbon dioxide levels
   b. Dissolved oxygen in the plasma
   c. Percentage of hemoglobin carrying oxygen
   d. Pao_2

CHAPTER 2 ANSWERS AND RATIONALES

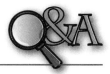

1. **d.**

   Rationale: Bronchovesicular breath sounds are windy sounds heard over the bronchi.

2. **a.**

   Rationale: Respiratory acidosis results in a high $Paco_2$.

3. **a.**

   Rationale: The kidneys reabsorb bicarbonate to buffer the increased acidity of the blood.

4. **c.**

   Rationale: Vesicular breath sounds are heard over the majority of the lung fields.

5. **c.**

   Rationale: Pulse oximetry measures the percentage of hemoglobin carrying oxygen as oxyhemoglobin.

QUICK LOOK AT THE CHAPTER AHEAD

Many systems are affected when respiratory disorders interfere with breathing, patency of the airways, and gas exchange. This chapter will review:

- Disorders of the upper respiratory tracts such as rhinitis, sinusitis, and pharyngitis

- Disorders of the lower respiratory tract such as asthma, chronic obstructive pulmonary disease (COPD), and respiratory failure

- Findings on assessment

- Diagnostic tests for specific respiratory disorders

- Collaborative treatment strategies for particular disorders to maximize ventilation and oxygenation

3

Management of Adults with Respiratory Disorders

TERMS
☐ acute respiratory failure
☐ asthma
☐ chronic obstructive pulmonary disease (COPD)
☐ emphysema
☐ hypoxemia
☐ pleural effusion
☐ pneumonia
☐ pulmonary embolism
☐ thoracentesis
☐ tuberculosis (TB)

CASE STUDY

Mrs. A is a 57-year-old woman who calls her physician's office because she "can not breathe." She has a history of asthma and hypertension. Yesterday, she helped her daughter clean the basement. Mrs. A found that her inhaler did not improve her breathing the previous night. The triage nurse, listening on the phone, hears Mrs. A stopping between words to catch her breath. The triage nurse recommends that Mrs. A have her husband drive her to the office immediately.

When she arrives, her vital signs are: temperature—100.5°F orally, respiration—32 breaths per minute, heart rate—96 beats per minute, and blood pressure 146/92 mmHg. Her oxygen saturation (Sao_2) is 90%. On examination, scattered wheezes are noted over both lung fields during inspiration and expiration with diminished breath sounds at the bases. Pulmonary function tests show a 30% decrease in her normal peak expiratory flow rate (PEFR). She is visibly anxious and breathing in rapid, shallow breaths. The physician sees her and recommends a nebulizer treatment with albuterol.

Important Questions to Ask

- What physiologic changes cause wheezing?
- Why is her PEFR decreased during an asthma attack?
- What could have caused this asthma attack?

When oxygenation is disturbed, all tissues are affected. Oxygen is basic to the metabolism of every cell in the body. The process of supplying oxygen to the cells begins with ventilation, the moving of air into and out of the respiratory tract. It continues with the diffusion of gases across the alveolar membrane and into the circulation. The oxygen arrives at the cell by perfusion, the circulation of blood throughout the body. In this chapter, respiratory disorders in the upper and lower respiratory tracts, as well as disorders of diffusion and perfusion, are reviewed. Interventions to maximize oxygenation will be discussed in Chapter 4.

 ## RESPIRATORY TRACT DEFENSES

The respiratory tract has many methods of defense against the neverending assault by the environment. The airways provide filtration of inspired air and protection of the respiratory tract, as well as humidification and temperature regulation. The first line of defense is air filtration in the nose. The nasal hairs and mucus trap many foreign particles. Obviously, mouth breathing circumvents this system and reduces its effectiveness. The sneezing reflex is initiated in the nose when irritation or particles stimulate the trigeminal nerve. The cough reflex also assists in expelling particles or mucus that is occluding or irritating the airways.

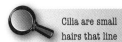 Cilia are small hairs that line the respiratory tract and constantly beat to move particles and mucus up the respiratory passages to where they can be expelled by coughing, sneezing, or swallowing.

More sophisticated methods of defense in the respiratory tract involve the mucociliary blanket. Cilia are small hairs that line the respiratory tract and constantly beat to move particles and mucus up the respiratory passages to where they can be expelled by coughing, sneezing, or swallowing. Dehydration, smoking, and certain drugs (e.g., atropine) can thicken sputum, rendering this defense mechanism less effective.

The mucus in the airways contains secretory immunoglobulins (IgA) that protect the respiratory tract against bacteria and viruses. Both B and T lymphocytes also protect the respiratory passages. Macrophages in the alveoli engulf and destroy foreign particles. Some particles, such as asbestos, may not be completely removed and can cause tissue changes over time, such as asbestosis or malignancy. Smokers are particularly susceptible to lung damage because much of the debris from habitual smoking remains in the lung tissue.

The large airways of the lower respiratory tract such as the bronchi also protect the lungs. Overreaction to irritants occurs in diseases such as asthma where narrowed airways are caused by bronchoconstriction and excessive mucous production. The smooth muscle surrounding the bronchi may constrict when irritants, such as dust and fumes,

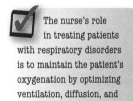 The nurse's role in treating patients with respiratory disorders is to maintain the patient's oxygenation by optimizing ventilation, diffusion, and perfusion.

are inhaled. When the bronchi are irritated, mucus production increases to encase foreign particles. These protective mechanisms may actually impede normal ventilation.

Despite the elaborate protective mechanisms that exist in the respiratory tract, disorders may develop as a result of multiple causes. Assaults on the respiratory tract by the environment include physical trauma, viral or bacterial infection, and altered cellular processes, such as emphysema or malignancy. The nurse's role in treating patients with respiratory disorders is to maintain the patient's oxygenation by optimizing ventilation, diffusion, and perfusion. Nursing care of patients with respiratory disorders requires the following:

- Understanding normal respiratory anatomy and physiology
- Distinguishing between different disorders of the upper and lower airways
- Assessment of the patient based on the knowledge of different signs and symptoms of respiratory disorders and their impact on the patient's functioning
- Developing nursing and collaborative care plans with appropriate long- and short-term goals with the patient
- Implementing the principles of oxygenation into the care plans
- Evaluating the effectiveness of the interventions
- Revising the treatment plan as necessary

This chapter will review disorders of the upper and lower airways, their clinical presentations, possible diagnostic studies, and collaborative treatment strategies to optimize ventilation and oxygenation.

 DISORDERS OF THE UPPER AIRWAYS

The nose, sinuses, and pharynx are the first passages through which air enters the respiratory tract. They provide many defenses against the environment, including air filtration, humidification, and warming. Unfortunately, the filtering abilities of the mucus membranes can lead to irritation and infection of these membranes by the captured intruders.

Acute Rhinitis

The most frequent infection in human beings is **acute rhinitis**. It is usually caused by the common cold virus or rhinovirus (see Table 3-1). There are more than 100 different rhinoviruses that can cause the annoying symptoms of runny and stuffy nose (rhinorrhea), malaise, sore throat, coughing, and sneezing. Colds are most frequent between

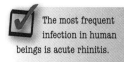
The most frequent infection in human beings is acute rhinitis.

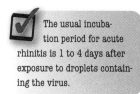
The usual incubation period for acute rhinitis is 1 to 4 days after exposure to droplets containing the virus.

Table 3-1 Symptoms of the Common Cold

1. Red, swollen nasal membranes
2. Mucoid to thin nasal discharge
3. Sneezing and coughing
4. Malaise, headache, and possibly low-grade fever
5. Decreased sense of taste and smell

November and March, with most adults having two to three colds per year. The usual incubation period for acute rhinitis is 1 to 4 days after exposure to droplets containing the virus.

Assessment

During the assessment, note the patient's breathing pattern, especially during speaking, noting any shortness of breath or change in breathing pattern. Clinical findings may include reddened nasal membranes and inferior turbinates, nasal discharge, and dry lips and mouth from mouth breathing. If the patient complains of a sore throat, this should lead to an examination of the posterior pharynx and possible throat culture to rule out beta-hemolytic streptococcal ("strep") infection (see Table 3-2). The patient's temperature and white blood cell count usually remain normal with a cold but may be elevated with a bacterial infection.

> The patient's temperature and white blood cell count usually remain normal with a cold but may be elevated with a bacterial infection.

Elderly patients and those with chronic respiratory disease are particularly prone to complications from the common cold, including sinusitis, bronchitis, and **pneumonia** (an infection of the lung tissues). These conditions may lead to dyspnea, productive cough, fever, hypoxemia, and disorientation.

> Elderly patients and those with chronic respiratory disease are particularly prone to complications from the common cold, including sinusitis, bronchitis, and pneumonia.

Note the color and consistency of nasal discharge in the assessment. Acute rhinitis from a cold virus initially produces clear, runny drainage followed by thicker, milky secretions. Yellow or greenish nasal discharge may indicate a secondary infection of the sinuses. Allergic reactions usually produce thin, clear, or mucoid nasal secretions. Postnasal drip is drainage of nasal secretions down the posterior nasal pharynx causing repeated swallowing and irritation. Other causes of nasal discharge

Table 3-2 How to Obtain a Throat Culture

1. Assemble equipment: tongue depressor, light source, sterile swab, and culture medium.
2. Explain procedure to patient and warn of gagging sensation when the swab is applied to back of throat.
3. In a seated position, have the patient tilt head back slightly and open mouth.
4. Depress tongue with a moistened tongue depressor. Avoid touching the walls of the mouth or throat.
5. Using a light source, visualize the posterior oropharynx, noting any areas of redness or exudate.
6. Put down the light source while maintaining the tongue depressor on the tongue and pick up the sterile swab. While the patient says "Ahhh" to elevate the soft palate, put the swab in the mouth without touching the tongue or walls of the mouth and brush the swab over the wall of the posterior pharynx and the tonsils, trying to reach areas of redness or exudate. Discard tongue depressor.
7. Put swab in appropriate culture medium per individual facility guidelines. Label specimen and send to appropriate laboratory. Wash hands. Document that a culture was obtained.
8. Tell patient that results will not be ready for 24 to 48 hours, depending on the lab and antibiotics that may be needed for treatment if the culture is positive. Some rapid strep tests may be ready in 10 minutes but are less accurate than a culture.

include sinusitis, drugs such as birth control pills and antihypertensives, as well as smoke and seasonal allergies.

Treatment

Treatment of acute rhinitis is directed at maintaining ventilation and minimizing symptoms (see Table 3-3). Acute rhinitis is a self-limiting condition that usually resolves in 7 to 10 days. Because the nasal discharge may occlude the airways, the following interventions are directed toward liquefying secretions:

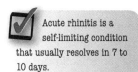
Acute rhinitis is a self-limiting condition that usually resolves in 7 to 10 days.

- Ensure adequate fluid intake (at least 2500 mL/day or one half the body weight in pounds equals the total ounces per day).
- Avoid dairy products that may thicken secretions.
- Humidify the air with a vaporizer, and use saline nasal drops to maintain moist nasal mucus membranes.

Table 3-3 Cold Prevention

1. Decrease droplet exposure by frequent hand washing, especially after blowing the nose or sneezing.
2. Use a tissue for blowing the nose, sneezing, and coughing; discard after each use.
3. Avoid using the drinking glasses and eating utensils of others with a cold.
4. Take vitamin C supplementation for possible antiviral effects.

- ◆ Allow adequate rest.
- ◆ Use over-the-counter medications such as antihistamines (chlorpheniramine or pseudoephedrine) to decrease nasal discharge.

Unfortunately, antihistamines may also dry out the mucous membranes, predisposing the patient to mucus stasis and a secondary bacterial infection. Over-the-counter sympathomimetics such as pseudoephedrine may be used to decrease mucus production by constricting the vasculature of the mucous membranes. Nasal drops, such as phenylephrine, produce vasoconstriction but should be limited to less than 72 hours of use because of the risk of rebound congestion (**rhinitis medicamentosa**). Echinacea (coneflower), an herbal remedy, is thought to be effective as an antimicrobial, but this treatment is still being investigated. Zinc lozenges are advertised as useful in decreasing the length of cold symptoms, but studies concerning the effectiveness of zinc have provided inconsistent results.

 Rhinitis medicamentosa is rebound nasal congestion after prolonged antihistamine use.

Nursing management of acute rhinitis usually occurs in the outpatient setting. Along with an assessment and diagnostic testing, such as a throat culture, the nurse teaches the patient about symptom management. She instructs the patient to seek further health care if the following occurs:

- ◆ Symptoms last more than 7 days.
- ◆ Temperature exceeds 100.5°F.
- ◆ Nasal discharge becomes yellow to green or is accompanied by face pain or headache.
- ◆ The patient has frequently recurring colds.

Allergic Rhinitis

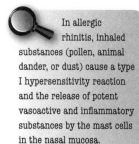

In allergic rhinitis, inhaled substances (pollen, animal dander, or dust) cause a type I hypersensitivity reaction and the release of potent vasoactive and inflammatory substances by the mast cells in the nasal mucosa.

A frequent cause of nasal discharge is allergic rhinitis. Unlike acute rhinitis in which a virus is responsible for the symptoms, **allergic rhinitis** is the result of environmental allergens. In allergic rhinitis, inhaled substances (pollen, animal dander, or dust) cause a type I hypersensitivity reaction. This leads to the release of potent vasoactive and inflammatory substances by the mast cells in the nasal mucosa. These substances produce vasodilation and increased capillary permeability in the mucus membranes, causing sneezing, watery eyes, and hypersecretion of thin mucus. It affects 10–20% of adults, most of whom have a family history of allergies, atopic dermatitis, asthma, or eczema.

Assessment

When assessing a patient with allergic rhinitis, ask the patient about occupation, smoke exposure, life stresses, alcoholic beverage intake, and drug exposure.

In cases of allergic rhinitis, the assessment focuses on the patient's symptoms, their relation to possible causative agents, their clinical course, and seasonal variations. When assessing a patient with allergic rhinitis, ask the patient about occupation, smoke exposure, life stresses, alcoholic beverage intake, and drug exposure. The most common symptoms of allergic rhinitis are nasal congestion with thin, clear discharge, frequent sneezing, itchy eyes with increased tearing, and pruritis. The physical examination may show pale, swollen nasal mucosa with swollen turbinates, watery nasal discharge, watery eyes with puffy eyelids, reddened conjunctiva, dark circles under the eyes (allergic shiners), and pharyngitis.

A diagnosis of allergic rhinitis may require further diagnostic tests, such as skin testing, serum immunologic studies, and nasal smear to identify the allergen and look at the number of eosinophils. A large number of eosinophils may indicate an allergic response; serum immunologic studies may also indicate an allergic response when the IgE, a serum immunoglobulin, is elevated. Skin testing involves the application of a dilute allergen into needle scratches or pricks in the upper inner aspect of the arm or back. Normal saline is used as a control on the opposite side. Fifteen minutes later the sites are assessed for a response. A flare (reddened area) or a wheal (a raised area) over a site more than 5 mm larger than the control would indicate an allergic response. Identification of the allergen provides a direction for treatment.

Treatment

Allergic rhinitis often occurs only during specific times of the year and is usually related to pollen exposure ("hay fever"). The most common offenders are grasses, ragweed, and wind-pollinated trees. Despite the name, hay does not contribute. Skin testing is useful in identifying pollen allergies. Total avoidance of pollen would be difficult at best. Treatment focuses on teaching the patient strategies to avoid pollen exposure (see Table 3-4).

Reduction of exposure to specific allergens may be difficult. Careful questioning of patients with allergic rhinitis may identify specific substances such as foods, food dyes, molds in cheese, wine, dried fruit, and some drugs that stimulate allergic responses. Once identified, the patient should avoid the offending foods and drugs. Decreasing exposure to other allergens such as animal dander may require removing the pet(s) from the household. Sensitivity to house dust and mites requires more involved steps to minimize exposure (see Table 3-5).

> Careful questioning of patients with allergic rhinitis may identify specific substances such as foods, food dyes, molds in cheese, wine, dried fruit, and some drugs that stimulate allergic responses.

If the offending substance(s) cannot be completely avoided or symptoms continue despite measures to avoid allergens, then medications may be useful in minimizing symptoms. Antihistamines are the most frequently used treatment for allergic rhinitis. They help decrease the nasal congestion, mucous production, and excessive tearing and pruritus. Tolerance to these drugs can occur, and patients should be taught to report changes in drug effectiveness so that another class of antihistamine may

Table 3-4 Reducing Exposure to Pollen

1. Stay indoors during times of high pollen count, especially in centrally air-conditioned homes where almost all pollen is filtered out by the system. Go outside only during or immediately after rainfall when the air has been cleared of pollen.
2. Avoid eating honey, which may contain pollen.
3. Drive with the windows closed.
4. Install an air filter in the house to capture pollen.

Table 3-5 Reducing Exposure to Allergens

1. Remove wall-to-wall carpeting and use hard floors, with washable throw rugs if desired.
2. Encase mattresses and pillows in airtight covers and change them yearly. Wash bedding three times a week.
3. Remove all feather-containing pillows and comforters. Use blankets and pillows made out of synthetic materials as they are less likely to harbor mites than feathers and wool.
4. Avoid sweeping. Dust gently with a damp cloth.
5. If possible, have someone else vacuum. Change the vacuum cleaner bag and filter regularly.
6. Remove dust-collecting furniture and draperies.
7. Reduce high humidity to decrease mite breeding. Do not use humidifiers or vaporizers.
8. Install a high-efficiency air filter.
9. Do not have pets. If that is not possible then do not allow pets in the bedroom and bathe them weekly.
10. Avoid cigarette smoke.

be initiated. Antihistamines may be used in conjunction with decongestants to alleviate symptoms without the drowsiness that may occur with antihistamines alone. Both cromolyn and glucocorticoid nasal sprays are useful in relieving nasal congestion by stabilizing mast cells in the nasal mucosa. They have a slow onset of action and may take 3 to 5 days to become effective. Prophylactic use of medications may be useful for seasonal allergies to minimize responses to known allergens such as pollen.

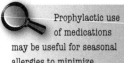
Prophylactic use of medications may be useful for seasonal allergies to minimize responses to known allergens such as pollen.

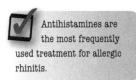
Antihistamines are the most frequently used treatment for allergic rhinitis.

If medication and exposure reduction are not effective in decreasing symptoms, then immunotherapy may provide some relief. Immunotherapy is a **desensitization** process involving subcutaneous injections of the known allergen in gradually increasing doses to increase the patient's tolerance to the substance. Because anaphylactic reactions can occur, desensitization treatments are done in a physician's office where emergency supplies are immediately available. Although the treatment may be effective in many patients, it is lengthy and expensive, requiring 2 to 5 years of treatment. Adherence to the lengthy process may be improved by teaching patients about the treatment plan and possible side effects, and accommodating the patient's schedule.

Nursing management of patients with allergic rhinitis usually occurs in the out-patient setting. Important components of the nurse's role include assessing symptoms and treatment effectiveness, teaching about avoidance to allergens, observing for secondary compli-

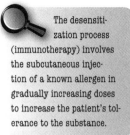

The desensitization process (immunotherapy) involves the subcutaneous injection of a known allergen in gradually increasing doses to increase the patient's tolerance to the substance.

cations, and encouraging adherence with the treatment plan. These interventions facilitate normal air passage through the nose, allowing the nasal passages to perform their important functions, minimize symptoms, and improve quality of life.

Sinusitis

An infection of the sinuses (**sinusitis**) may be a bacterial infection or secondary to a viral exposure. Bacteria, viruses, fungi, and allergic reactions may all cause sinusitis. Acute sinusitis usually develops after a primary viral infection or the common cold. The normal drainage paths from the sinuses to the nasopharynx are blocked by swollen mucous membranes and exudate, and thick sputum and bacteria begin to grow. Exudate and white blood cells fill the sinus, causing pressure and pain.

Assessment

The most common presenting symptom of sinusitis is facial pain and headache. The area over the sinus may be swollen and tender to palpation. There may also be toothaches if the maxillary sinuses are involved and a headache if the frontal or ethmoid sinuses are involved. The physical assessment of the nasopharynx will reveal reddened mucosa in the nasal passages with yellow to green exudate.

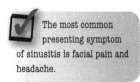

The most common presenting symptom of sinusitis is facial pain and headache.

Treatment

Most cases of sinusitis present in the outpatient setting. Symptoms such as fever and facial swelling may indicate more diffuse infection requiring intravenous antibiotics. The treatment for acute sinusitis includes humidification with a vaporizer to help drain the sinuses, oral antibiotics for

10 to 14 days, and topical vasoconstrictors such as phenylephrine for, at most, 7 days. It is important to teach the patient about finishing the entire course of antibiotics even if he or she is feeling better. This will prevent reinfection with resistant organisms.

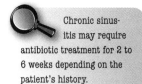

Chronic sinusitis may require antibiotic treatment for 2 to 6 weeks depending on the patient's history.

Chronic sinusitis may require antibiotic treatment for 2 to 6 weeks depending on the patient's history. If the sinusitis does not respond to antibiotics, then surgical intervention may be required to open the sinus passages and improve ventilation and drainage of the sinus.

Other Disorders of the Nose

Normal ventilation through the nose may be interrupted by nasal fractures, septal deformities, **nosebleeds** (epistaxis), tumors, and polyps. Nasal fractures are the most common fracture of the facial bones. (Refer to the section on facial trauma later in this chapter.) Septal deformities, such as a deviated septum, may impede airflow. They may result from trauma or developmental deformities and are usually asymptomatic. Restricted airflow through one or both nasal passages or chronic sinusitis caused by the deviated septum blocks the sinus opening and may indicate the need for surgical correction.

Nosebleed, or epistaxis, occurs commonly and may result from trauma (including nasal fracture and nose picking), infections such as sinusitis and rhinitis, drying of the mucous membranes, bleeding disorders, malignancies of the nose or paranasal sinuses, hypertension, and some systemic infections such as scarlet fever.

Nosebleed or **epistaxis** occurs commonly and may result from trauma (including nasal fracture and nose picking), infections such as sinusitis and rhinitis, drying of the mucous membranes, bleeding disorders, malignancies of the nose or paranasal sinuses, hypertension, and some systemic infections such as scarlet fever. The diagnosis is obvious from the clinical exam. Treatment involves applying gentle pressure to the nose for 5 to 10 minutes while the patient remains seated with his head tilted forward to prevent aspiration of blood or clots. If this method does not stop the bleeding, topical medications like tetracaine should be applied to vasoconstrict the capillaries in the nasal mucosa. If the bleeding continues, the bleeding site needs to be located and cauterized chemically (silver nitrate) or electrically, or the nasal passage needs to be packed to apply direct pressure to the bleeding site. Chronic or recurrent nosebleeds may indicate a bleeding tendency and a need for further evaluation.

Nasal polyps are grape-like masses of swollen nasal mucosa. They may block the nasal passages, impede drainage of the sinuses, and promote sinusitis. Polyps are benign growths that may result from chronic sinusitis and allergic rhinitis. The treatment involves topical treatment with corticosteroids using a nasal inhaler. Nursing management involves teaching the patient about the medications using a nasal inhaler and evaluating the effectiveness of the treatment. Surgical treatment may be required to remove the polyps as they tend to recur.

Other growths in the nose may be benign or malignant. The most common benign growth in the nasal passage is a **papilloma**. The most common malignancy is a squamous cell tumor. Patients with intranasal growths show symptoms of a unilateral airway ob-

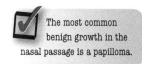

The most common benign growth in the nasal passage is a papilloma.

struction, bloody discharge, numbness, or swelling. Surgical excision may be required to determine the pathology of the growth and plan the treatment course.

Pharyngitis

Acute inflammation of the pharynx, **pharyngitis,** may be caused by viral or bacterial infections. Pharyngitis, or a sore throat, may cause pain, especially when swallowing, and tender lymph glands in the neck. Patients may also have a fever and malaise.

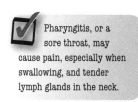

Pharyngitis, or a sore throat, may cause pain, especially when swallowing, and tender lymph glands in the neck.

Clinical findings of pharyngitis include mild to severe redness of the pharynx with or without swollen tonsils. Exudate may or may not be present on the tonsils or posterior oropharynx. In viral infections of the pharynx, there is usually no exudate but the pharynx is reddened with a "cobblestone" ap-

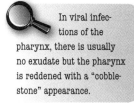

In viral infections of the pharynx, there is usually no exudate but the pharynx is reddened with a "cobblestone" appearance.

pearance. In bacterial infections, the pharynx and tonsils are reddened, and a white to yellow exudate may be present over these areas. Cervical lymphadenopathy may also be present.

Assessment

Assessment includes asking the patient about the onset and duration of symptoms, checking the vital signs for fever, and obtaining a throat culture to rule out beta-hemolytic streptococcal infection (see Table 3-2). Strep infections may have serious consequences such as acute glomerulonephritis and rheumatic fever.

Treatment

Treatment of strep infections includes antibiotic therapy, warm saline gargles, a soft diet, rest, analgesics for pain relief, throat lozenges, and plenty of fluids (2 to 4 L per day). Teach patients to finish the course of antibiotics, even though they may be feeling better, to prevent reinfection with antibiotic-resistant organisms. Patients should call their health care provider if they are still having symptoms or fever after 3 days of antibiotic treatment.

Oropharyngeal Cancer

Malignancies of the mouth, tongue, or pharynx often involve complex medical and nursing care. Screening for oral cancers should be done in the following groups of people who are at high risk:

- Chronic use of cigarettes
- Age over 40 years old
- Use of chewing tobacco
- Regular use of alcohol

The most common presentations of oropharyngeal cancers are a painless red or white lesion in the oropharynx and cervical lymphadenopathy. The most common malignancy of the oropharynx is squamous cell carcinoma.

Assessment

Patients receiving treatment for head and neck cancers require specialized assessments before, during, and after treatment. All patients who will be receiving radiation therapy or chemotherapy to the head and neck should have a thorough dental examination prior to beginning their treatment. It will be difficult or even impossible to do certain dental procedures, such as extractions, after radiation treatment because it can destroy the blood vessels in the jawbone. Salivary glands may also be destroyed by radiation therapy, predisposing the patient to a dry mouth (**xerostomia**), altered taste perceptions, accelerated tooth decay, difficulty chewing, swallowing, and speaking.

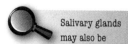

Salivary glands may also be destroyed by radiation therapy, predisposing the patient to a dry mouth (xerostomia), altered taste perceptions, accelerated tooth decay, difficulty chewing, swallowing, and speaking.

Treatment

Medical treatment for oropharyngeal cancers is often complex, involving surgery, radiation therapy, and chemotherapy. Surgery involves excision of the lesion, surrounding tissue, and, perhaps, lymph nodes. Nursing care for patients with oropharyngeal cancers is also complex and may include the following:

- Maintaining a patent airway
- Ensuring adequate nutrition
- Teaching patient about mouth care
- Controlling treatment side effects
- Providing alternative methods of communication
- Recognizing changes in body image and self-esteem that may occur after treatment

One common side effect of treatment for head and neck cancers is **mucositis**, the breakdown, ulceration, and infection of the oral mucosa. It may be quite painful requiring a break during treatment. Mucositis develops because the cells that line the oral cavity have a rapid turnover rate. The cancer treatment

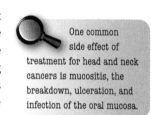

One common side effect of treatment for head and neck cancers is mucositis, the breakdown, ulceration, and infection of the oral mucosa.

affects rapidly dividing cells and can kill normal cells in the mucosa, as well as malignant cells. The damaged lining can ulcerate and become susceptible to infection.

A common infection in patients who are being treated for malignancies or are immunocompromised is oral **candidiasis,** or thrush. **Candidiasis** is the infection of mucous membranes with *Candida albicans* and creates distinctive whitish patches on the oral mucosa that may be quite painful. Antifungal agents such as fluconozole are used to treat these infections.

Treatment for mucositis involves preventative dental care, thorough mouth care, frequent assessment of the oral cavity, and topical and/or systemic analgesia. Current treatments include antibiotic therapy for bacterial infections, antifungal agents, antiulcer medications (misoprostol), and amino acid (glutamine) mouthwashes. Teaching patients about oral care prior to treatment will minimize side effects and promote early detection of problems (see Table 3-6). (Nursing care of the oncology patient receiving chemotherapy and radiation therapy is reviewed later in this chapter).

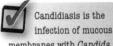

Candidiasis is the infection of mucous membranes with *Candida albicans*.

Laryngitis

Laryngitis is an acute or chronic inflammation of the mucus membranes lining the larynx and sometimes the vocal cords themselves. It occurs most frequently as a result of viral infection but may also be related to other respiratory infections such as bronchitis and influenza. Hoarseness and unnatural diminution of the voice may occur due to chronic overuse of the voice, exposure to inhaled irritants such as cigarette smoke or volatile gases, allergic reactions, or endotracheal intubation.

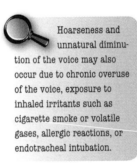

Hoarseness and unnatural diminution of the voice may also occur due to chronic overuse of the voice, exposure to inhaled irritants such as cigarette smoke or volatile gases, allergic reactions, or endotracheal intubation.

Table 3-6 Care of the Mouth During Cancer Treatment

1. Brush teeth gently after every meal and before bed with a soft toothbrush rinsed in warm water to further soften the bristles, or use a sponge toothbrush.
2. Do not use mouthwashes that contain alcohol as they can dry out the mucosa.
3. Eat soft foods that are warm, not too hot or too cold, and avoid spicy foods.
4. Avoid alcohol and all tobacco products.
5. Use a saliva substitute to keep the mouth moist if dryness is a problem.

Assessment

Assessment of the patient with acute laryngitis focuses on the symptoms of hoarseness, difficulty swallowing (**dysphagia**), and any other symptoms of respiratory infections. Laryngeal examination is performed indirectly with a laryngeal mirror or directly with a fiber-optic laryngoscope. When any disorder other than acute laryngitis is suspected or hoarseness lasts more than 2 weeks, patients should be referred to an otolaryngologist.

Treatment

The primary treatment of laryngitis is voice rest. Nursing management of the patient with laryngitis involves teaching the patient about voice rest, increased fluid intake (2 to 4 L per day), topical lozenges, and steam inhalation (such as sitting in a steamy shower or use of a humidifier) to relieve some of the symp-

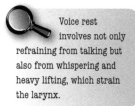

Voice rest involves not only refraining from talking but also from whispering and heavy lifting, which strain the larynx.

toms. Voice rest involves not only refraining from talking but also from whispering and heavy lifting, which strain the larynx. Antibiotics may be ordered if other respiratory infections like bronchitis are suspected. Avoidance of inhaled irritants, such as cigarettes or noxious fumes, is important in treating chronic laryngitis. Recurrent bouts of laryngitis that do not respond to conventional treatment require further medical evaluation.

Vocal Cord Nodules and Polyps

Vocal cord nodules are frequently seen in people who use their voice frequently and loudly, such as singers and actors. Vocal cord polyps develop as a result of chronic voice abuse or inhalation of irritants such as ciga-

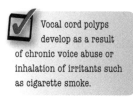

Vocal cord polyps develop as a result of chronic voice abuse or inhalation of irritants such as cigarette smoke.

rette smoke (see Figure 3-1). Symptoms in both cases include hoarseness and a breathy voice quality.

Assessment

Assessment of patients with symptoms of chronic hoarseness should be performed by an otolaryngologist. Direct or indirect laryngoscopy and possibly biopsy may be necessary to identify the source of the symptoms.

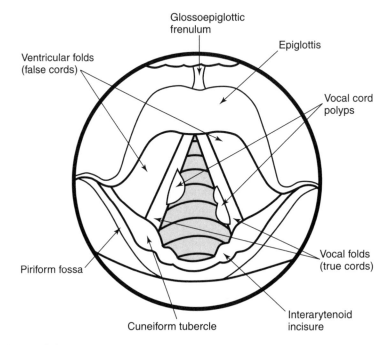

Figure 3-1 Vocal cord polyps.

Treatment

Treatment for vocal cord nodules and polyps involves surgical removal and voice therapy. Malignancy needs to be ruled out in both cases, especially in cases of chronic cigarette abuse. The nurse focuses on teaching the patient how to prevent voice abuse and methods of smoking cessation. If surgical removal of the polyp or nodule is done, then complete voice rest will require the patient to use alternative methods of communication such as picture boards, slate, and alphabet boards for 2 weeks. Preoperative education of the patient and family is important because most of these procedures are done on an ambulatory basis, putting the burden of the communication challenges on the family.

Vocal Cord Paralysis

Vocal cord paralysis may result from neck or chest tumors, central nervous system tumors, trauma, or viral illness. Other causes include prolonged intubation, total thyroidectomy, lung tumors, aortic aneurysms, and an enlarged right atrium. The patient with vocal cord paralysis presents with a diminished or hoarse voice and possibly difficulty breathing and swallowing. Identification of the cause is vitally important to protect the airway.

 The patient with vocal cord paralysis presents with a diminished or hoarse voice and possibly difficulty breathing and swallowing. Identification of the cause is vitally important to protect the airway.

Assessment

To accurately assess the patient with vocal cord paralysis, direct laryngoscopy is necessary to visualize the vocal cords. Nursing care focuses on airway protection. Putting the patient in a high Fowler's position and suctioning as necessary to remove secretions facilitates the maintenance of a patent airway. **Stridor**, coarse loud sounds when breathing, may indicate difficulty in moving air through the paralyzed cords and emergency intubation or tracheotomy may be necessary.

Treatment

Treatment focuses on maintaining the airway even at the expense of the voice. Patients are taught supraglottic swallowing (i.e., taking a deep breath and holding it prior to swallowing). This maneuver allows the larynx to elevate and the epiglottis to close, preventing food and fluids from entering the lower respiratory tract during swallowing. Because patients with vocal cord paralysis are at high risk for aspiration, they must be carefully assessed for aspiration pneumonia.

Laryngeal Trauma

Laryngeal trauma can occur from blunt force, fracture, or from prolonged endotracheal intubation. Symptoms may be an obvious laceration or **hemoptysis**; swelling and laceration; or symptoms of hoarseness, dyspnea, **aphonia**, and subcutaneous emphysema. Nursing care focuses on maintaining a patent airway, frequent evaluation of vital signs and pulse oximetry, and observation for symptoms of increased respiratory difficulty such as stridor, tachypnea, dyspnea, and restlessness. Respiratory distress resulting from laryngeal trauma may require emergency intubation. Prolonged intubation may result in further laryngeal damage, and may necessitate the creation of a tracheostomy to bypass the larynx.

Respiratory distress resulting from laryngeal trauma may require emergency intubation.

Facial Trauma

One of the most common injuries seen in emergency rooms is facial trauma. Whether from physical fights, automobile accidents, falls, or sports injuries, the bones in the face are susceptible to fracture. Nasal fractures are the most common facial injury. Patients complain of pain, tenderness, and swelling over the nose and may have epistaxis and rhinorrhea. The nurse should quickly assess the adequacy of the airway and any other more serious trauma. A history of the event that caused the accident is important, including details about the patient's response to the injuries, especially

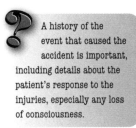 A history of the event that caused the accident is important, including details about the patient's response to the injuries, especially any loss of consciousness.

any loss of consciousness. Blows to the head that are forceful enough to break facial bones may also cause head trauma. The nurse should be alert to signs of head trauma and increasing intracranial pressure.

 Blows to the head that are forceful enough to break facial bones can also cause head trauma. The nurse should be alert to signs of head trauma and increasing intracranial pressure.

Assessment

Physical assessment may reveal **ecchymosis** (bluish discoloration of the skin caused by extravasation of blood into the subcutaneous tissues), swelling, asymmetry, and bony fragments if a compound fracture occurred. Palpation of the area may reveal unusual mobility of the nasal bones or displacement, and crepitus.

Treatment

Treatment of nasal fractures involves reducing the fracture if displacement occurred, ice packs, and analgesics. Care for the nasal fracture includes ice packs for 20 minutes of each hour for the first 24 hours. This reduces swelling and hematoma formation. Closed reduction of a displaced nasal fracture usually returns the bones to their normal position, and packing may be inserted to stabilize the area. If there was not any displacement of the nasal bones, placement of a cast over the dorsum of the nose may protect it from further trauma.

Nursing management includes evaluating the patient for serious injuries such as airway obstruction and/or head trauma that may have occurred with the nasal fracture. Patients are instructed not to blow their nose or pinch the nostrils together, as this could force air into the subcutaneous tissues. The swelling and hematoma should resolve in 2 to 3 weeks. Patients should avoid situations where reinjury could occur, such as contact sports.

Maxillofacial Fractures

Maxillofacial fractures are more serious than nasal fractures. Rapid assessment of the patient is required. Hemorrhage and airway obstruction are the two most common life-threatening complications. The nurse presumes that cervical injuries are present with maxillofacial fractures until X-rays are negative because the force required to cause maxillofacial trauma is sufficient to cause a cervical spine injury. Bone chips may perforate the dura, causing cerebrospinal fluid (CSF) leaks. The patient may perceive CSF leaks as a salty postnasal drip or rhinorrhea. The fluid in the nose should be checked for glucose by dipstick, which is present in CSF but not in nasal mucus.

> The nurse presumes that cervical injuries are present with maxillofacial fractures until X-rays are negative because the force required to cause maxillofacial trauma is sufficient to cause a cervical spine injury.

Treatment

Treatment of maxillofacial fractures involves maintaining a patent airway, controlling bleeding, protecting the cervical spine, and treating the head injuries. Nursing management involves trauma care: maintaining a patent airway with suctioning if needed, elevating the head of the bed (if injuries allow) to decrease bleeding, observing for head injuries and CSF leaks, assessing for orbital injuries, and evaluating changes in vision and eye movement. Patients with jaw fractures who require **intermaxillary fixation** need ongoing care after discharge to assess oral hygiene and nutritional status. Intermaxillary fixation is the wiring together of the upper and lower jawbones by a series of stainless steel wires and elastics.

Cancer of the Head and Neck

Caring for patients with head and neck cancer may be one of the greatest challenges for nurses. The disease and treatment may leave the patient with difficulty eating, swallowing, breathing, and speaking. Surgical excision may change the patient's body, altering his appearance and body image. Treatment depends on a multidisciplinary team to identify the tumor, decide the appropriate treatment(s), support the patient during treatment, and return the patient to his optimum functioning.

Squamous cell carcinomas account for 90% of head and neck tumors. The average patient is a male and over 50 years. Over 85% of all patients with head and neck cancer have a history of tobacco or alcohol use. Patients with these risk factors should have a careful

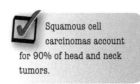

Squamous cell carcinomas account for 90% of head and neck tumors.

oral exam annually. Head and neck tumors usually remain confined to the region and then spread in an orderly fashion along the associated lymphatic chains. Early detection of tumors while they are still relatively small and confined can greatly improve the prognosis. Even when the cancer has spread to the lymph nodes, a cure is possible.

Head and neck tumors may present in a variety of ways. Oral cancers may be detected by a dentist, a healthcare provider during routine assessment, or by the patient (see Table 3-7). Oral cancers usually begin with red patches (**erythroplasia**) or whitish patches (**leukoplakia**) on the mucous membrane. Nasal tumors may cause facial swelling, numbness, facial pain, and epistaxis. Patients with oropharyngeal cancer may complain of hoarseness, a lesion in the mouth, pain when swallowing, unilateral ear pain (from destruction of the glossopharyngeal nerve), and fullness in the face. Because of the va-

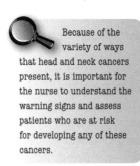

Because of the variety of ways that head and neck cancers present, it is important for the nurse to understand the warning signs and assess patients who are at risk for developing any of these cancers.

riety of ways that head and neck cancers present, it is important for the nurse to understand the warning signs and assess patients who are at risk for developing any of these cancers.

Table 3-7 Warning Signs of Head and Neck Cancer

1. Oral lesion or sore that does not heal in 2 weeks
2. Persistent or unexplained oral bleeding
3. Color changes (red, white, black, or brown) on the mouth or tongue
4. Difficulty swallowing
5. Persistent hoarseness or changes in voice quality
6. Persistent or recurrent sore throat that does not respond to treatment
7. A lump in the mouth, throat, or neck
8. Pain in the mouth, lips, throat, neck, or under the dentures

Assessment

The first contact that a nurse may have with a patient with head and neck cancer is during the assessment. Sensitive questioning about tobacco (all forms) and alcohol use is important. Calculate the number of packs per year of cigarette use with the formula in Chapter 2. Ask about other risk factors to potential carcinogens, such as occupational exposure (woodworkers, asbestos exposure, and petroleum workers). Review the course of the presenting symptoms and note their onset and duration.

In patients with suspected head and neck cancers, ask about risk factors to potential carcinogens, such as tobacco products and occupational exposure (woodworkers, asbestos exposure, and petroleum workers).

Treatment

The treatment course for head and neck cancers varies depending on the location and stage of the disease, the physician's recommendation, and the patient's desires. The treatment course for head and neck cancers is determined by the stage of the disease. Tumors are biopsied to determine the histology, and follow-up CAT scans or MRIs are used to assess tumor size and local spread. Head and neck tumors are staged according to the TNM system. T indicates the size and site of the primary tumor, N denotes the number and size of local lymphatic spread, and M is used to indicate the presence of distant metastases.

Head and neck tumors are staged according to the TNM system. T indicates the size and site of the primary tumor, N denotes the number and size of local lymphatic spread, and M is used to indicate the presence of distant metastases.

Many tumors of the head and neck require some surgery to biopsy and remove the tumor. More extensive surgery or radiation therapy is required to treat the tumor bed and the associated lymph nodes that may have disease. Chemotherapy has an increasing role in advanced cancers. Because there are so many different tumors and treatments, this section will focus on the patient with laryngeal cancer.

Laryngeal cancer is the most common head and neck cancer, 95% of which is squamous cell carcinomas. The cancer may occur in the true vocal cords, the epiglottis, the pyriform sinus, or the postcricoid area. Patients usually present symptoms of hoarseness, pain, a lump in the neck, or difficulty swallowing.

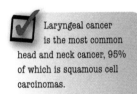

Laryngeal cancer is the most common head and neck cancer, 95% of which is squamous cell carcinomas.

Early stages of cancer in the vocal cord and epiglottis are treated with radiation therapy. Daily radiation treatments for 6 to 7 weeks can be tiring for the patient. The treatments themselves are not painful, but the side effects can cause many difficulties for the patient as the treatment progresses. Because radiation affects all anatomic structures within the treatment field, the pharynx, larynx, and esophagus may all be affected. Side effects of radiation therapy appear as the treatment progresses and the total dose of radiation to the area increases. Side effects include skin reactions, **esophagitis** (inflammation of the lining of the esophagus with pain on swallowing), laryngitis, and pharyngitis. If the oropharynx is in the treatment field, then the patient may experience xerostomia (dry mouth), decreased taste, and possibly infections of the oropharynx. Mucositis may be very painful and may make it difficult for the patient to eat and swallow. The challenge for nurses is to maintain optimum nutrition, control pain, and watch for treatment reactions.

Surgical treatment of laryngeal cancer depends on the stage of the tumor. More advanced glottic cancers with cartilage invasion may require complete **laryngectomy** with a radical neck dissection to remove the associated lymph nodes. A complete laryngectomy is performed when previous treatment with radiation or chemotherapy and radiation therapy have failed (see Figure 3-2). After the laryngectomy, the patient can no longer speak in the normal way. Later, a tracheoesophageal fistula may be surgically created into which a one-way valve can be inserted for speech. Other methods of creating speech are by eructation or esophageal speech and the use of an **electrolarynx**. When a tracheostomy is created, an opening

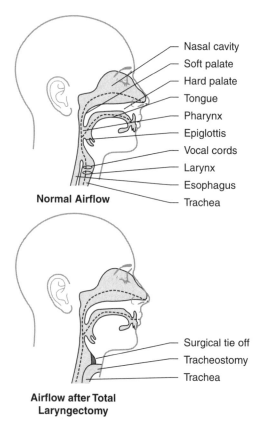

- Nasal cavity
- Soft palate
- Hard palate
- Tongue
- Pharynx
- Epiglottis
- Vocal cords
- Larynx
- Esophagus

Normal Airflow

- Trachea

- Surgical tie off
- Tracheostomy
- Trachea

**Airflow after Total
Laryngectomy**

Figure 3-2 Altered airflow after total laryngectomy.

is made from the trachea to the anterior neck to maintain the airway. The pharynx is sutured to the esophagus to permit swallowing.

DISORDERS OF THE LOWER RESPIRATORY TRACT

Disorders of the lower respiratory tract may be acute or chronic processes. Acute processes include brief infections such as pneumonia and chronic processes include emphysema and asthma. Chronic conditions often have a disease course marked with remissions and exacerbations. The nursing care for acute and chronic respiratory disorders is a collaborative process with the nurse, the physician, and the respiratory therapist all contributing to the development of the best care plan for the patient. In this section, acute infections (influenza, acute bronchitis, pneumonia, and tuberculosis) will be reviewed first followed by diseases of chronic airflow limitation (asthma, chronic bronchitis, and emphysema), acute respiratory failure, adult respiratory distress syndrome (ARDS), pulmonary vascular disorders (pulmonary embolus and pulmonary hypertension), pleural effusion, lung cancer, and chest trauma including pneumothorax. (Specific interventions to maintain oxygenation such as oxygen therapy, tracheostomy, mechanical ventilation, thoracentesis, and chest tube maintenance and endotracheal suctioning are reviewed in Chapter 5.)

Influenza

Influenza is a viral infection of the respiratory tract. It usually occurs in epidemics during the fall and winter. Influenza may be a serious infection, particularly in those over 65 years of age, immunocompromised patients, and those with chronic lung and heart disease. There are three common types of the influenza virus: A, B, and C, as well as numerous subtypes. The incubation period is 1 to 4 days after exposure to droplet nuclei spread by coughing or sneezing. The presenting symptoms fall into three syndromes: a rhinotracheitis, a viral respiratory infection, and a viral pneumonia. The presentation depends on the type of droplet exposure. Fine droplet exposure inhaled into the nasal passages may produce a **rhinotracheitis**. A larger exposure of viral-laden droplets directly into the lower airways may produce a viral respiratory infection or **pneumonia**. Basic hygiene (hand washing, covered sneezes, and coughs) may decrease the spread of influenza.

 Influenza may be a serious infection, particularly in those over 65 years of age, immunocompromised patients, and those with chronic lung and heart disease.

Assessment

Assessment of the patient requires an understanding of the normal course of influenza versus other respiratory tract disorders. The first symptoms of influenza are often abrupt onset of fever, chills, and malaise followed by a profusely runny nose (rhinotracheitis), muscle aches, and headache. The symptoms of **rhinotracheitis** peak in 3 to 5 days and resolve spontaneously in 7 days. Secondary complications may develop after the acute infection and may be related to bacterial infections that may include sinusitis, **otitis media** (infection of the middle ear), bacterial pneumonia, and bronchitis. These secondary bacterial infections occur just as the patient is starting to feel better or when symptoms are prolonged after the normal influenza course.

The symptoms of **influenza pneumonia** are more severe and can rapidly progress to hypoxemia and even death. The symptoms of cough, fever, chills, and malaise come on abruptly and can be quite severe.

Treatment

Treatment for influenza is usually symptomatic including antipyretics, decongestants, fluids, and rest. Amantadine, an antiviral drug, may be used to shorten the course of an influenza infection or for prophylaxis. Prolonged courses of influenza indicate additional assessment, especially in the elderly or otherwise compromised patients.

Prolonged courses of influenza (greater than 2 weeks of symptoms) indicate the need for additional assessment, especially in the elderly or otherwise compromised patients.

Treatment of patients with influenza includes rest, extra fluids, and acetaminophen for high temperatures (greater than 101°F). Acetaminophen is preferred over aspirin as an analgesic and antipyretic because of the risk of **Reye's syndrome**, a rare complication of influenza that causes liver failure and encephalitis. It is seen more often when aspirin is used during an influenzal illness, particularly in children.

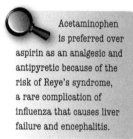
Acetaminophen is preferred over aspirin as an analgesic and antipyretic because of the risk of Reye's syndrome, a rare complication of influenza that causes liver failure and encephalitis.

Many influenza infections can be prevented by use of a vaccine. At-risk individuals should be vaccinated annually in the fall. The vaccine is reformulated each year to include the most common strains of the influenza virus from the previous year's data. Populations at high risk for complications from influenza include people over 65 years of age; residents of nursing homes and chronic care facilities; patients with chronic heart, lung, metabolic, or immunologic problems; and children or adults receiving chronic aspirin therapy (because of the risk of Reye's syndrome). The influenza vaccine should not be given to individuals with an allergy to egg whites. Side effects to the vaccine are infrequent and include redness and tenderness at the vaccination site and, rarely, malaise and fever.

 The influenza vaccine should not be given to individuals with an allergy to egg whites.

Acute Bronchitis

Acute bronchitis is the inflammation of the large airways in the lower respiratory tract. It may be caused by bacteria, viruses, or exposure to inhaled irritants. Bronchitis can be classified as acute or chronic. Chronic bronchitis will be reviewed later in the chapter.

 The most common infective agents in acute bronchitis are *Staphylococcus aureus*, *Pneumococcus*, and *Haemophilus influenza*.

Acute bronchitis may result from a previous infection with a virus (i.e., influenza) predisposing a patient to a secondary bacterial infection. The most common infective agents in acute bronchitis are *Staphylococcus aureus, Pneumococcus,* and *Haemophilus influenza*. The bacteria are usually passed from the nasopharynx to the bronchi by small amounts of aspirant. The organisms cause an inflammatory response in the bronchi with swelling and excessive mucus production.

 Symptoms of acute bronchitis include a productive cough, fever, malaise, substernal pain especially when coughing, and auscultatory crackles and wheezes.

Assessment

Symptoms of acute bronchitis include a productive cough, fever, malaise, substernal pain especially when coughing, and auscultatory crackles and wheezes. Wheezes may indicate some degree of bronchoconstriction. A dry cough often progresses to a productive cough with purulent and/or blood-streaked sputum. Acute bronchitis can progress to a severe illness with high fever, dyspnea, and cyanosis requiring hospitalization.

Treatment

Treatment is based on the clinical findings and includes antibiotics, extra fluids, humidity, rest, acetaminophen for fever and pain, and sometimes oxygen therapy. Cough suppressants should be used cautiously because excessive secretions need to be cleared from the lungs. Expectorants (such as guaifenesin) may be useful in relieving chest congestion. Cigarette smokers are encouraged to stop smoking, as this further irritates the lining of the bronchi.

Pneumonia

Pneumonia is an inflammatory process of the parenchymal structures of the lung, such as the bronchioles and alveoli, and may impair gas exchange. Bacteria, viruses, fumes, and even gastric contents can cause pneumonia. Pneumonia is classified by location, infectious agent, and other factors.

Normally, respiratory defense mechanisms such as the cough reflex and the mucociliary blanket protect the lower airways. Some factors that can impair the effectiveness of these defense mechanisms are immunodeficiency, smoking, viral diseases, and loss of the cough reflex due to neuromuscular disease or anesthesia. Although antibiotics have decreased the mortality associated with pneumonia, it is still a leading cause of death in adults in the United States. In 2003, a new deadly form of pneumonia emerged, **severe acute respiratory syndrome (SARS)**.

Assessment

Pneumonia may present with a variety of symptoms depending on the type and location. Signs and symptoms include cough, fever, pleuritic chest pain, and adventitious lung sounds. Older adults with pneumonia may present with confusion and lethargy rather than fever and cough. The cough may be dry or productive. On auscultation, there may be decreased breath sounds and adventitious sounds such as wheezes or crackles over the affected area.

 Older adults with pneumonia may present with confusion and lethargy rather than fever and cough.

Chest X-ray reveals pulmonary infiltrates in cases of pneumonia. Other diagnostic tests include sputum for culture and sensitivity, white blood cell count (and differential), pulse oximetry, arterial blood gases (ABG), and possibly bronchoscopy.

Pneumonia is classified according to the anatomic distribution and the causative agent. Acute bacterial pneumonia has one of two anatomic

Lobar Pneumonia   Bronchial Pneumonia

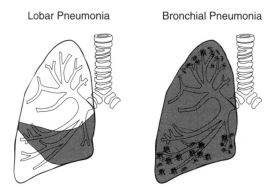

Figure 3-3 Lobar and bronchial pneumonia.

patterns: either lobar or bronchial pneumonia (see Figure 3-3). **Lobar pneumonia** is so named because a chest X-ray reveals inflammation of a lobe of the lung. Approximately 90% of all forms of **lobar pneumonia** are caused by *Streptococcus pneumoniae*. The symptoms of lobar pneumonia are rapid onset of malaise, chills, high fever, and **leukocytosis** (e.g., increased white blood cell count). Initially, the cough may produce watery sputum, and the breath sounds may be diminished due to congestion in the alveolar walls. Later, the sputum becomes rusty colored or purulent. Pleuritic pain, especially on deep respiratory movements, may be present.

Bronchial pneumonia differs from lobar pneumonia in both the presentation and the course of the illness. On chest radiography, a bronchial pneumonia appears as patchy consolidation in several lobules. It is usually the extension of a preexisting bronchitis. Bronchial pneumonia tends to be a disease of the very young, the very old, and the immunocompromised. It presents insidiously with a low-grade fever, cough, crackles, and leukocytosis. Many different organisms can cause bronchial pneumonia, including the previously mentioned *Streptococcus*

> ✓ Bronchial pneumonia tends to be a disease of the very young, the very old, and the immunocompromised.

> ✓ Approximately 90% of all forms of lobar pneumonia are caused by *Streptococcus pneumoniae*.

> 🔍 Many different organisms can cause bronchial pneumonia, including the previously mentioned *Streptococcus pneumoniae*, as well as *Staphylococcus aureus*, *Haemophilus influenzae*, and *Pseudomonas aeruginosa*.

pneumoniae, as well as *Staphylococcus aureus*, *Haemophilus influenzae*, and *Pseudomonas aeruginosa*. **Nosocomial pneumonia** is pneumonia that develops within 48 hours of admission to a healthcare facility.

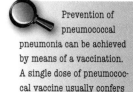

Prevention of pneumococcal pneumonia can be achieved by means of a vaccination. A single dose of pneumococcal vaccine usually confers immunity for 5 to 7 years.

Treatment

The treatment for either lobar or bronchial pneumonia is antibiotics, rest, extra fluids, and sometimes oxygen therapy. For debilitated patients, care should be taken to wash hands with either soap or alcohol gel and use respiratory equipment between patients so as to prevent nosocomial spread of bacteria. Prevention of pneumococcal pneumonia can be achieved by means of a vaccination. A single dose usually confers immunity for 5 to 7 years. Pneumococcal vaccination is recommended for individuals with chronic respiratory, cardiac, and immunologic disorders, diabetes mellitus, and those with a history of alcoholism. Healthy adults over 65 years of age may also benefit from being vaccinated.

Treatment may also involve oxygen supplementation and intubation, and mechanical ventilation as indicated by the diagnostic testing. **Positive end-expiratory pressure (PEEP)** may be added in severe cases to prevent alveolar collapse and improve gas exchange. (See Chapter 4 for more information on PEEP.)

BOOP: Idiopathic Bronchiolitis Obliterans

Idiopathic bronchiolitis obliterans with organizing pneumonia (**BOOP**) is one type of bronchiolitis obliterans, an inflammatory disease of the small airways. Organizing pneumonia refers to unresolved pneumonia with persistent alveolar exudates and fibrosis of the airways. BOOP is a nonspecific reaction to bronchial injury characterized by the proliferation of granulation tissue in the airways, particularly the terminal bronchioles.

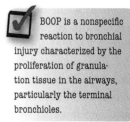

BOOP is a nonspecific reaction to bronchial injury characterized by the proliferation of granulation tissue in the airways, particularly the terminal bronchioles.

BOOP most commonly occurs between the ages of 40 and 70 and occurs equally among men and women. Although there is no known cause, BOOP has been associated with collagen vascular disease such as rheumatoid arthritis and Crohn's disease, and specific situations such as bone marrow transplantation.

Assessment

The presenting symptoms of BOOP are usually flu-like in nature, including fever, persistent and nonproductive cough, dyspnea, anorexia, and weight loss. On physical assessment, auscultation may reveal crackles. Chest X-rays show patchy airspace opacities. CAT scan of the chest may reveal areas of consolidation, a nonspecific finding. Bronchoscopy may be normal or reveal slightly inflamed airways. Blood tests show an increased sedimentation rate and C-reactive protein. A definitive diagnosis requires thoracotomy and biopsy.

Treatment

Treatments vary depending on the patient's condition and may include oxygen therapy, corticosteroids, and bronchodilators. BOOP is very responsive to corticosteroid therapy but may recur when steroids are tapered. Newer treatments with immunosuppressive drugs are under investigation.

Tuberculosis

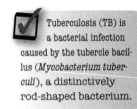

Tuberculosis (TB) is a bacterial infection caused by the tubercle bacillus (*Mycobacterium tuberculi*), a distinctively rod-shaped bacterium.

Tuberculosis (TB) is a bacterial infection caused by the tubercle bacillus (***Mycobacterium tuberculi***), a distinctively rod-shaped bacterium. Once called *consumption*, patients with tuberculosis often spent years isolated in sanatoriums until the disease was considered cured. TB is now better understood and treatment can be completed on an out-patient basis for most patients.

Tuberculosis occurs most commonly in the lungs but can affect other organs. It is characterized by pulmonary infiltrates and granuloma formation with fibrosis and cavity formation. It occurs twice as often in men and is four times more common in nonwhites than whites. TB is spread via airborne droplets from an infected person coughing, sneezing, or speaking. The risk of infection increases with increased exposure such as in families living in close proximity. The tubercle bacillus is inhaled and lands in the alveoli, particularly in the upper lobes, and the body begins an inflammatory response. The response causes vasodilation and increased vascular permeability. Fluids, white blood cells (WBC), and macrophages leak into the area infected by the **tubercle bacillus**. Later, an immune response mediated by T cells results in a walled-off area around the infection called a **tubercle** or granuloma (see Figure 3-4). This immune response can be detected 3 to 12 weeks after infection by a skin

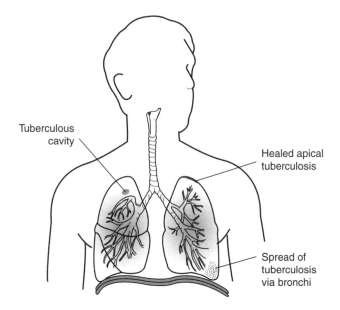

Figure 3-4 Tuberculosis.

test with a purified protein derivative (PPD). Bacilli within the tubercle may remain viable for many years, even decades.

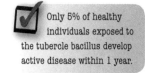

Only 5% of healthy individuals exposed to the tubercle bacillus develop active disease within 1 year.

Most individuals who are exposed to the tubercle bacillus do not develop the active TB. Only 5% of healthy exposed individuals develop active disease within 1 year. The disease often becomes dormant with exposed individuals never developing active TB. However, it may activate later in life due to age or an immunocompromised condition. Individuals infected with human immunodeficiency virus (HIV) are more at risk for development of tuberculosis after exposure than those without HIV. Other populations at risk for tuberculosis include the following:

- Individuals in close contact with a newly diagnosed patient
- Blacks and Hispanics between 25 and 40 years old
- Individuals with multiple sexual partners
- Recent immigrants from Africa, Asia, Mexico, and South America
- Gastrectomy patients
- Individuals with diabetes, malnutrition, and/or cancer

The walls of the tubercle are made of a cheesy white substance called casein. The bacteria within the tubercle begin to destroy the surrounding lung tissue, causing a caseation necrosis. The bacteria may stay within the tubercle, secluded from the rest of the lung and body, or the walls of the tubercle may liquefy and the bacteria will multiply and spread directly into other chest structures or indirectly, via lymphatic channels, to other parts of the body (**miliary tuberculosis**).

Many older people have walled-off lesions in their lungs from earlier tuberculosis infections. Early in the 1900s, 80% of adults were infected with tuberculosis before the age of 30. Although the tubercle may remain intact and the disease dormant for years, even decades, the bacillus may become active again if the host becomes immunocompromised due to age, immunodeficiency, steroid use, or diabetes (secondary or reactivated tuberculosis). Nursing home patients are 10 times more likely to contract the disease. Individuals with weakened immune systems from disease or immunosuppressants and homeless persons are at increased risk for active TB.

Assessment

Nursing care of the patient with tuberculosis begins with an accurate assessment. The following are the most common symptoms of tuberculosis:

+ Cough
+ Fever
+ Night sweats
+ Anorexia and weight loss

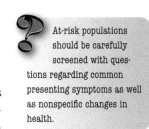
At-risk populations should be carefully screened with questions regarding common presenting symptoms as well as nonspecific changes in health.

Symptoms may be present for months prior to the patient seeking health care. Persistent cough (usually productive), hemoptysis, and pleuritic chest pain are the most suggestive symptoms, but nonspecific changes in health such as malaise, loss of appetite, weight loss, or just the loss of a sense of well-being may be present. At-risk populations should be carefully screened with questions regarding common presenting symptoms as well as nonspecific changes in health.

It is important to ask the patient if he or she has ever been tested for TB and what the results were at that time. The nurse should inquire about immediate members of the family or household who might have TB. The nurse should also ask the patient about recent travel to developing countries where TB is more common (e.g., Asia, Africa, and South America).

On examination, the nurse may note dullness to percussion over the affected portion of the lung, a sign of consolidation of the infected lung tissue. On auscultation, there may be bronchial breath sounds, crackles, or whispered petroliloquy.

Diagnostic testing for TB may require several tests to distinguish TB from other respiratory disorders. The standard skin test uses purified protein derivative (PPD). The nurse injects 5 units (0.1 mL) of PPD intradermally (not subcutaneously) and the patient must return to have the area around the injection site read in 48 to 72 hours. The area of induration (not just redness) is measured in millimeters at the greatest diameter. One practical method for reading the site is using a ballpoint pen and running it across the skin just before the

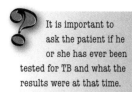 It is important to ask the patient if he or she has ever been tested for TB and what the results were at that time.

 The nurse injects 5 units (0.1 mL) of PPD intradermally (not subcutaneously) and then the patient must return to have the area around the injection site read in 48 to 72 hours.

 A positive reaction to a PPD is an indurated area at the injection site of 10 mm or greater at the site.

area of induration until resistance is met and then lifting the pen off the skin. This motion is repeated on the opposite side and the distance between the pen marks is measured in millimeters. A positive reaction to a PPD is an indurated area at the injection site of 10 mm or greater at the site. Any reaction over 5 mm should be considered positive in patients with HIV, those patients who have close contacts with others with TB, or a previous chest X-ray that shows an old TB infection. All positive skin tests must be reported to the local or state health departments. It is important to tell patients that a positive skin test does not mean that they have tuberculosis but that they have been exposed to the bacillus.

Patients with positive TB skin tests are referred for further diagnosis and treatment. A chest X-ray, physical exam, sputum cultures (three early morning samples), and blood tests are done. Chest X-ray may reveal nodular lesions, patchy infiltrates, cavity formation, and calcium deposits. CT scan and MRI may be used to evaluate lung damage or confirm a diagnosis.

Sputum cultures, as well as cultures from other tissues such as cerebrospinal fluid, pleural fluid, urine, and drainage from abscesses, may show heat sensitive, aerobic, acid-fast bacilli.

Treatment

Treatment for tuberculosis depends on whether the disease is latent or active, age of the patient, comorbid conditions, and the strain of the TB. Latent disease is treated with isoniazid daily or twice weekly for 9 months.

Patients with a diagnosis of active tuberculosis and those who have contact with others with active TB and are at risk for development of the disease are treated with a combination of drugs. The most common medications for treating TB are isoniazid (INH), rifampin (RIF), pyrazinamide (PZA), ethambutol (EMB), and streptomycin (SM). One drug, isoniazid or INH, is used for prophylactic treatment after exposure to known infected individuals. INH should be taken with food to decrease stomach upset. Rifampin cases urine to turn orange and may make oral contraceptives less effective.

 INH (isoniazid) should be taken with food to decrease stomach upset.

Initially, four drugs are used to treat active TB to prevent the development of multiple-drug resistant (MDR) strains of TB. MDR strains of tuberculosis have emerged recently in the HIV-positive population. Multiple drugs are used for extended treatment (12 months) in cases of known or suspected MDR TB. Fluoroquinolones are often added to the regimen for MDR TB.

> ☑ Rifampin causes urine to turn orange.

 Rifampin may make oral contraceptives less effective.

If the patient had a positive skin test but no other manifestation of TB, he is put on a course of INH prophylaxis for 6 to 9 months. This long treatment may be more difficult to justify to asymptomatic patients. The lifetime chance of developing full-blown TB in an immunocompetent person is 10%. The issue becomes one of public health and safety, especially with the increasing numbers of multiple drug resistant TB strains and individuals who are HIV-positive. Individuals who are HIV-positive and have a positive skin test have a 7% chance per year of developing full-blown TB. It is important to emphasize that adherence with the regimen is important because the patient may develop active TB and be contagious even though he or she does not have any symptoms. Common side effects of INH therapy are peripheral neuritis, hepatitis, and hypersensitivity. Patients are advised not to drink alcohol while taking INH.

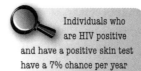
Individuals who are HIV positive and have a positive skin test have a 7% chance per year of developing full-blown TB.

Nursing care of the patient with tuberculosis involves not only administration of medications or observed therapy but also careful monitoring of adverse events including nausea, peripheral neuritis, and elevated liver enzymes caused by drug-induced hepatitis.

For patients with active pulmonary TB, hospitalization, isolation, and combined antimicrobial therapy are necessary. The patient should be in respiratory isolation with negative air pressure to minimize air (and bacillus) flow out of the room. If the patient leaves the room, a specialized mask should be worn. The door should be closed at all times. Provide a covered trash receptacle for used tissues. Isolation should be maintained for at least 2 weeks after initiating antimicrobial therapy and until the patient is showing clinical response to treatment (decreasing bacillus count in sputum). This may be difficult for the patient and his family, and alternative methods of socialization and recreation should be suggested. Some creativity on the part of the nurse and patient may yield interesting solutions to this problem: videotaped movies, computer games, telephones, and so on. Nurses should encourage a healthy diet with small frequent meals to conserve energy. The patient's weight should be monitored weekly. Pyroxidine (B6) supplements may be added to prevent INH-induced peripheral neuropathies.

Pyroxidine (B6) supplements may be added to prevent INH-induced peripheral neuropathies.

Patients are followed periodically throughout their treatment for TB to ensure adherence, follow their response to treatment, and monitor side effects of treatment. Nonadherence is the cause of most treatment failures. If the patient and his family understand the disease and treatment, they are more apt to adhere and complete the drug regimen. For patients whose adherence to the medication regimen is a concern, such as alcoholics, "observed therapy" or **directly observed treatment (DOT)** may be a solution. With DOT, the patient makes regular appointments to take his medication as the nurse watches (usually a four-drug regimen 3 times a week). Patients are followed with regular sputum smears to evaluate the effectiveness of treatment as evidenced by decreasing numbers of bacilli in the sputum.

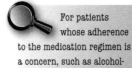

For patients whose adherence to the medication regimen is a concern, such as alcoholics, "observed therapy" or directly observed treatment (DOT) may be a solution.

Chronic Obstructive Disorders of the Lung

The term *chronic obstructive disorders* is used to describe conditions that impede airflow through the pulmonary airways. This group can be further broken down into the chronic obstructive pulmonary disease (COPD) and

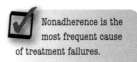

Nonadherence is the most frequent cause of treatment failures.

asthma. COPD causes changes to the airways that do not improve over several months. Asthma, which was previously included in this group, is now considered separately because the changes in the airways are reversible. Chronic bronchitis and emphysema will be reviewed together because they share many of the same causative factors and treatments.

Chronic Obstructive Pulmonary Disease

Chronic obstructive pulmonary disease is increasing in prevalence in the United States and around the world. In the United States over 16 million people are afflicted with COPD, and it is now the fourth leading cause of death (after cardiovascular diseases, cancer, and cerebrovascular disease). It is expected to become the third leading cause of death by 2020. The cost in terms of direct health care and diminished quality of life is astronomical.

The term *chronic obstructive disorders* is used to describe conditions that impede airflow through the pulmonary airways.

Several risk factors are linked to the development of COPD. Without doubt, the number one cause is cigarette smoking. Other established risk factors are occupational dust exposure (silica, cotton, chemical fumes) and congenital enzyme deficiencies. These other factors are only minor contributors compared to cigarette smoking. What

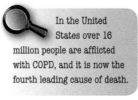

In the United States over 16 million people are afflicted with COPD, and it is now the fourth leading cause of death.

smokers mistakenly call "smoker's cough" is related to the changes in COPD. Nurses can help to prevent COPD by teaching school-age children about the harmful effects of smoking, educating their patients about smoking cessation (see Table 3-8), and encouraging the use of masks for individuals who work in high-risk environments.

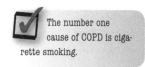

The number one cause of COPD is cigarette smoking.

COPD is characterized by limitation of expiratory airflow that is not fully reversible. Although the changes to the airways that are clumped

Table 3-8 Smoking Cessation

1. Ask your smoking patient about his smoking status and interest in quitting. It is more productive to find out his reasons for quitting (e.g., health, family pressure, cost, and smoking-related illnesses in friends or family).
2. Boost his motivation by telling him about the harmful effects of smoking. Use his symptoms as a reason to quit. Explain that his symptoms (e.g., cough, dyspnea, and sore throat) may be caused by cigarettes and that quitting may relieve them.
3. Make a plan with your smoking patient to quit smoking. Set a date for stopping. Enlist a smoking buddy to help the patient adhere to his goals. Use an informal contract signed by the patient and his buddy.
4. Follow-up with your patient, as most smokers need several attempts before they finally quit. Common withdrawal symptoms include cravings, irritability, insomnia, difficulty sleeping, and constipation. Explain that each attempt at quitting is a learning experience that will help the patient to successfully quit the next time.
5. Offer the following strategies for dealing with nicotine withdrawal symptoms:
    *   Cravings—These last 1 to 3 minutes. Chew a carrot or sugar-free gum, take slow, deep breaths, and engage in another activity.
    *   Irritability—Avoid stressful situations during quitting; use relaxation exercises or hypnosis.
    *   Temptation—Avoid smokers or tell them that you are trying to quit and to smoke elsewhere; throw away all cigarettes; change routine to avoid smoking.
    *   Pharmacology aids—These include nicotine gum, the patch, an inhaler, clonidine, and bupropion.
6. Help your patient stay on track with follow-up phone calls, posting honor rolls of quitters, and supplying patient education materials.
7. Refer your patient to established smoking cessation programs in his community (contact the local offices of the American Cancer Society and the American Lung Association for referrals).

together as COPD include several diseases, this section will review the two most common forms of COPD: chronic bronchitis and emphysema (see Table 3-9).

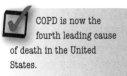

COPD is now the fourth leading cause of death in the United States.

Chronic bronchitis is characterized by a hypersecretion of mucus and chronic cough. In COPD, a productive cough is defined as being present for at least 3 months of the year for 2 years in a row. Infections develop secondarily as a result of mucus stasis. Most

Chronic bronchitis is characterized by a hypersecretion of mucus and chronic cough.

patients with chronic bronchitis are cigarette smokers and have a cough all year round. The changes associated with chronic bronchitis are not manifested until late middle age and occur most often in men.

Table 3-9 Different Manifestations of Chronic Bronchitis and Emphysema

	Chronic Bronchitis	Emphysema
Onset of symptoms	> 35 years	> 50 years
Smoking history	Usually	Usually
Skin color	Pale to cyanotic	Pink
Respiratory rate	Increased	Increased
Dyspnea	Predominant symptom	May be absent in early stages
Cough	Chronic	Absent or mild
Sputum	Copious, mucopurulent	Absent or minimal
A-P diameter	Normal to slight increase	Increased
Auscultation	Wheezes, rhonchi	Diminished breath sounds, prolonged expiration, wheezes
Percussion	Normal	Hyperresonant
Blood gases	Hypoxemia, hypercapnia	May be normal until late stages
Other findings	Infections, right heart failure	Weight loss

The physiologic changes in chronic bronchitis start a cycle of airway obstruction and destruction with hypertrophy of the mucus-secreting glands with excessive mucus production, a decrease in ciliated epithelial cells, and a decrease in mucociliary clearance. With excessive mucus and decreased effectiveness of the mucociliary blanket, there is mucus stasis, which invites inflammation and infection. Chronic inflammation in COPD causes scarring and ulceration of the epithelial lining of the pulmonary airways. It is also thought that the chemicals in cigarette smoke cause an inflammatory response that activates neutrophils. The neutrophils produce enzymes that break down elastin in the bronchoalveolar walls. Airways are stenosed or collapsed and fewer alveoli are ventilated. Air is trapped in the alveoli, resulting in decreased diffusion of oxygen and carbon dioxide. The Pao_2 declines and the $Paco_2$ increases. The decreased Pao_2 results in pulmonary vasoconstriction and pulmonary hypertension. The increased pulmonary pressures put a strain on the right side of the heart and result in right-sided heart failure or pulmonary heart disease (**cor pulmonale**).

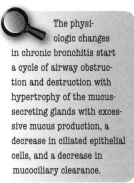

The physiologic changes in chronic bronchitis start a cycle of airway obstruction and destruction with hypertrophy of the mucus-secreting glands with excessive mucus production, a decrease in ciliated epithelial cells, and a decrease in mucociliary clearance.

Emphysema is characterized by loss of lung elasticity, narrowed bronchioles, and abnormal dilation of the terminal air spaces caused by the destruction of the alveolar walls (without evidence of fibrosis). Dilation of the airspaces results in hyperinflation of the lungs, air trapping, and increased total lung capacity. The physiologic changes associated with emphysema are thought to be caused by the destruction of elastin in the alveolar walls by enzymes (elastases and proteases) released by neutrophils. Some alveoli deteriorate and form **bullae** (larger air-filled spaces), while others remain enlarged but lose their elasticity. Although the number one cause of emphysema is cigarette smoking, certain genetic disorders such as **alpha-1-antitrypsin deficiency** have been linked to the elastin destruction seen in emphysema. Smoking may also decrease the amount of alpha-1-antitrypsin, resulting in increased destruction of elastin. Patients develop dyspnea after more than one-third of their lung tissue is destroyed. Cough is rare and nonproductive in emphysema.

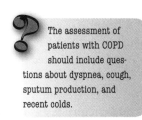

The assessment of patients with COPD should include questions about dyspnea, cough, sputum production, and recent colds.

Assessment

The patient with COPD requires careful questioning about risk factors and an understanding of the physical changes that occur in COPD. The nurse should always ask about current and previous smoking

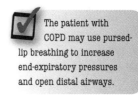

The patient with COPD may use pursed-lip breathing to increase end-expiratory pressures and open distal airways.

habits and attempts to quit. The nurse encourages honesty with a non-judgmental attitude and matter-of-fact questions. The assessment of patients with COPD should include questions about dyspnea, cough, sputum production, and recent colds. The nurse notes any postural changes in respiratory rate. The patient may be propping himself up on a table or elbows to increase the effectiveness of the accessory muscles used in breathing. The respiratory rate may be increased and expiration may be prolonged. The patient with COPD may use pursed-lip breathing to increase end-expiratory pressures and open distal airways. The chest may have an increased anterior-posterior diameter (barrel chest) with decreased chest movement and increased abdominal movement during breathing.

The terms *blue bloater* and *pink puffer* were once used to differentiate between patients with chronic bronchitis and emphysema. These phrases only partly describe the differences because many patients with COPD have components of both diseases. The physiologic changes of each diseaese cause a different responsiveness to hypoxia. Patients with chronic bronchitis were described as blue bloaters because the increased secretions and airway obstruction caused hypoxemia, cyanosis (blue), and peripheral edema from right-sided heart failure (bloater). Patients with emphysema have less surface area for ventilation and perfusion but are well compensated (pink) with hyperventilation (puffer).

Several tests are used to diagnose COPD. A thorough history and physical examination, pulmonary function tests, chest radiography, and laboratory tests are all used to diagnose COPD. Spirometry is the most frequently used pulmonary function test. It indicates whether an airway obstruction exists but does not discriminate between the different causes. The most specific spirometric test for airflow reduction is the forced expiratory volume in 1 second (FEV_1). An FEV_1 below 80% of expected without a significant decrease in forced vital capacity (FVC) is considered diagnostic of COPD.

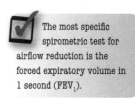

The most specific spirometric test for airflow reduction is the forced expiratory volume in 1 second (FEV_1).

(See Chapter 2 for a description of spirometry.) In chronic bronchitis there may also be an increased residual air volume (RV) from air trapped within the alveoli. The total lung capacity (TLC) may be increased in emphysema.

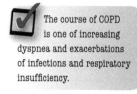

The course of COPD is one of increasing dyspnea and exacerbations of infections and respiratory insufficiency.

Arterial blood gases may show changes in advanced disease. The Pao_2 decreases and the $Paco_2$ increases with the kidneys compensating by retaining bicarbonate (HCO_3^-). The pH may be normal if the kidneys have sufficiently compensated for the acidosis caused by the high $Paco_2$. The hypoxemia (decreased Pao_2) and hypercapnia (increased $Paco_2$) seen in chronic bronchitis may not exist in emphysema because the increased respiratory rate compensates for the decrease in alveolar surface area. The hemoglobin may increase as a compensatory mechanism in chronic bronchitis to increase the oxygen-carrying capacity of the blood.

The course of COPD is one of increasing dyspnea and exacerbations of infections and respiratory insufficiency. Many patients with COPD have clinical features of both COPD and emphysema. They may first seek medical attention later in life as their dyspnea increases or they have repeated respiratory infections. The increasing dyspnea makes eating difficult, with subsequent weight loss, malnutrition, and dehydration. Patients with chronic bronchitis may have a worsening cough particularly in the morning. As the disease progresses, patients may have decreased activity tolerance, increased dyspnea, weight loss, and declining mental acuity and, later, respiratory failure and heart failure.

Treatment

Treatment can facilitate the health and quality of life of patients with COPD. The goals of treatment are to alleviate the acute symptoms and prevent complications. The treatment of COPD includes the following:

- Bronchodilators (e.g., ipratropium and albuterol or salmeterol via metered-dose inhalers) to improve airflow
- Corticosteroids (to decrease inflammation) if bronchodilators are not sufficient
- Low-flow oxygen if the Pao_2 is less than 55 mmHg or the Sao_2 is less than 88%. It can also be used during exercise or at night for patients with nocturnal hypoxemia.

- Long-acting bronchodilator like theophylline if the patient does not improve with combination therapy. Theophylline serum levels and side effects must be monitored to prevent toxicity.
- Antibiotics to treat infections as most exacerbations are triggered by bacterial infections

Nurses can facilitate the physical health and psychosocial functioning of patients with COPD. Nursing care focuses on the impact of physiologic changes on the patient's functioning. The chronic dyspnea can influence activity tolerance and capability for self-care. Coughing and shortness of breath can disturb sleep and contribute to chronic feelings of fatigue. The extra work of breathing in COPD can increase calorie requirements, but eating and swallowing may be limited by dyspnea. Certain medications such as theophylline can cause nausea and vomiting, contributing to decreased intake. Feelings of anxiety and suffocation can occur because of chronic hypoxia. The patient may also feel powerless as the disease progresses despite efforts to comply with the treatment regimen. Family members may have to take on new roles as the patient's activity tolerance declines. COPD is a chronic and progressive disease with many implications for the family as well as the patient.

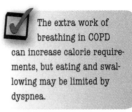

The extra work of breathing in COPD can increase calorie requirements, but eating and swallowing may be limited by dyspnea.

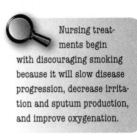

Nursing treatments begin with discouraging smoking because it will slow disease progression, decrease irritation and sputum production, and improve oxygenation.

Remember that many patients with COPD rely on the hypoxemic drive to stimulate respiration. Administer oxygen cautiously, watching for decreased respiratory rate, signs of respiratory failure, and/or decreased mental acuity.

COPD affects many aspects of the patient's life, and nurses can help the patient and the family adjust to the changes. (See the bibliography for sources of extensive care plans for patients with COPD). Nursing treatments begin with discouraging smoking because it will slow disease progression, decrease irritation and sputum production, and improve oxygenation. Nursing interventions for the patient with COPD also include the following:

1. Teach effective breathing patterns such as pursed-lip and diaphragmatic breathing; use a high Fowler's position and tables to

"prop" on. (Rationale: Effective breathing patterns improve ventilation of the alveoli by maintaining intrathoracic pressure at the end of exhalation.)

2. Improve airway clearance by encouraging the patient to cough or "huff" every 1 to 2 hours, humidify inspired air, drink 10 glasses of fluid per day, and to use nebulizer treatments, bronchodilators, expectorants, and postural drainage therapy (PDT) as ordered. (Rationale: Interventions should improve airway clearance and remove mucus from airways allowing better ventilation.)

3. Improve gas exchange by using all the above interventions plus incentive spirometry every 1 to 2 hours, and low-flow oxygen therapy (1 to 2 L/min as ordered to maintain a PO_2 of 55 mmHg). Remember that many patients with COPD rely on the hypoxemic drive to stimulate respiration. Administer oxygen cautiously, watching for decreased respiratory rate, signs of respiratory failure, and/or decreased mental acuity. (Rationale: Low-flow oxygen therapy and incentive spirometry help increase the tidal volume and oxygen available for gas exchange.)

4. Educate patients to take medications as ordered by their healthcare provider. These may include an inhaled anticholinergics (e.g., ipratropium), either alone or with an inhaled short-acting beta-agonist (e.g., albuterol), or a long-acting beta-agonist (e.g., salmeterol). (Rationale: Medications taken as directed can increase airway diameters, decrease mucus production, and decrease the incidence of exacerbation.)

5. Encourage adequate nutritional intake by monitoring meals and weight, serve easily chewed foods in small portions, and allow rest periods to minimize fatigue. (Rationale: Shorter eating periods and smaller portions are not as tiring and may increase total intake.)

6. Prevent infections with influenza vaccination (annually) and pneumococcal vaccination (one time, reassess in 5 years). Teach patients to watch for changes in sputum (yellow to green or more copious amounts) or increased temperature, and report these findings to their healthcare provider. Avoid crowded areas, take antibiotics as ordered, and clean respiratory equipment properly. (Rationale: Patients with COPD are more susceptible to infections.)

7. Evaluate activity tolerance, and help patient and family plan daily activities to minimize fatigue. Use breathing techniques and supplemental oxygen as needed. Activities should be spaced over the day and avoided for 30 minutes after eating when patients tend to be fatigued. Activities can be gradually increased as tolerated by the patient. Patient should coordinate activity with pursed-lip breathing on exhalation during the work part of an activity. (Rationale: Paced activities allow the patient rest periods, minimizing dyspnea and fatigue.)

8. Teach family to assess patient's orientation and report changes such as drowsiness and confusion to the healthcare provider. (Rationale: Disorientation may signal hypoxemia, and indicate the need for further assessment and intervention by the healthcare provider.)

9. Teach patient and family about COPD: emphasize healthy behaviors, smoking cessation, and the signs of potential problems. Encourage the patient to use local organizations such as the American Lung Association. (Rationale: Patients and families who understand COPD can actively participate in their care, feel more in control, and adhere with treatment regimens.)

10. Promote healthy sleep patterns by evaluating sleep patterns, discouraging daytime naps and beverages with caffeine, and using techniques to optimize oxygenation, including position and supplemental oxygen as ordered. Evaluate patients for obstructive sleep apnea (e.g., snoring, choking, and gasping during sleep) as the incidence of such increases in COPD patients. (Rationale: Patients experience less fatigue and have more energy for their life activities.)

11. Decrease feelings of powerlessness by evaluating the patient's perceptions about heath, incorporating the patient in decision making, and explaining that exacerbations are part of COPD. (Rationale: Patients who feel more in control feel less powerless to their disease process and are more adherent to their treatment plan.)

Asthma

Increasing numbers of Americans are suffering from **asthma**. As many as 17 million peo-

> Medications taken as directed can increase airway diameters, decrease mucus production, and decrease the incidence of exacerbation.

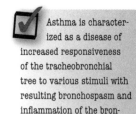

ple of all ages are afflicted with asthma and over 5000 people a year die from this chronic, inflammatory disease. Asthma is characterized as a disease of increased responsiveness of the tracheobronchial tree to various stimuli with resulting **bronchospasm** and inflammation of the bronchial mucosa. Episodes are variable in severity, and the changes in airflow are often reversible.

> Asthma is characterized as a disease of increased responsiveness of the tracheobronchial tree to various stimuli with resulting bronchospasm and inflammation of the bronchial mucosa.

Asthma can be divided into two types: intrinsic and extrinsic. **Intrinsic asthma** is considered a nonallergic type of asthma where bronchospasm is the reaction to nonallergic factors. Intrinsic factors include emotional stress, changes in humidity and temperature, exposure to noxious fumes, and coughing. In adults, intrinsic asthma may occur as a result of a respiratory tract infection. **Extrinsic asthma** occurs as a response to an allergen or trigger to which the patient is hyperresponsive. It is thought that extrinsic asthma is mediated by immunoglobulin (IgE). Extrinsic asthma appears more often in children and may disappear during adolescence. It is also associated with other hereditary allergies such as eczema and seasonal rhinitis.

The classic symptoms of wheezing and dyspnea in asthma are caused by a variety of cellular responses. Although the exact etiology of asthma is not known, there are many causative agents or triggers. Some of the more common triggers include the following:

- Air pollutants (cigarette smoke, industrial pollution, and formaldehyde)
- Perfumes
- Cold, dry air or abrupt weather changes
- Allergens (feathers, animal dander, dust mites, pollen)
- Foods, especially those with sulfites (wine, beer, salad, dried fruits, eggs)
- Viral infections
- Gastroesophageal reflux disease
- Stress
- Anxiety
- Exercise
- Wood and vegetable (flour) dust

> Asthma can be divided into two types: intrinsic and extrinsic. Intrinsic asthma is considered a nonallergic type of asthma where bronchospasm is the reaction to a virus in the upper respiratory tract or to cold air or exercise. Extrinsic asthma occurs as a response to an allergen or trigger to which the patient is hyperresponsive.

- Assorted chemicals and enzymes (solvents, rubber and latex, paints, laundry detergents)
- Medications such as aspirin, other nonsteroidal anti-inflammatory drugs, and beta-blockers
- Food additives such as monosodium glutamate (MSG) and tartrazine (yellow dye)
- Endocrine factors (menses, pregnancy, and thyroid disease)

A trigger, whether intrinsic or extrinsic, causes a complex series of pathophysiologic responses during an asthma attack. An asthma attack can be divided into an early and late response. The early response is characterized by bronchospasm as the mast cells in the bronchial walls are stimulated to release histamine, which in turn triggers constriction of the smooth muscle in the bronchial walls, swelling of the mucus membranes, and increased mucus production. The early response lasts about 90 minutes.

The late response occurs when the lung's immune system reacts to the trigger. This occurs 3 to 4 hours later and can last up to 12 hours. Eosinophils and mast cells produce a variety of chemical mediators such as prostaglandins, leukotrienes, brady-kinin, and platelet activating factor. The immune mediators in asthma cause sustained inflammation of the bronchial walls with increased vascular permeability, edema, increased mucus production, and heightened responsiveness to the trigger. The next exposure to the trigger may cause a brisker response, beginning a vicious cycle of trigger and response. Prolonged inflammation

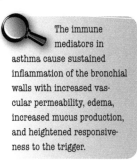

The immune mediators in asthma cause sustained inflammation of the bronchial walls with increased vascular permeability, edema, increased mucus production, and heightened responsiveness to the trigger.

may subsequently damage the pulmonary tissues, causing thickening of the membranes, destruction of the ciliated cells, and hypertrophy of the mucus glands (see Figures 3-5 and 3-6).

Assessment

Initial assessment of a patient with asthma often occurs during an asthma attack. The classic symptoms of an **asthma attack** are dyspnea, wheezing, paroxysmal cough, and tightness in the chest. Patients are often very anxious and have increased respiratory and heart rates. In patients with severe asthma, the attacks may actually occur during sleep (nocturnal asthma).

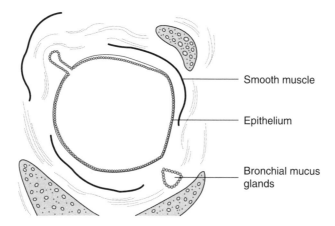

Figure 3-5 Normal bronchiole.

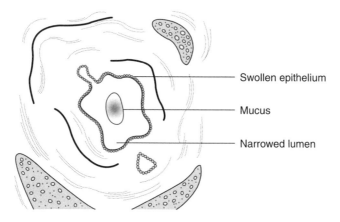

Figure 3-6 Bronchiole in asthma.

Asthma attacks may vary in severity in the same patient. A severe asthma attack may be associated with loud wheezing, use of accessory muscles, and distant breath sounds on auscultation. The breathlessness may be so severe as to make the patient speak in one- or two-word responses. Asthma attacks can be fatal, and the mortality rate is increasing despite better understanding of the disease process. Ominous signs in patients with asthma include decreased wheezing, inaudible breath sounds, cyanosis, fatigue, and inability to lie down. Be aware of these signs and assess patients for respiratory and heart failure.

Ominous signs in patients with asthma include decreased wheezing, inaudible breath sounds, cyanosis, fatigue, and inability to lie down.

A diagnosis of asthma is based on clinical presentation, history, physical examination, pulmonary function tests, and pulse oximetry and/or arterial blood gas measurements. The nurse is often the first contact for the patient experiencing an asthma attack, and a calm attitude and reassuring manner can help decrease the patient's anxiety. The history should include the course of this attack, previous episodes of shortness of breath, age of onset, precipitating factors, and how the symptoms influence the patient's functioning.

> The history should include the course of this attack, previous episodes of shortness of breath, age of onset, precipitating factors, and how the symptoms influence the patient's functioning.

Pulmonary function tests, particularly peak expiratory flow rate (PEFR), FVC, maximum mid-expiratory flow (MMEF), and FEV will show decreased values during an asthma attack and improve after treatment. The PEFR measures the rate of airflow with a forced expiration. Small, inexpensive PEFR meters can be used at home by patients to monitor respiratory status, measure treatment effectiveness, and evaluate possible attacks (see Figure 3-7). Daily

> A written action plan for appropriate treatment at specific PEFR levels improves patient management of asthma and prevents emergency department visits and hospitalizations.

PEFR monitoring is recommended for patients with moderate to severe asthma. A written action plan for appropriate treatment at specific PEFR levels improves patient management of asthma and prevents emergency department visits and hospitalizations.

Arterial blood gas values and pulse oximetry are also used to reveal the extent of the hypoxemia and possible need for hospitalization. Typically, the ABGs will reveal hypoxemia and respiratory alkalosis as a result of the increased respiratory rate. If the asthma worsens, the acid–base balance shifts to respiratory acidosis due to carbon dioxide retention and hypoxemia.

Other laboratory tests to diagnose asthma include the methacholine provocation tests, allergy testing, sputum stain for eosinophils, chest X-rays, possibly sinus X-rays, and rhinoscopy. The provocation tests are

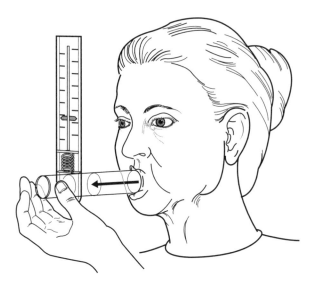

Figure 3-7 Peak flow meter.

done in a hospital setting and a trigger such as methacholine (a beta-agonist) or cold air is used, and then pulmonary function tests measure the bronchial response to the trigger. The patient is then treated with a bronchodilator to relieve the bronchospasm.

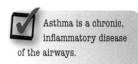

Asthma is a chronic, inflammatory disease of the airways.

Treatment

The guidelines for the treatment and management of asthma published by the National Heart, Lung, and Blood Institute (NHLBI) detail the primary objectives of therapy as the following:

1. Maintain normal activity levels (including exercise).

2. Maintain normal (or near normal) pulmonary function.

3. Prevent chronic and troublesome symptoms.

4. Prevent recurrent exacerbations of asthma.

5. Provide optimal drug therapy while minimizing adverse effects from asthma medications.

6. Meet patient and families' expectations regarding asthma care.

Asthma is a chronic, inflammatory disease of the airways. Inflammation of the airways is a major factor in respiratory symptoms and disease chronicity. The four stages are mild (episodic), moderate (one to two times a week), severe, and status asthmatic. Treatment of all stages involves nonpharmacologic and pharmacologic methods. Nonpharmacologic methods are aimed at preventing attacks and intervening early during an attack. These methods include the following:

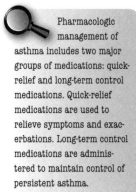

Pharmacologic management of asthma includes two major groups of medications: quick-relief and long-term control medications. Quick-relief medications are used to relieve symptoms and exacerbations. Long-term control medications are administered to maintain control of persistent asthma.

1. Education of patients about the disease

2. Identification of triggers in the environment

3. Eradication of triggers such as cigarette smoke, dust mites, and animal dander (see Table 3-5)

4. Teaching relaxation techniques such as controlled breathing

5. Administration of immunotherapy through a desensitization program to block IgE response

Pharmacologic management of asthma includes two major groups of medications: quick-relief and long-term control medications. Quick-relief medications are used to relieve symptoms and exacerbations. Long-term control medications are administered to maintain control of persistent asthma.

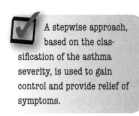

A stepwise approach, based on the classification of the asthma severity, is used to gain control and provide relief of symptoms.

Asthma is classified based on the clinical features of the disease: presence of daily symptoms, limitations to physical activity, frequency of exacerbations, use of quick-relief medications, pulmonary functioning (PEFR), and presence of nighttime symptoms.

A stepwise approach, based on the classification of the asthma severity, is used to gain control and provide relief of symptoms. It is recommended that patients be started at a higher step to achieve control of symptoms and then "step down" to a lower level of treatment versus a step-up approach where treatment is aimed at the patient's level and then increased if relief is not achieved.

The four steps are:

Step 1: Mild intermittent

Step 2: Mild persistent

Step 3: Moderate persistent

Step 4: Severe persistent

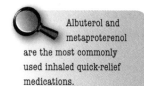

Albuterol and metaproterenol are the most commonly used inhaled quick-relief medications.

Bronchodilators, most commonly short-acting, inhaled beta$_2$-agonists, are quick-relief medications that act primarily to relax bronchial smooth muscle and dilate the airways. Albuterol and metaproterenol are the most commonly used inhaled quick-relief medications. Anticholinergics such as ipratropium are used to increase the effects of bronchodilators.

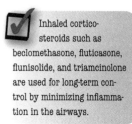

Inhaled cortico-steroids such as beclomethasone, fluticasone, flunisolide, and triamcinolone are used for long-term control by minimizing inflammation in the airways.

Beta$_2$-agonists are usually administered via inhalation with a metered-dose inhaler (MDI) but may also be administered subcutaneously and orally (see Figure 3-8). Correct use of the MDI is essential for accurate administration of the medication into the lungs, and spacers are often

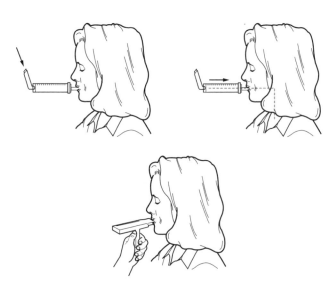

Figure 3-8 Metered dose inhaler.

used to make the coordination of inhalation and release of medication easier (see Table 3-10).

Long-term control medications are indicated for mild persistent, moderate persistent, and severe persistent asthma. They can be divided into the corticosteroids, leukotriene modifiers, methylxanthines, and cromolyn. Corticosteroids provide anti-inflammatory and immunosuppressive effects to relieve bronchial edema. Inhaled corticosteroids such as beclomethasone, fluticasone, flunisolide, and triamcinolone are used for long-term control by minimizing inflammation in the airways. An MDI with a spacer is used for the administration of inhaled corticosteroids to provide more direct steroid administration into the lungs without the residual drug in the mouth. Residual steroids on the oral mucosa can predispose the patient to thrush infections. Systemic corticosteroids such as prednisone and methylprednisolone are reserved for moderate to severe exacerbations to speed recovery and reestablish control during periods of deterioration. Leukotriene modifiers, such as montelukast, are used as prophylaxis and for chronic treatment of asthma.

Theophylline, a methylxanthine, is a bronchodilator administered orally or intravenously (as aminophylline). Time-released oral formula-

> Systemic corticosteroids such as prednisone and methylprednisolone are reserved for moderate to severe exacerbations to speed recovery and reestablish control during periods of deterioration.

Table 3-10 Correct Use of a Metered-Dose Inhaler (MDI)

1. Remove the cap from the MDI.
2. Shake MDI.
3. Place index finger on top of canister and thumb on bottom of mouthpiece.
4. Take a breath in and out slowly.
5. Place inhaler about 1 inch in front of open mouth.
6. At the beginning of inhalation, press down on the canister and at the same time, begin to inhale slowly and deeply.
7. Hold breath 5 to 10 seconds.
8. Wait 1 to 2 minutes and repeat as directed.
9. Rinse out mouth and spit out (if steroid inhaler is used).
10. If using a spacer, follow directions except place lips around spacer mouthpiece.
11. Rinse inhaler in warm water to clean.

tions help to minimize toxicity and side effects and achieve more stable blood levels. Theophylline toxicity is fairly common and includes nausea, vomiting, dizziness, rapid pulse, twitching, insomnia, and seizures. Blood levels need to be monitored to maintain drug levels within a safe yet effective range.

Cromolyn is an anti-inflammatory drug in a different class from corticosteroids. Cromolyn stabilizes the mast cells, thereby preventing the release of histamine, a potent bronchoconstrictor. Cromolyn may be given by inhalation or in a nasal spray to stabilize the nasal mucosa in allergic rhinitis, and it is used prophylactically before exposure to a known trigger. Cromolyn, inhaled corticosteroids, and leukotriene modifiers are never used during an acute asthma attack.

> Cromolyn, inhaled corticosteroids, and leukotriene modifiers are never used during an acute asthma attack.

Nursing management of the patient with asthma requires extensive education of the patient and family. For patients with mild to moderate asthma, education about asthma, environmental triggers, medications and their side effects, and treatment follow-up can control the disease and prevent attacks. Written guidelines provide patients with the steps to follow if their symptoms progress and directions for when to seek treatment if their medications are not relieving their symptoms.

 For patients with mild to moderate asthma, education about asthma, environmental triggers, medications and their side effects, and treatment follow-up can control the disease and prevent attacks.

Nursing Care of Patients with Asthma

Nursing care for the patient with mild to moderate asthma includes teaching about the following:

- Monitor PEFR per the NHBLI guidelines for 2 to 4 weeks to obtain a "personal best" average.
- Follow the "zone system" (green, yellow, red) for taking medications. Green for a PEFR 80% to 100% of personal best and no symptoms; use maintenance medications. Yellow for a PEFR of <50% to 80%; use rescue medication plan. Red for PEFR of <50%; use bronchodilator, and if no improvement in 10 to 15 minutes, call a healthcare provider or go to an emergency room.

- Take medications in the correct order: beta-agonists first, followed by steroids. Use the MDI correctly. Use bronchodilator 30 minutes before exercise if this a known trigger.
- Use inhaled beta$_2$-agonists to relieve wheezing during an attack. Do not use steroids, leukotriene modifiers, or cromolyn during an attack (rescue medications). If the beta$_2$-agonist does not relieve symptoms in 10 to 15 minutes, go to the emergency room or contact your healthcare provider.
- Identify and eliminate environmental triggers, such as animal dander, dust mites, feather pillows and puffs, and cigarette smoke. Clean regularly with a damp cloth. Clean furnace and air conditioners annually. Wash all bedding in hot water (see Table 3-5).
- Reduce stress and anxiety. Get enough sleep and rest. Try relaxation techniques.
- Avoid medications such as aspirin and nonsteroidal anti-inflammatory drugs (NSAIDs) that may precipitate attacks, and avoid antihypertensives that contain an angiotensin-converting enzyme (ACE) because these drugs may worsen a cough associated with bronchoconstriction.
- Minimize respiratory infections that may precipitate an attack by avoiding crowds and infected people, engaging in frequent hand washing, and receiving the influenza vaccine annually.
- Continue activity at a normal level, avoiding possible triggers such as cold air.
- Drink an adequate amount of fluid (2.5 to 3 L per day) to liquefy secretions.
- Seek emergency care if medications fail to control symptoms; nails or lips are gray or blue; difficulty breathing, walking, or talking; declining PEFR rates (falls into red zone <50% of the personal best).

Severe asthma and status asthmaticus are potentially life-threatening conditions that need close care and follow-up. Symptoms of severe asthma include frequent attacks with nocturnal awakenings that result in limited activity levels. **Status asthmaticus** is a severe, prolonged asthma attack that does not respond to conventional treatment. Patients are seen in the emergency room for careful evaluation of respiratory function and treatment with oxygen therapy, and in-

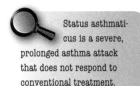
Status asthmaticus is a severe, prolonged asthma attack that does not respond to conventional treatment.

travenous medications such as aminophylline and epinephrine, inhaled beta$_2$-agonists, and/or antibiotic therapy for presumed infection. Patients may be quite anxious and fatigued from the work of breathing. Pulse oximetry and arterial blood gases help to determine whether respiratory failure is imminent and whether endotracheal intubation with mechanical ventilation is necessary. Usually, the medications and supplemental oxygen reverse the wheezing, and the patient recovers. In 1% to 3% of cases of status asthmaticus, mechanical ventilation may be required. Respiratory failure may progress to acidemia with cardiac dysrhythmias and may result in death.

Asthma is a treatable disease, and most patients do well with the appropriate medications and elimination of triggers. Education about asthma and a written treatment plan give patients and their families the ability to manage asthma. The healthcare team can provide resources if home management is not effective.

Acute Respiratory Failure

Acute respiratory failure occurs when the lungs cannot maintain arterial oxygenation and/or eliminate carbon dioxide. Acute respiratory failure is defined as gas exchange that is inadequate to meet the metabolic needs of the body. Impaired gas exchange leads to decreased oxygenation of the body tissues. Patients with acute respiratory failure are often seriously ill and require intensive care and support.

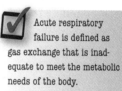
Acute respiratory failure is defined as gas exchange that is inadequate to meet the metabolic needs of the body.

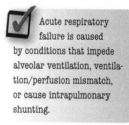
Acute respiratory failure is caused by conditions that impede alveolar ventilation, ventilation/perfusion mismatch, or cause intrapulmonary shunting.

There are many different causes of acute respiratory failure, and the presentation depends on the underlying condition. In patients with normal lung tissue, acute respiratory failure produces high levels of carbon dioxide in the blood (hypercapnia) and lower levels of oxygen (hypoxia). But in patients with COPD, acute respiratory failure may only be signaled by a deteriorating condition and hypoxia because these patients normally have higher levels of carbon dioxide.

Acute respiratory failure is caused by conditions that impede alveolar ventilation, ventilation/perfusion mismatch, or cause intrapulmonary shunting. Alveolar hypoventilation may result from an airway obstruction and causes increased levels of alveolar carbon dioxide.

Ventilation/perfusion (V/Q) mismatch is the most common cause of hypoxemic respiratory failure. In normal lungs, the areas of the alveoli that are aerated also have an adequate blood supply, allowing gas exchange to take place. The V/Q ratio is one way to compare the pulmonary ventilation to the pulmonary circulation. Ventilation without perfusion occurs when there is adequate ventilation but the circulation to alveoli is blocked (for example, pulmonary embolism). Perfusion without ventilation occurs when the oxygen does not reach the perfused alveolar membrane. This occurs when secretions and edema block airways and impede gas exchange at the alveolar membrane (see Figure 3-9).

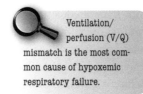
Ventilation/perfusion (V/Q) mismatch is the most common cause of hypoxemic respiratory failure.

V/Q mismatch exists when there is normal pulmonary blood flow with insufficient ventilation or insufficient blood flow and normal ventilation. Intrapulmonary shunting occurs when blood passes from the right side of the heart to the left side of the heart without being oxygenated.

Conditions that may cause acute respiratory failure include the following:

- COPD
- Pulmonary embolism
- Bronchitis/bronchospasm
- Cor pulmonale (heart failure)
- Pulmonary edema

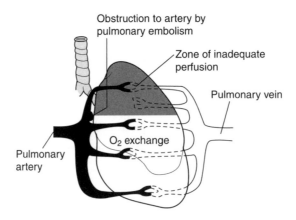

Figure 3-9 Ventilation/perfusion mismatch in pulmonary embolism.

- Atelectasis
- Central nervous system depression or disease (head trauma, opioid overdose, tumor, hemorrhage, anesthesia)
- Pneumothorax (trauma, flail chest)
- Ventilatory failure (acute respiratory distress syndrome [ARDS], massive pneumonia, cystic fibrosis, sleep apnea)
- Disorders of the muscles and nerves (multiple sclerosis, Guillian-Barré syndrome, myasthenia gravis, polio, amylotrophic lateral sclerosis [Lou Gehrig's disease])

The entire respiratory system (the lungs, the central nervous system, the heart, the respiratory muscles, and the airways) is involved in oxygenation. Disorders in any of these components of the respiratory system can lead to respiratory failure. Acute respiratory failure is associated with imbalances including **hypovolemia** (depleted intravascular volume), metabolic acidosis, respiratory alkalosis, **hyperkalemia** (high serum potassium) and **hypervolemia** (excessive intravascular volume).

 Acute respiratory failure is defined as gas exchange that is inadequate to meet the metabolic needs of the body.

Signs and symptoms of acute respiratory failure are the result of compensatory mechanisms from many body systems.

In patients with COPD, acute respiratory failure may only be signaled by a deteriorating condition and hypoxia.

Assessment

Signs and symptoms of acute respiratory failure are the result of compensatory mechanisms by many body systems. Increased respiratory rate (tachypnea) and signs of labored breathing (use of accessory muscles in the abdomen and shoulders, flared nostrils, and pursed-lip breathing) are classic symptoms of respiratory failure. The hallmark signs of respiratory failure are hypoxemia and hypercapnia.

Hypoxemia is defined as an arterial oxygen concentration of less than 60 mmHg. Patients with hypoxemia are usually dyspneic and may be anxious, disoriented, confused, and delirious. Other signs of hypoxemia are central cyanosis, tachypnea, tachycardia, hypertension, and tremors. **Hypercapnia** is defined as an arterial carbon dioxide concentration ($Paco_2$) greater than 50 mmHg. Patients are hypercapneic because they are hypoventilating.

Respiratory failure affects the cardiovascular system. The sympathetic nervous system is stimulated with resulting tachycardia to improve cardiac output. Peripheral vasoconstriction results in cool, pale, clammy skin. If respiratory failure progresses, the myocardium is deprived of oxygen and the blood pressure and heart rate drop and potentially life-threatening arrhythmias may develop.

Respiratory failure disrupts the blood supply to the central nervous system (CNS). Patients may experience changes to the sensorium. Initially, patients may feel anxious but continued hypoxia may produce confusion and delirium. Headache may result from prolonged hypercapnia as higher carbon dioxide levels and acidemia produce vasodilation in the brain. If elevation of carbon dioxide levels continues, patients may experience seizures and slip into a coma.

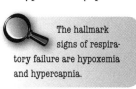

The hallmark signs of respiratory failure are hypoxemia and hypercapnia.

Physical assessment of the patient with respiratory failure begins with observing the rate, depth, and character of the respirations. The patient in respiratory failure may use accessory muscles in the chest and abdomen as seen by retraction of the intercostal spaces and suprasternal area, and the contraction of abdominal muscles during respiration. Breath sounds may be diminished or absent over the affected area of the lung.

Treatment

Treatment for acute respiratory failure includes addressing the underlying cause, maintaining an open airway, and ensuring alveolar ventilation. The goal of treatment in hypoxemic respiratory failure is to ensure adequate oxygenation to the vital organs (brain, heart, and lungs).

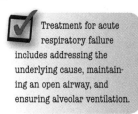

Treatment for acute respiratory failure includes addressing the underlying cause, maintaining an open airway, and ensuring alveolar ventilation.

Oxygen therapy is given to patients in acute respiratory failure with careful monitoring. The treatment goal is to maintain an Sao_2 of at least 90% and/or a Pao_2 of 60 mmHg without causing oxygen toxicity. Oxygen is delivered via Venturi mask to control oxygen concentrations. If conservative treatment fails to maintain oxygenation, if the patient becomes exhausted, or if respiratory arrest occurs, then intubation and mechanical ventilation may be required. Positive end expiratory pressure (PEEP) may be added to prevent airway and alveolar collapse and improve gas exchange. (See Chapter 4 regarding interventions to maintain oxygenation.)

Other treatments to improve oxygenation include pharmacologic agents, chest physiotherapy, and suctioning. Bronchodilators are used to open airways and are usually administered via inhalation but may also be given intravenously (i.e., theophylline). Antibiotics and corticosteroids may be added to treat underlying infection and inflammation. In the case of pulmonary embolism, treatment may include anticoagulants. Intravenous fluids are given to correct dehydration or, in the case of fluid overload, diuretics may be administered. Chest physiotherapy includes postural drainage, percussion, and vibration of the chest wall to mobilize secretions and improve aeration. When coughing is insufficient to clear secretions, suctioning may be required to maintain airway patency.

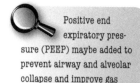

Positive end expiratory pressure (PEEP) maybe added to prevent airway and alveolar collapse and improve gas exchange.

Patients with acute respiratory failure have varying courses depending on the underlying disease. The goals of treatment are to maintain adequate oxygenation and pulmonary ventilation and treat the underlying condition. Nursing care of the patient with acute respiratory failure involves careful monitoring of vital sign changes, implementing interventions to improve oxygenation, administering appropriate medications, and assessing response to treatment.

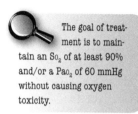

The goal of treatment is to maintain an So_2 of at least 90% and/or a Pao_2 of 60 mmHg without causing oxygen toxicity.

The following is an outline of nursing care of patients in acute respiratory failure:

1. Monitor vital signs every 15 minutes.
   - Watch for tachypnea, tachycardia, and check temperature hourly, especially if infection in suspected. (Rationale: Increasing heart rate or respiratory rate could be indicative of increasing respiratory failure.)
   - Check for pulsus paradoxus (a drop in systolic blood pressure greater than 10 mmHg during inspiration).
   - Monitor arterial blood gases every 30 minutes or as ordered.
   - Watch for decreasing Pao_2 or increasing $Paco_2.$
   - Watch for decreasing pH (acidemia) or increasing pH if compensation by the kidneys has occurred with bicarbonate retention. (Rationale: Arterial blood gas values guide treatment and indicate patient response to interventions.)

- Observe for restlessness or anxiety. (Rationale: Increasing restlessness may signal falling O_2 levels.)
- Encourage the patient to cough every 15 to 30 minutes. (Rationale: Secretions may block airways and prevent ventilation of the alveoli.)
- If the patient with COPD is retaining carbon dioxide, encourage deep breathing and exhalation through pursed lips. (Rationale: Patients with COPD may need hypoxemia to drive the respiratory rate and may not inhale deeply if their O_2 levels rise with supplemental oxygen.) As the patient improves he or she may be allowed short rest periods.
- Auscultate breath sounds every hour or more often if vital signs change.
  - Notify physician of increasing crackles and dyspnea.
  - Notify physician of diminished breath sounds. (Rationale: Detection of deteriorating respiratory status will focus interventions in a timely manner.)
- Administer supplemental O_2 to maintain a Pao_2 above 60 mmHg and Sao_2 over 90%. Frequently assess the inspired oxygen (Fio_2) levels, ABGs, and pulse oximetry. Intubation and mechanical ventilation may be required if Pao_2 levels continue to fall below 60 mmHg despite reasonable oxygen concentrations. (Note: Cautiously administer oxygen at 1 to 2 L per minute in patients with COPD, and increase as necessary based on the ABGs and pulse oximetry so as not to override the patient's hypoxic drive). (Rationale: Continuous assessment of respiratory status allows changes in interventions to maintain adequate oxygenation.)
- If the patient is intubated, maintain ventilator settings at ordered parameters.
- Keep a resuscitation bag at the bedside.
- Monitor electrocardiogram (ECG) for arrhythmias.
- Use sedatives and hypnotics cautiously in patients who are in acute respiratory failure but not mechanically ventilated, as such agents may depress respiratory drive. Ventilated patients require sedation but continue to need support, as they may be conscious and frightened.

2. Create an accepting environment for the patient, but be aware of the possibility that increasing anxiety and restlessness may indicate worsening hypoxia.
   - Stay with patient if he is dyspneic, as he may be frightened.

- Reassure patient during episodes of breathlessness. Avoid repeating the word "relax," as it may minimize the patient's experience or even provoke anger. (Rationale: Anxiety may increase oxygen demand.)
- Gently remind the patient to take slow breaths.
- Reorient the confused patient.
- Pace activities to patient's energy level and tolerance, providing rest periods as needed.
- Allow visitors when appropriate for short periods so as not to make the patient tired. Make sure visitors do not have signs of colds or infections. (Rationale: Hypoxemia and dyspnea will both make the patient anxious, and support and reassurance from significant others is invaluable.)

3. Remind the patient to cough every 15 to 30 minutes using whatever technique best clears the airways.
- Elevate the head of the bed so the patient is in high Fowler's or semi-Fowler's position and change position every 1 to 2 hours.
- Use percussion, vibration, and postural drainage to facilitate movement of mucus.
- Increase fluid intake (if allowed) or administer intravenous fluids to keep secretions liquid.
- Administer bronchodilators prior to percussion and vibration to dilate airways and improve movement of secretions.
- Provide humidified air to aid in liquefying secretions.
- Obtain sputum for culture and sensitivity, if ordered.
- Provide frequent mouth care.

4. Monitor temperature every hour if fever is present.
- Administer antibiotics as ordered.
- Screen all visitors with colds or potential infections. (Rationale: Patients with respiratory failure are susceptible to infections. Careful monitoring of temperature and other signs of infection will direct treatment.)

5. Monitor intake and output and obtain daily weights.
- Follow hemoglobin and hematocrit for signs of fluid overload.
- Watch for neck vein distention, tachycardia, and tachypnea as signs of right-sided heart failure.
- Encourage 2 L/day of fluids unless patient is retaining fluid or is in heart failure.

- Maintain intravenous access for fluid and medication administration.
- Maintain nutritional status with small, frequent, high-protein meals; limit salt intake in patients with COPD and heart failure as it could increase fluid retention and increase the risk of heart failure. (Rationale: The work of breathing greatly increases with respiratory failure, and the patient may not be able to consume sufficient calories, requiring parenteral nutrition. Patients are at risk for fluid overload and heart failure because of increased pressure in the pulmonary vasculature.)

Adult Respiratory Distress Syndrome

Adult respiratory distress syndrome (ARDS) is a severe, life-threatening condition that occurs as a complication of a variety of clinical disorders, from sepsis to trauma. ARDS is manifested by dyspnea, severe hypoxemia, decreased lung compliance, and noncardiac pulmonary edema. ARDS is a form of pulmonary edema that is also known as shock lung, wet lung, and stiff lung. Despite the advancements in technology and the understanding of ARDS, this is a deadly syndrome with a mortality rate above 50% if not detected and treated quickly.

ARDS is a deadly syndrome with a mortality rate above 50% if not detected and treated quickly.

The onset of ARDS is often quite sudden and nursing care requires an understanding of patients at risk and watching for early signs of respiratory failure. Clinical presentations of ARDS vary depending on the precipitating event, but usually appear within 24 to 48 hours of the event. Certain disorders that put patients at risk for developing ARDS include the following:

- Trauma—Massive bodily injury; increased intracranial pressure from head trauma, tumor, or cerebral vascular accident
- Sepsis—Infection, septicemia (particularly gram-negative sepsis), pneumonia
- Shock—Hemorrhagic, septic, or anaphylactic shock
- Toxins—Inhaled noxious gases and smoke, oxygen toxicity, drug overdose
- Hemolytic disorders—Disseminated intravascular coagulation (DIC), multiple blood transfusions

- Complications of cardiopulmonary bypass
- Aspiration—Gastric contents, near drowning
- Fat and amniotic fluid emboli
- Pancreatitis

ARDS develops as a result of damage to the lungs by chemical mediators. Many different mediators have been identified as causative agents including platelet-activating factor, histamines, serotonin, bradykinin, and tumor necrosis factor (TNF). The process begins as an inflammatory reaction following injury with the release of histamine, serotonin, and bradykinin. These substances are responsible for inflammation and damage to the alveolar capillary membrane causing fluids to shift into the interstitial space. Liquids and proteins leak out of the capillaries causing pulmonary edema. Decreased blood flow, increased fluid within the alveoli and decreased production of surfactant lead to alveolar collapse and impaired gas exchange and severe hypoxemia. With less alveolar surface area available for gas exchange, a ventilation/perfusion mismatch develops (the circulation is adequate but the ventilation is impaired). The terminal airways become compressed by the edema and lung compliance decreases. The chemical mediators cause damage to the alveolar epithelium. The cascade of events ends in fibrosis, scarring of the lungs, and refractory hypoxemia despite supplemental oxygen. ARDS can be fatal unless intensive interventions are initiated to maintain oxygenation.

> ARDS develops as a result of damage to the lungs by chemical mediators including platelet-activating factor, histamines, serotonin, bradykinin, and tumor necrosis factor (TNF).

 ARDS can be fatal unless intensive interventions are initiated to maintain oxygenation.

Assessment

Careful assessment of patients at risk for ARDS is essential for early detection and treatment. Signs and symptoms may include the following:

1. Rapid onset of tachypnea and dyspnea

2. Tachycardia

3. Increasing anxiety, restlessness, and agitation (due to worsening hypoxemia)

ARDS develops over four stages. In stage I, patients develop dyspnea in the hours or days following injury. Auscultation may reveal decreased breath sounds. In stage II, respiratory distress may become more pronounced with increasing respiratory rate, increasing heart rate, and restlessness. The patient may have a dry cough or frothy sputum. Auscultation may reveal crackles at the bases of the lungs. In stage III, there is marked respiratory distress with tachypnea, tachycardia, and labile blood pressure. The skin may be cool, clammy, and cyanotic. There are diminished breath sounds on auscultation and possibly crackles and rhonchi. Stage IV is severe ARDS with decreased respiratory and heart rates, loss of consciousness, and cardiovascular collapse.

Diagnostic testing includes arterial blood gas analysis and chest X-ray. Pulmonary artery catheterization may be needed to monitor pulmonary edema and identify the cause. The three main features of ARDS that distinguish it from other respiratory disorders are:

- Diffuse, bilateral patchy infiltrates on chest X-ray
- No improvement in arterial oxygenation with supplemental oxygen
- No signs of heart failure

Early in the course of ARDS, the breath sounds and chest X-ray may be normal because the edema is in the interstitial spaces. Initially, arterial blood gases show a low $Paco_2$ due to compensatory hyperventilation. As the alveolar surface area available for gas exchange decreases, the $Paco_2$ increases, Pao_2 decreases, and acidosis develops. Supplemental oxygen does not improve the arterial oxygen concentration. The increasing fluid in the alveoli and lung interstitium soon becomes apparent on the chest X-ray as diffuse bilateral pulmonary infiltrates.

The three main features of ARDS that distinguish it from other respiratory disorders are:

- Diffuse, bilateral patchy infiltrates on chest X-ray
- No improvement in arterial oxygenation with supplemental oxygen
- No signs of heart failure.

Treatment of ARDS revolves around identification and treatment of the underlying cause and supportive respiratory care.

Treatment

Treatment of ARDS revolves around identification and treatment of the underlying cause and supportive respiratory care. Many patients with ARDS require endotracheal intubation

Patients with ARDS respond poorly to increased concentrations of oxygen.

and mechanical ventilation to support adequate oxygenation. If the patient is ventilated he or she will require intensive nursing and supportive care. Sedation will be required at regular intervals to reduce restlessness.

Patients with ARDS respond poorly to increased concentrations of oxygen. The Pao_2 may not correspond to the amount of Fio_2. This is called the gradient between the alveolar and arterial oxygen content. Patients with ARDS often need progressively higher concentrations of oxygen to maintain an adequate Pao_2. Airway management with intubation and mechanical ventilation allows for greater control of ventilation and oxygenation if other noninvasive treatments fail to improve oxygenation. Two methods of increasing the arterial oxygen levels are positive end expiratory pressure (PEEP) and continuous positive airway pressure (CPAP). PEEP enhances oxygenation by keeping airways and alveoli open at the end of expiration. High-frequency jet ventilation may also be used. Pressures in the pulmonary vasculature are monitored with pulmonary artery catheters. Antibiotics are used to treat any underlying infection. Blood transfusions and intravenous colloids are infused to maintain the circulating blood volume and improve the oxygen-carrying capacity of the blood.

Nursing Care of the Patient with ARDS

Nursing management of the patient with ARDS begins with the identification of patients who are at risk and continued assessment for early detection of this syndrome. The following types of intensive nursing care are required for patients with diagnosed ARDS:

1. Monitor vital signs, arterial blood gases, or sensorium frequently, and notify the physician immediately. Tachypnea and restlessness may be the earliest signs of impending ARDS. A minimal rise or a dropping Pao_2, despite treatment with a high flow rate (8 to 10 L per min) of oxygen, or a rise in the $Paco_2$, may be early clinical signs of respiratory failure. Early treatment may prevent the development of full-blown ARDS.

2. Maintain the patient's oxygenation despite increasing demands for oxygen. The prone position or semi-Fowler's position may improve alveolar ventilation and oxygen diffusion. Deliver humidified oxygen through a tight-fitting mask possibly with continuous positive airway pressure (CPAP). Repeat ABGs, Sao_2, pulmonary catheter measurements, and vital signs frequently. If the patient

requires intubation, check ventilator settings regularly. Suctioning will be required to maintain the patency of the tube and airways.

3. Maintain fluid balance by monitoring vital signs, pulmonary catheter pressures, intake and output, and daily weights. Pulmonary capillary wedge pressures may increase during ARDS as a result of hypoxemia triggering pulmonary vasoconstriction. The goal of fluid replacement is to maintain an adequate circulating volume and maximize the oxygen-carrying capability of the blood. Monitor electrolyte levels frequently.

4. Sedate the patient as ordered to decrease restlessness. Provide special precautions to maintain patient safety and prevent falls. Intubated patients require special interventions to prevent complications from sedatives and neuromuscular blocking agents. Provide careful eye care to protect the corneas from drying and abrasion. Perform passive range of motion exercises to preserve mobility. Rotate positions and provide skin care to prevent breakdown.

Lung Cancer

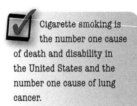

Cigarette smoking is the number one cause of death and disability in the United States and the number one cause of lung cancer.

The incidence of lung cancer has increased steadily for men and women for several decades. Although the rate for men has stabilized recently, the rate for women is now almost equal to men. The typical patient with lung cancer is a male, 55 to 60 years of age, with a smoking history. Most lung cancer results from chronic inhalation of carcinogens, particularly cigarette smoke. It is important to emphasize that cigarette smoking is the number one cause of death and disability in the United States and the number one cause of lung cancer. Occupational exposure to carcinogens can occur from sources such as asbestos, petroleum products, carbon-containing products, coal dust, and radiation exposure. Occupational exposure accounts for only a small proportion of lung cancer, and tobacco smoking is the overwhelming cause of most lung cancers.

Assessment

Most patients are asymptomatic when their lung cancers are discovered, perhaps on a routine preoperative chest X-ray (see Figure 3-10). They may present with hemoptysis, dyspnea, chest pain, or pleuritic pain. Common symptoms include the following:

- Cough
- Hoarseness
- Wheezing
- Dyspnea
- Hemoptysis
- Chest pain
- Fever
- Weakness
- Weight loss
- Anorexia
- Shoulder pain
- Gynecomastia (large cell)
- Hypercalcemia

Regardless of the stage of the disease, less than 20% of all patients with lung cancer are cured of their disease.

Patients with metastatic disease (i.e., cancer that has spread from the original tumor to other parts of the body) may have more systemic symptoms such as weight loss, fatigue, malaise, and anorexia. The prognosis

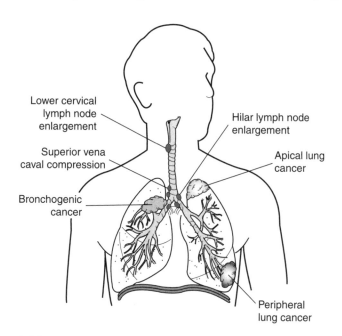

Lower cervical lymph node enlargement

Hilar lymph node enlargement

Superior vena caval compression

Apical lung cancer

Bronchogenic cancer

Peripheral lung cancer

Figure 3-10 Clinical features of lung cancer.

is poor for patients with metastatic lung cancer. Regardless of the stage of the disease, less than 20% of all patients with lung cancer are cured of their disease.

The diagnosis is made by chest X-ray, lung biopsy, sputum cytology, bronchoscopy, mediastinoscopy, MRI, and/or CAT scan. There are four different classifications of lung cancer:

- Squamous cell carcinoma (25–35%)
- Adenocarcinoma (25–35%)
- Small cell or oat cell carcinoma (10–25%)
- Large cell or mixed carcinoma (5–20%)

Small cell or oat cell carcinoma is considered separately because it is highly malignant and tends to metastasize early. Bronchogenic cancer can arise centrally at the hilar area (i.e., the hilum is where the main stem bronchus splits into the right and left bronchi) or more peripherally in the bronchioles. The pathology of the tumor is useful in determining the appropriate treatment.

Staging of lung cancer is done with the TNM system (tumor, nodes, and metastases). There are four stages, with stage I being the smallest, most localized tumor and stage IV being advanced disease. Unfortunately, 80% of patients with lung cancer have advanced disease at the time of diagnosis. Lung cancer can grow quietly for years in the soft spongy tissue of the lungs. There are no pain receptors in lung tissue to signal tumor growth or invasion. The rich blood and lymphatic supply in the lungs feeds the tumor and provides a pathway for the tumor cells to spread throughout the body.

> Staging of lung cancer is done with the TNM system (tumor, nodes, and metastases).

Advanced lung cancer presents with a variety of symptoms that may be different from the tumor's pulmonary origins. The tumor can press against or destroy the recurrent laryngeal nerve, causing hoarseness. The lung cancer may have already metastasized to the bones, causing pain in distant sites. It may have spread to the bones in the vertebral column causing spinal cord compression with symptoms of weakness and numbness in the extremities. The bone metastases and altered renal function may cause symptoms of hypercalcemia (muscle weakness, anorexia, nausea, constipation, and lethargy). The superior vena cava may be compressed by a tumor, resulting in facial and arm swelling. In the syndrome of inappropriate antidiuretic hormone (SIADH), the tumor produces antidiuretic hormone (ADH), causing increased urine production and hypovolemia and hyponatremia.

Treatment

The treatment of lung cancer is determined by the histology, location, and extent of the tumor, as well as the lymph node involvement and the presence of metastases. Lung cancer may metastasize to other sites in the lungs, to

> ✓ The treatment of lung cancer is determined by the histology, location, and extent of the tumor, as well as the lymph node involvement and the presence of metastases.

the brain, bones, and liver. The patient's pulmonary and cardiac status also affects decisions about treatment, including surgery. Surgery is not curative in most cases of lung cancer.

Nonsmall-cell lung cancer in the earliest stages (I and II) may be treated surgically. If the patient has sufficient respiratory capacity, the surgeon can perform a **lobectomy** (removal of the affected lobe) or **pneumonectomy** (removal of the lung). Surgery is not usually curative if the disease is advanced at the time of diagnosis. Chemotherapy and radiation therapy may be used together or separately to treat the disease. Radiation therapy may also be used to treat nonoperable cancers and metastases in the bone and brain.

Nursing Care of the Patient with Lung Cancer

The role of nursing in lung cancer treatment begins with prevention. Education programs in the schools are essential to preventing smoking in the young. Community programs can encourage smoking cessation in established smokers by teaching the effects of cigarette smoke and offering cessation programs. Nurses need to educate the public about the risks of smoking and the effects of secondhand smoke, especially on children. Increasingly, lung cancer has become a dis-

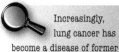

> Increasingly, lung cancer has become a disease of former smokers. Smoking cessation greatly reduces the risk of developing lung cancer but does not eliminate it. Former smokers need to be carefully assessed for symptoms of lung cancer.

ease of former smokers. Smoking cessation greatly reduces the risk of developing lung cancer but does not eliminate it. Former smokers need to be carefully assessed for symptoms of lung cancer.

Nursing care of the patient with a lung cancer diagnosis will vary depending on the treatment course and the progression of the disease. Patients undergoing surgical treatment, such as a **thoracotomy** (a surgical opening into the thoracic cavity) for lobectomy or pneumonectomy, need acute care before, during, and after their surgery (see Table 3-11).

Complications may occur after thoracic surgery. Potential problems during the postoperative period include **atelectasis** (collapse of alveoli) caused by general anesthesia, poor cough effort, and stasis of secretions; **pleural effusion** (abnormal accumulation of fluid in the intrapleural space) related to the surgical disruption of normal pleural fluid drainage and malignant processes; and **lung abscess** (localized inflammation and infection in the lung) related to infection and tumor necrosis.

Patients with lung cancer may require chemotherapy to improve their survival time, to treat symptoms of their disease, or to prevent complications. Cytotoxic drugs may be used alone or in conjunction with radiation therapy and surgery to shrink lung tumors and metastases. Multiple drugs are often used to increase the tumor cell kill. Some cytotoxic drugs are delivered intravenously and others orally. The intravenous drugs may be delivered by different types of catheters, including central venous catheters and implanted infusion devices.

Cytotoxic drugs primarily affect the ability of the cell to replicate. This is a beneficial effect if the cell is malignant, but this same effect may be detrimental to normal cells. Since cytotoxic drugs can affect both normal and malignant cells, there are often side effects from chemotherapy. The drugs used in chemotherapy have their greatest effect on cells that are rapidly dividing (e.g., in the hair follicles, bone marrow, skin, lining of the gastrointestinal tract and, of course, malignant cells). The most common side effects are hair loss (alopecia), bone marrow suppression with **leukopenia** (low white blood cell count), **thrombocytopenia** (low platelet count), nausea and vomiting, and mucositis (stomatitis), the breakdown of the lining of the gastrointestinal tract with oral ulcers and diarrhea.

> The drugs used in chemotherapy have their greatest effect on cells that are rapidly dividing (e.g., in the hair follicles, bone marrow, skin, lining of the gastrointestinal tract and, of course, malignant cells).

Radiation therapy is commonly used to treat primary lung tumors and metastatic disease to the brain and bones. Radiation therapy may be used in conjunction with chemotherapy and before or after surgery. The treatments themselves are painless and are delivered to a specific site. The side effects of radiation therapy are mostly site specific (i.e., only the treated area will have side effects). For example, if only a portion of the lung and

Table 3-11 Nursing Care of the Patient Undergoing a Thoracotomy

1. Explain what the patient may experience during the perioperative period (anesthesia, recovery room, chest tubes, incision, catheter, intravenous, etc). Describe preoperatively what the patient can do to facilitate healing and prevent complications (e.g., deep breathing and coughing, using the incentive spirometer as indicated, asking for pain medication, ambulating with assist, splinting the incision, maintaining nutritional intake as soon as possible after surgery, increasing activity as allowed, balancing rest and activity, quitting smoking).

2. Discuss the need for pain medication preoperatively, and try to reduce the anxiety related to the pain experience (increased anxiety levels can increase pain). Administer pain medications or encourage patient to use patient-controlled analgesia (PCA) when uncomfortable so that he or she can cough effectively. Provide nonpharmacologic methods of pain relief (massage, position changes, diversional activities, relaxation techniques), teach patient how to splint the incision with a pillow during position changes and activity, secure drainage tubes, and report unrelieved pain to the physician.

3. Decrease anxiety levels by working with the patient in a supportive, gentle manner. Assess the patient's anxiety level and areas of concern, reassure him that you will do all you can to answer his questions and help him or her during the hospitalization, try to maintain the same caregivers on each shift, report excessive anxiety to the physician, and administer antianxiety medications as ordered.

4. Promote solid respiratory recovery with the following interventions: Assess the patient's airway, ventilation, and oxygenation; obtain vital signs every 15 minutes immediately postoperation; and then gradually decrease the frequency. Auscultate for breath sounds, encourage the patient to cough, deep breathe, and use the incentive spirometer every 1 to 2 hours. Assist the patient into the semi-Fowler's position when blood pressure is stable to improve the effectiveness of coughing and ventilation. Help the patient splint the incision during activity, including coughing. Maintain patency of drainage tubes; use nursing interventions and medications to reduce pain. Deliver oxygen therapy as ordered, and monitor O_2 saturation and arterial blood gases as ordered. Observe for complications such as increased drainage on the dressing, sudden increase in chest tube drainage, decreased or absent breath sounds, subcutaneous emphysema or any change in vital signs (tachypnea, hypotension, tachycardia). Consult surgeon whenever the patient's status is questionable.

thorax is treated, then the side effects will be skin reaction within the treatment portal and esophagitis if the stomach is in the field. Possible systemic side effects of radiation therapy are fatigue and anorexia.

Nursing Care of Patients with Lung Cancer

- Explain the treatment plan and potential side effects with the patient and family.
- Teach patient about self-care during treatment: surgery, chemotherapy, and/or radiation therapy. Discuss medications for symptom control, adequate nutritional intake, strategies for managing fatigue, and medications to avoid to minimize bleeding (due to decreased platelet count).
- Prevent infection by teaching the patient to avoid crowds and infected people, use good oral hygiene after meals and before bed, wash hands frequently, care for the skin gently, use excellent sterile technique when caring for intravenous access devices, take axillary temperatures only, avoid sharing eating utensils, cook meat well and wash fruit and vegetables, and report to healthcare provider any fever, bleeding, and changes in skin, mouth, cough, or urine.
- Instruct patient on ways to manage fatigue, balance rest and activity, modify daily activities, and avoid fatiguing situations.
- Assess nutritional intake by encouraging adequate fluid intake (8–10 glasses or 2 L/day if not contraindicated) monitoring weight and intake, minimize nausea by teaching patient to eat cool, dry foods when nausea is present, eat small meals with liquids between meals, rest and allow a family member to prepare meals, avoid offensive odors, clean mouth regularly, and use antiemetics as necessary.
- Assess patient's pain (location, intensity on a pain scale, aggravating factors), maintain comfort, and minimize pain using nonpharmacologic and pharmacologic methods as necessary.
- Teach patient receiving radiation treatments about skin care in the radiation field. Wash skin in treatment field gently with mild soap and lukewarm water if tattoos are used (no washing if skin markings are used to mark the treatment area), pat dry, and hydrophilic moisturizers (no petroleum-based products, deodorants, or powders), cornstarch as needed to minimize friction, no scratching or rubbing skin, no tape, no bras, keep area open to air as much as possible, avoid sun exposure, and use electric shavers.

Pulmonary Embolism

A **pulmonary embolus** is a blockage of a pulmonary artery by foreign matter from a peripheral vein, such as clot, fat emboli, or air. A pulmonary embolus causes swelling and necrosis of lung tissue distal to the occluded artery. Pulmonary emboli may arise in the deep veins as a result of phlebitis in the extremities. Often, the patient has a history of **deep vein thrombosis** (**DVT**). Certain factors predispose patients to DVT including prolonged bed rest or extended periods of immobility (car or plane rides) and dehydration. These factors lead to venous stasis, endothelial injury in the veins, and **hypercoagulability**. Many disorders may increase the risk of pulmonary embolism. Conditions that predispose patients to pulmonary emboli include the following:

* Phlebitis
* Atrial fibrillation
* History of DVT, thromboembolism, phlebitis, vascular insufficiency
* History of hypercoagulability
* Prolonged immobility
* Major trauma
* Surgery (particularly of the legs, pelvis, abdomen or thorax) and anesthesia
* Long bone fracture (fat emboli)
* Certain types of cancer (pancreatic and colorectal cancers)
* Use of high-dose estrogen supplements
* Intravenous drug abuse (talc emboli)

Although a large embolus can cause occlusion of a main pulmonary artery that is rapidly fatal, smaller emboli produce varied symptoms related to their size and location in the pulmonary vasculature. The abrupt onset of chest pain, dyspnea, and sometimes cough is a common presentation of **pulmonary embolism**. Hemoptysis (blood tinged sputum) is present in 20–30% of cases.

Assessment

Patients with pulmonary embolism usually present with dyspnea as a first symptom. They may also have tachycardia, chest pain,

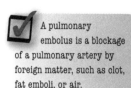
A pulmonary embolus is a blockage of a pulmonary artery by foreign matter, such as clot, fat emboli, or air.

and hemoptysis. A large embolism may quickly produce cyanosis, shock, syncope, and distended jugular veins. On auscultation, crackles and a pleural friction rub may be heard over the area of infarction.

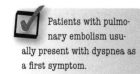

Patients with pulmonary embolism usually present with dyspnea as a first symptom.

Diagnostic testing is needed to rule out other causes of the symptoms and establish a diagnosis of pulmonary embolus. Chest X-ray is used to rule out other pulmonary diseases and may show areas of atelectasis or diaphragm elevation, prominence of a pulmonary artery, or a wedge-shaped infiltrate. Lung scans may show perfusion defects beyond the occluded pulmonary artery. Electrocardiograms (EKGs) rule out cardiac sources of chest pain and may show distinct changes with massive pulmonary emboli. Ar-

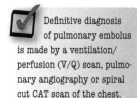

Definitive diagnosis of pulmonary embolus is made by a ventilation/ perfusion (V/Q) scan, pulmonary angiography or spiral cut CAT scan of the chest.

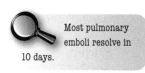

Most pulmonary emboli resolve in 10 days.

terial blood gas analysis sometimes reveals a decreased PaO_2 and $PaCO_2$. Definitive diagnosis of pulmonary embolus is made by a ventilation/perfusion (V/Q) scan, pulmonary angiography or spiral cut CAT scan of the chest. A V/Q mismatch is caused by adequate ventilation but inadequate perfusion of the lung tissue distal to the pulmonary embolus.

Treatment

The treatment of pulmonary embolus is aimed at preventing further tissue damage and maintaining adequate pulmonary circulation. Most pulmonary emboli resolve in 10 days. Treatment includes anticoagulants (heparin, enoxaparin, dalteparin, fondaparinux, and then long-term warfarin therapy) and thrombolytics (streptokinase or tissue plasminogen activator, the so-called clot busters), and supplemental oxygen.

Nursing Care of Patients with Pulmonary Embolus

Because the functioning of the lung tissue blood distal to the embolus may be impaired, nursing care requires frequent assessment of the patient's oxygenation, as shown in the following outline:

- ◆ Monitor vital signs frequently, including oxygen saturation, respiratory rate, pulse, blood pressure, and arterial blood gases as ordered. ABGs may reveal hypoxemia and respiratory alkalosis.

- Administer oxygen as ordered via nasal cannula or mask.
- Anticoagulation with heparin is usually begun intravenously for rapid anticoagulation. Monitor partial thromboplastin (PTT) and prothrombin levels (PT) levels. Low-molecular-weight heparins and/or factor Xa inhibitors are administered subcutaneously. Long-term anticoagulation with warfarin is begun during hospitalization but takes up to 7 days to reach the necessary INR levels (international normalization ratio). Precautions are taken to prevent excessive bleeding (e.g., longer compression of venipuncture sites).
- Maintain adequate hydration to minimize hypercoagulability.
- Evaluate legs for swelling, change in color and pain. Never vigorously massage the legs of a patient with deep vein thrombosis and/or pulmonary embolism.
- Watch for increasing dyspnea, tachypnea, or hemoptysis and notify the physician immediately. Prepare for endotracheal intubation and transfer to the intensive care unit.

 Never vigorously massage the legs of a patient with deep vein thrombosis and/or pulmonary embolism.

Pulmonary Hypertension

Pulmonary hypertension is a condition of chronically elevated pulmonary artery pressure (PAP). Primary (idiopathic) pulmonary hypertension refers to higher than normal

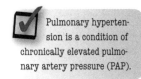
Pulmonary hypertension is a condition of chronically elevated pulmonary artery pressure (PAP).

PAP (greater than 30 mmHg systolic or greater than 18 mmHg mean PAP) and increased pulmonary vascular resistance without an obvious cause. **Primary pulmonary hypertension** has no known cause but is seen in familial patterns and may be related to collagen vascular disorders. It occurs most commonly in women between the ages of 20 and 40 years, and it may be fatal within 3 to 4 years.

Secondary pulmonary hypertension is the result of cardiac diseases and/or pulmonary disease. Cardiac diseases include left-sided heart failure, ventricular septal defect, and patent ductus arteriosus. Pulmonary disorders that may cause pulmonary hypertension include COPD, alveolar hypoventilation, and vascular obstruction (i.e., pulmonary embolism). Decreased ventilation may cause hypoxemia and increased pulmonary vascular resistance, resulting in pulmonary hypertension.

Assessment

Patients with pulmonary hypertension usually report a pattern of increasing dyspnea with exertion and fatigue and weakness. Physical assessment may reveal tachycardia, tachypnea with mild exertion, and decreased blood pressure. Changes in mental status such as restlessness, agitation, and confusion may result from hypoxemia. Signs of right-sided heart failure such as jugular vein distention, peripheral edema, and ascites may be present. Examination of the thorax reveals decreased diaphragmatic excursion with ventilation and decreased breath sounds and/or loud, turbulent breath sounds. Cardiac auscultation may demonstrate a systolic ejection murmur, a split S2, and an S3 or S4.

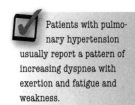

Patients with pulmonary hypertension usually report a pattern of increasing dyspnea with exertion and fatigue and weakness.

Diagnostic testing is necessary to determine the cause of the symptoms. Arterial blood gas analysis usually reveals hypoxia. Pulmonary function tests may show decreased flow rates and increased residual volumes in COPD or reduced total lung capacity in restrictive diseases such as asthma. Pulmonary artery catheterization is useful in measuring pulmonary artery pressures, PAP, and possibly pulmonary artery wedge pressures (PAWP). Echocardiography and radionuclide imaging may be useful in determining cardiac origins of pulmonary hypertension

Treatment

The treatment of pulmonary hypertension is dependent on the cause of the disorder. Supplemental oxygen, pharmacologic agents, and lifestyle changes may all be required to treat the disorder and maintain optimum functioning. Supplemental oxygen is often used to correct hypoxemia. Medications for pulmonary hypertension include the following:

- Digoxin to increase cardiac output
- Diuretics to decrease intravascular volume
- Calcium channel blockers and beta-adrenergic blockers to decrease cardiac workload
- Bronchodilators to open airways

Nursing Care of the Patient with Pulmonary Hypertension

Patients with pulmonary hypertension require regular monitoring both in the hospital and at home. While inpatient care focuses on optimizing cardiac and pulmonary functioning and determining the best interventions, out-patients need to learn self-care techniques to monitor their condition and maximize functioning. Nursing interventions include the following:

* Assess cardiopulmonary status including pulse, respiratory rate, blood pressure, and oxygen saturation. Auscultate heart and breath sounds, being alert for changes that may indicate heart failure. Take frequent measurements (every 2 hours) of PAP and PAWP if patient has pulmonary catheter in place.
* Monitor intake and output, including daily weights. Institute fluid restrictions if necessary. Teach patient about dietary restrictions, daily weights for at-home care including parameters for calling the healthcare provider.
* Pace patient activities to avoid overexertion and hypoxia. Use supplemental oxygen as ordered. Encourage patients to organize activities at home with rest periods.
* Administer medications as ordered and monitor for adverse effects. Teach patient about medication regimen including guidelines for calling the healthcare provider.

Pleurisy

Pleurisy is an inflammation of the pleural membranes. There are actually two pleural membranes: the parietal pleura, the membrane that lines the thoracic cage, and the visceral pleura, the membrane that covers the lungs. A potential space, the pleural space, lies between the two membranes and is filled with a thin layer of pleural fluid, allowing the lungs to expand smoothly within the thorax. When either membrane becomes irritated, the roughened surfaces grate on each other, causing pain.

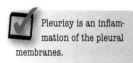
Pleurisy is an inflammation of the pleural membranes.

Assessment

Patients usually describe pleural pain as sharp, worsening with deep inhalation. The pain is often low and unilateral. On auscultation, there may be a pleural friction rub over the affected area. There is no diagnostic test for pleurisy, and the diagnosis is arrived at by clinical presentation.

Treatment

Treatment often includes antibiotics and pain medication.

Nursing Care of the Patient with Pleurisy

Nursing management of the patient with pleurisy includes both pharma-cologic and positional interventions to minimize pain. Teach the patient to splint the chest with a pillow during coughing or moving. Throat loz-enges may decrease the urge to cough and moisten the throat, minimiz-ing painful coughing.

Pleural Effusion

> A small pleural effusion (200 to 300 cc) may not cause any symptoms, but large amounts (up to 5000 cc) can cause dyspnea, cough, pleuritic chest pain, and even shifting of the trachea to one side.

A **pleural effusion** is a collection of fluid in the pleural space. This potential space can fill with pleural fluid if the normal drainage routes are blocked or it can fill with pus or blood. **Pleural effusion**s are caused by dis-eases that change the formation and absorp-tion of pleural fluid, as in congestive heart failure (transudative pleural effusion), or when the pleural linings are diseased, as in lung cancer (exudative pleural effusion). A small pleural effusion (200 to 300 cc) may not cause any symptoms, but large amounts (up to 5000 cc) can cause dyspnea, cough, pleuritic chest pain, and even shifting of the trachea.

Assessment

With large effusions, the chest exam may reveal dullness to percussion over the effusion and decreased or bronchial breath sounds on ausculta-tion. Chest X-ray is often diagnostic but ultrasound, CAT scan, and MRIs may be useful in making the diagnosis.

Treatment

The treatment depends on the underlying condition causing the pleural effusion. **Thoracentesis**, the insertion of a needle into the pleural space to drain the fluid or air, often relieves the pressure and associated dys-pnea (see Figures 3-11 and 3-12). Laboratory analysis of the fluid may reveal the cause of the pleural effusion (e.g., infection or malignancy). Antibiotics and chest tube drainage may be required to treat the pleural effusion (see Table 3-12).

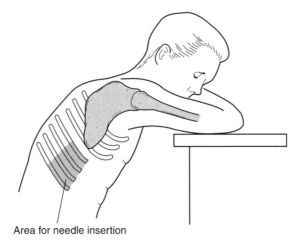

Area for needle insertion

Figure 3-11 Nursing care of the patient undergoing a thoracotomy.

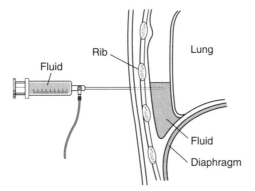

Rib
Lung
Fluid
Fluid
Diaphragm

Figure 3-12 Thoracentesis insertion.

Pneumothorax

A **pneumothorax** is an accumulation of air in the pleural space. The air enters the space usually as the result of a break in the visceral pleura surrounding the lung (see Figure 3-13). The break might be the result

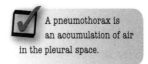

A pneumothorax is an accumulation of air in the pleural space.

of a tuberculosis infection, a ruptured emphysematous bulla, trauma, or a surgical disruption. With a spontaneous pneumothorax, the onset

Table 3-12 Nursing Care of the Patient Undergoing Thoracentesis

1. Explain the procedure to the patient and obtain an informed consent. Let the patient know that a local anesthetic will be used to numb the area where the needle is inserted. The procedure takes a few minutes, and a chest X-ray will be obtained afterward (see Figure 3-12).
2. Assess the patient's vital signs and respiratory status before the procedure, including breath sounds and So$_2$.
3. Position the patient on the side of the bed with arms over a bedside table and a pillow for comfort.
4. Remind the patient not to talk or move during the procedure.
5. Stay with the patient and reassure him about the progress of the procedure. (Note: Coughing is a common response to removal of pleural fluid.)
6. Place a dressing over the puncture site.
7. Send any specimens from the thoracentesis to the laboratory as ordered.
8. Reassess the patient's vital signs and breath sounds after the procedure.
9. Send the patient for a chest X-ray if ordered.

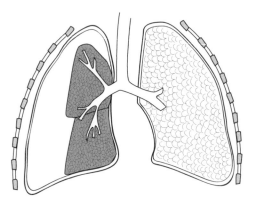

Figure 3-13 Pneumothorax.

is sudden with severe sticking pain and dyspnea. On examination, the chest may expand asymmetrically, and there might be fullness in the intercostal spaces. **Subcutaneous emphysema** (air in the subcutaneous tissues) follows puncture of the chest wall with air leaking out of the chest into the subcutaneous tissue.

Auscultation reveals absent breath sounds, and percussion demonstrates tympanic resonance over the air-filled portion of the chest. Diagnosis is made by chest X-ray. A large pneumothorax can be life-threatening if the air pressure continues to build, shifting the mediastinal contents to the opposite side with kinking of the great vessels and compression of the heart. Cardinal signs of a **mediastinal shift** include deviation of the trachea away from the injured lung, severe dyspnea, distended neck veins, and progressive cyanosis (see Figure 3-14).

> Cardinal signs of a mediastinal shift include deviation of the trachea away from the injured lung, severe dyspnea, distended neck veins, and progressive cyanosis.

One cause of a **mediastinal shift** is a tension pneumothorax. In cases of **tension pneumothorax**, the visceral pleura is damaged, allowing air to escape into the pleural space during inspiration while trapping air in the pleural space during expiration. Pressure can quickly build, causing a **mediastinal shift** and become life-threatening if not relieved. Thoracentesis and/or chest tube insertion are needed to relieve pressure in the pleural space. Chest tube placement with closed chest drainage is instituted to drain air and fluid and maintain normal pressures in the pleural space. (See Chapter 4 for more information regarding closed chest drainage and thoracentesis).

Nursing Management of the Patient with Pneumothorax

Nursing management of the patient with a pneumothorax involves regular assessment of the patient's vital signs, oxygen saturation, and breath

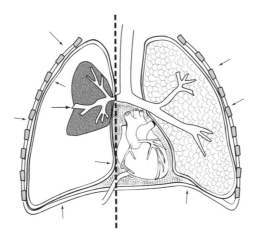

Figure 3-14 Tension pneumothorax with mediastinal shift.

sounds. Patients are often dyspneic and anxious, requiring emotional support and reassurance during chest tube placement and decompression of the pneumothorax. Oxygen should be administered as ordered to maintain adequate So_2 while not decreasing CO_2 drive if the patient has COPD. Antibiotics are usually given to prevent infection or treat underlying conditions.

Chest Injuries

Chest injuries require rapid assessment of the patient and immediate treatment. Chest injuries are usually categorized as blunt or penetrating injuries. Most blunt chest injuries occur as the result of motor vehicle accidents. Penetrating injuries occur from gunshot and stab wounds, and the severity of the wound is determined by the location and size of the penetration. Gunshot wounds are usually more serious as the bullet damages large areas of tissue with resultant rapid blood loss. Frequently, trauma to the head and abdomen may have occurred at the same time as the chest injury.

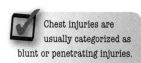

Chest injuries are usually categorized as blunt or penetrating injuries.

Assessment

Rapid assessment of the patient with traumatic injuries follows the ABCs: airway, breathing, and circulation. Patients with blunt injuries often have other injuries including myocardial contusion, rib and sternal fractures with potential complications such as hemorrhage, pneumothorax, hemothorax, and flail chest. Pneumothorax, as previously described in this chapter, results from an accumulation of air in the pleural space. **Hemothorax**, the accumulation of blood in the pleural space and cavity, results from laceration of blood vessels in the thorax by fractured ribs or penetrating wounds. **Flail chest** is usually the result of multiple rib fractures, causing a portion of the chest to "cave in" during inhalation. The movement of the chest during ventilation results in **paradoxical breathing**, that is the chest wall puffing out over the injured area during exhalation and collapsing inward during inhalation. This is usually extremely painful, and the area of the injury is often bruised. Flail chest can cause a **tension pneumothorax** with mediastinal shift that can be life-threatening.

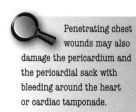

Penetrating chest wounds may also damage the pericardium and the pericardial sack with bleeding around the heart or cardiac tamponade.

A penetrating chest wound may pierce the thorax and the lung. A "sucking" chest wound develops with air being noisily sucked into the chest through the wound during inspiration and blowing out of the wound during expiration. The internal chest structures may also move back and forth during breathing with an open chest wound because of alternating intrathoracic chest pressure, causing a **mediastinal flutter**. Immediate treatment is necessary for mediastinal flutter before life-threatening hemodynamic changes develop.

Injury to the lung underneath the damaged chest wall (**pulmonary contusion**) is often present. Pulmonary contusion can result in collapsed alveoli, interstitial hemorrhage, and atelectasis. Penetrating chest wounds may also damage the pericardium and the pericardial sack with bleeding around the heart or **cardiac tamponade**. This life-threatening condition decreases the ability of the heart to pump effectively.

Assessment of chest injuries begins with the history of the traumatic event. Physical assessment may reveal bruising, swelling, penetrating wounds, and/or pain over fractured ribs. Percussion usually demonstrates dullness over **hemothorax** (an accumulation of blood and fluid in the pleural cavity) and tympany over pneumothorax. Auscultation may reveal decreased breath sounds over affected areas and muffled heart sounds if cardiac tamponade is present.

Diagnostic tests are needed to determine the severity of the injuries and the necessary treatment. Chest X-rays are used to detect rib and sternal fractures, pneumothorax, flail chest, atelectasis, pulmonary contusions, and hemothorax. CAT scans, echocardiography, esophageal ultrasound, and cardiac and lung scans are used to determine the extent of the injuries including aortic laceration and rupture, diaphragmatic rupture, and lung contusions.

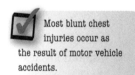

Most blunt chest injuries occur as the result of motor vehicle accidents.

Flail chest can cause tension pneumothorax with mediastinal shift that can be life-threatening.

Treatment

Treatment is based upon the specific injuries. Common chest injuries include rib fractures, flail chest, pneumothorax, hemopneumothorax, and pulmonary contusion. Rib fractures are the most common thoracic injuries. Causes of these fractures include trauma and those caused by sneezing or coughing. Severe coughing can cause rib fracture in the elderly and also in patients with osteoporosis or metastatic cancer. Simple fractures do not usually damage internal organs, like the heart and lungs. Treatment of a rib fracture includes analgesics to lessen pain, teaching the patient how to splint the area with a pillow during movement, and coughing and observation in case a pneumothorax develops later.

Treatment for blunt and penetrating chest injuries depends on the extent of the injury. Blunt injuries involve control of bleeding and stabilization of flail chest, if present. Mainte-
nance of a patent airway is essential, and if hypoxia worsens, intubation and mechanical ventilation with positive pressure ventilation may be required. The patient would also be treated for any other complications such as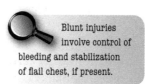
hemorrhage, pneumothorax, and shock. Antibiotics are used to prevent infection, and pain medication is usually prescribed.

Blunt injuries involve control of bleeding and stabilization of flail chest, if present.

Surgical intervention is usually required for penetrating chest injuries to control bleeding and repair damaged tissues. Chest tube placement is often required to stabilize intrathoracic pressure and drain air and fluid from the pleural cavity.

Nursing Care for Patients with Chest Injuries

Patients with chest injuries require rapid assessment, frequent monitoring, and ongoing reassurance:

- Immediately assess the ABCs: airway, breathing, and circulation.
- Assess breathing patterns and breath sounds including depth of respirations, use of accessory muscles, and chest movement. Also check Sao_2.
- Check pulses and blood pressure frequently, including color and temperature of skin to assess for hypovolemia and impending shock.
- Check for blood loss including *under* the patient.
- Assess for signs of mediastinal shift including deviated tracheal position, increasing dyspnea, and paradoxical breathing.
- Obtain a history of the causative injury, if possible, and report to authorities as defined by law.
- Prepare patient for surgical procedures including thoracentesis, chest tube placement, or thoracic surgery.
- Reassure patient frequently.

Atelectasis

Atelectasis is a common complication of bronchial obstruction, compression of lung tissue, or loss of surfactant. It is the incomplete expansion of part or all of a lung distal to a blockage of the airways (see Figure 3-15). It is a common complication of general anesthesia, but may also result from the following:

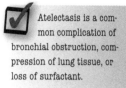

Atelectasis is a common complication of bronchial obstruction, compression of lung tissue, or loss of surfactant.

- Intrabronchial obstruction from secretions, foreign bodies, or bronchospasm
- Extrabronchial obstruction from tumors and pleural effusion
- Endobronchial disease, such as carcinoma

The most common findings of atelectasis are decreased chest expansion and breath sounds over the affected area. There may be retraction of the intercostal spaces over the affected area. Symptoms may progress to hypoxia, dyspnea, and tachypnea if a large portion of the lung is compressed or collapsed. The patient may or may not complain of any symptoms depending on the degree and the cause of the obstruction.

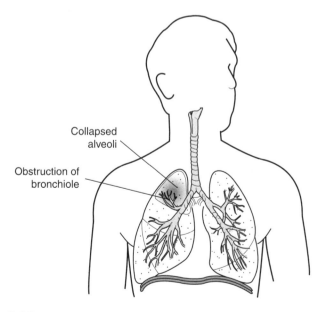

Collapsed alveoli

Obstruction of bronchiole

Figure 3-15 Atelectasis due to obstruction.

Older patients are particularly prone to atelectasis because of decreased tidal volumes, lung capacity, lung elasticity, and chest expansion. Older patients undergoing general anesthesia require careful assessment of their pulmonary functioning and special attention to pulmonary hygiene after surgery.

> Older patients are particularly prone to atelectasis because of decreased tidal volumes, lung capacity, lung elasticity, and chest expansion. Older patients undergoing general anesthesia require careful assessment of their pulmonary functioning and special attention to pulmonary hygiene after surgery.

The incidence of atelectasis increases after surgery. Pain, narcotics, and immobility can result in retention of thickened bronchial secretions, which can obstruct the airways.

Nursing Care of Patients with Atelectasis

Nursing interventions to prevent and reverse atelectasis in all patients include the following:

- Turn the patient every 1 to 2 hours, especially when obtunded, immobilized, or on bed rest.
- Encourage the patient to use the incentive spirometer every 1 to 2 hours, holding the inspiration for 5 seconds before exhaling (to increase alveolar expansion).
- Promote thinning of secretions by encouraging good fluid intake (eight glasses or at least 2 L of fluid a day (if not contraindicated) and humidification of oxygen or air.
- Encourage mobility and ambulation as soon as possible.
- Assist the patient with coughing and deep breathing every 1 to 2 hours.
- Administer antibiotics as ordered to prevent or treat pneumonia.
- Administer narcotics carefully, as they can decrease tidal volumes, respiratory rate, and the cough reflex.

CASE STUDY RESOLUTION

Mrs. A responded well to the albuterol treatment with a decreased respiratory rate (22 breaths per minute) and diminished wheezing. Her Sao_2 improved to 96%. Mrs. A was given a prescription for antibiotics (clarithromycin) and an inhaled steroid (flunisolide) to use after her broncho-dilator (metaproterenol). The nurse reviewed situations and substances to avoid (such as dust) and gave her a handout to take home. Mrs. A went home with her husband.

The answers to the questions in the introduction are as follows:

- What physiologic changes cause wheezing?

Asthma is characterized by bronchoconstriction with inflammation and increased mucus production. As air travels through the narrowed respiratory passages, it makes the wheezing sound.

- Why is her PEFR decreased during an asthma attack?

The peak expiratory flow rate (PEFR) is decreased because the narrowed airways restrict the flow of air out of the lungs. Many patients with moderate to severe asthma use peak flow meters at home to monitor their lung function. Mrs. A's PEFR is at 70% of her personal best. Following the zone therapy guidelines, Mrs. A treats her asthma with her rescue medication plan.

- What could have caused this asthma attack?

Mrs. A was cleaning her daughter's basement the day before the attack. Dust and mold can be sources of airway irritation for patients with asthma. The dust may have triggered the inflammatory response and a flare-up of her asthma. She also has a low-grade fever that could signal an infection.

CHAPTER 3 MULTIPLE-CHOICE QUESTIONS

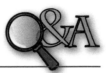

1. All of the following would decrease exposure to allergens except:
   a. Encase mattresses and pillows in airtight covers.
   b. Install wall-to-wall carpeting.
   c. Avoid dusting and vacuuming.
   d. Humidify air in the house.

2. Individuals at high risk for oropharyngeal cancers are:
   a. Under 40 years old
   b. Have a history of dental cavities
   c. Mouth breathers
   d. Tobacco and alcohol users

3. Tuberculosis can be detected by Mantoux test or PPD:
   a. 3 to 12 weeks after infection
   b. After tubercle formation
   c. 1 week after inflammation
   d. 6 to 12 months after exposure

4. Emphysema differs from chronic bronchitis in the following way:
   a. In chronic bronchitis, the terminal airspaces are dilated.
   b. In emphysema, there is destruction of the alveolar walls.
   c. Only patients with emphysema experience dyspnea and cough.
   d. Mucus production is less in chronic bronchitis.

5. The pathophysiologic changes seen in adult respiratory distress syndrome (ARDS) are caused by:
   a. High levels of supplemental oxygen and mechanical ventilation
   b. Infection by virulent bacteria
   c. Inflammatory mediators in the lung
   d. Increased CO_2 levels and respiratory acidosis

CHAPTER 3 ANSWERS AND RATIONALES

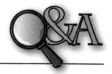

1. **b.**

   Rationale: Installation of wall-to-wall carpeting may actually trap more allergens in the environment.

2. **d.**

   Rationale: Excessive exposure to alcohol and tobacco has been associated with an increased risk for oropharyngeal cancers.

3. **a.**

   Rationale: Tuberculosis can be detected by Mantoux test or PPD 3 to 12 weeks after infection.

4. **b.**

   Rationale: In emphysema there is destruction of the alveolar walls; whereas, in chronic bronchitis there is hypersecretion of mucous.

5. **c.**

   Rationale: In adult respiratory distress syndrome (ARDS), inflammatory mediators in the lung increase capillary permeability and stimulate the release of neutrophils.

Respiratory disorders interfere with the maintenance of airways, patterns of breathing, clearance of secretions, and exchange of gases. Treatments are required to maintain and enhance oxygenation. This chapter will review the following topics:

- General health and policy issues for respiratory health

- Improving physical mobility

- Breathing and coughing exercises

- Mobilizing secretions

- Maintaining airway patency

- Closed chest drainage

- Oxygen therapy

- Mechanical ventilation

4

Common Interventions to Improve Oxygenation

TERMS
- [ ] incentive spirometry
- [ ] chest physical therapy
- [ ] nasal cannula
- [ ] mechanical ventilation
- [ ] endotracheal tube
- [ ] tracheostomy
- [ ] closed chest drainage
- [ ] extubation
- [ ] continuous positive airway pressure
- [ ] positive end-expiratory pressure

CASE STUDY

Mr. J, a 47-year-old male, is at the emergency room with a 10-day history of flu-like symptoms: fever, aches, loss of appetite, a productive cough with yellowish green sputum, and increasing shortness of breath. His only significant past medical history is a 30-pack year of cigarette smoking. The physical exam reveals a slightly anxious, diaphoretic, pale, well-nourished man who is leaning forward on the bedside table. Vital signs: temperature—102.4°F, apical pulse (AP)—112 and regular, BP—148/86 on the right arm and 152/90 on the left, respiration rate (RR)—28 breaths per minute and slightly labored, and Sao_2 is 89% on room air. Lung sounds: scattered expiratory wheezing throughout both lung fields; crackles—anteriorly from the left sternal border fourth intercostal space (ICS) to the sixth ICS at the midaxillary line, and posteriorly from T5 down. Crackles decrease but do not disappear with coughing or deep breathing. The nurse practitioner examining the patient makes the decision to admit him and writes orders to initiate oxygen therapy via nasal cannula at 2 L/min.

Improving oxygenation involves promoting ventilation, assisting diffusion of gases, and facilitating the perfusion of oxygen throughout the body. In this chapter, nursing interventions and collaborative strategies to enhance oxygenation will be reviewed with a special focus on incorporating collaborative interventions into the patient's nursing care.

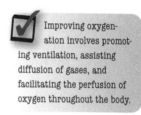 Improving oxygenation involves promoting ventilation, assisting diffusion of gases, and facilitating the perfusion of oxygen throughout the body.

While some interventions to improve respiratory health are performed in the acute and intensive care settings, others may be incorporated into the patient's care at home. Because every patient is unique, it is important to customize the interventions to the patient's abilities, lifestyle, and to the underlying disease process.

 ## GENERAL RESPIRATORY HEALTH AND POLICY

Promoting respiratory health begins with promoting healthy lifestyles. Respiratory health is maintained by exercise, clean air, and a competent cough reflex (see Table 4-1). Exercise is an important part of promoting respiratory and cardiovascular health. During exercise, ventilation

Table 4-1 Facilitating Respiratory Health

1. Exercise regularly—30 minutes, three to four times per week.
2. Do not smoke or use tobacco products.
3. Avoid secondhand smoke.
4. Support legislation to control and eliminate pollution.
5. Ensure adequate ventilation of wood stoves and furnaces.
6. Reduce exposure to noxious fumes at home and at work.

improves as the lungs expand more fully, and perfusion is enhanced by the increased cardiac output.

Part of promoting healthy ventilation is advocating for clean air in the environment, whether it is in the atmosphere or home and work environments. The quality of atmospheric air is often measured as the air quality index. Vulnerable people, such as those with respiratory disorders such as asthma or chronic obstructive pulmonary disease (COPD), should avoid going outside when the air quality index is poor. Of primary concern to healthcare providers are the risks associated with cigarette smoking. Nurses are in position to teach their patients and the community about the hazards of cigarette smoking. Of particular concern is the rising incidence of smoking in adolescence. Educational programs increasingly begin in grade schools to educate children about the dangers of smoking before adolescence. The risks associated with secondhand smoke should also be emphasized to adults so they can protect their children and limit their exposure to secondhand smoke.

> Vulnerable people, including those with respiratory disorders such as asthma or chronic obstructive pulmonary disease (COPD), should avoid going outside when the air quality index is poor.

Occupational hazards need to be evaluated in the nursing assessment. As described in Chapter 2, exposure to certain chemicals, asbestos, dust, and fumes at work puts patients at risk for respiratory problems. Policies at the local and federal levels are directed at reducing occupational exposure to hazardous materials, encouraging adequate ventilation in work sites, and requiring the use of protective apparatus.

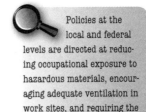
Policies at the local and federal levels are directed at reducing occupational exposure to hazardous materials, encouraging adequate ventilation in work sites, and requiring the use of protective apparatus.

When a patient's health is compromised by age, lifestyle, surgery, or disease, respiratory functioning may be disrupted. Advanced interventions to improve oxygenation require a collaborative approach. Nurses, physicians, and respiratory therapists work together to enhance ventilation, diffusion, and oxygenation through a variety of approaches. In this chapter, the following strategies for improving oxygenation will be reviewed:

- Improving physical mobility
- Breathing and coughing exercises
- Mobilizing secretions
- Maintaining airway patency
- Closed chest drainage
- Oxygen therapy
- Mechanical ventilation

IMPROVING PHYSICAL MOBILITY

When a patient's ability to move is compromised, maintaining physical and respiratory functioning becomes an important nursing intervention. Pain, surgical incision, medications, and age may make it difficult for the patient to move and breath. Chest expansion and alveolar inflation are diminished during immobility and may result in atelectasis, inadequate gas exchange, or even pneumonia.

> Chest expansion and alveolar inflation are diminished during immobility and may result in atelectasis, inadequate gas exchange, or even pneumonia.

The best position for maximum chest expansion is upright. Encourage able patients to ambulate three times a day to enhance ventilation and maintain cardiovascular conditioning. Patients undergoing surgery should be ambulated postoperatively as soon as allowed by the surgeon and at least three times a day thereafter. Premedication of the postoperative patient with an analgesic (30 to 45 minutes before the activity) will improve mobility and depth of inhalation. For the bedridden patient, the semi-Fowler's or high Fowler's position allows maximum chest expansion. In the patient with chronic airflow limitation (CAL), the orthopnea position or tripod position may provide relief from dyspnea and enhance ventilation. The tripod position involves having the patient sit at the bedside with a table in front of him or her, allowing for propping of the elbows on the table while compressing the lower chest.

If the patient is bedridden, he or she should be turned from side to side every 2 hours to improve chest expansion on the upward side and increased perfusion of the lung on the dependent side. Occasionally the prone position is used to improve oxygenation in ventilated patients who continue to deteriorate despite other interventions.

Patients with chronic respiratory disorders such as emphysema may have an impaired ability to oxygenate their blood and a decreased capacity to exert themselves. With less oxygen in the blood, less is available for the cells when activity increases the oxygen demands of the tissues. Deep breathing and coughing exercises (discussed later in this chapter) may be used to increase oxygenation and maintain airway patency.

Respiratory diseases such as emphysema or chronic bronchitis change the structure and the functioning of the respiratory tract. The diaphragm becomes flattened, reducing the ability of the chest to expand. Air becomes trapped in distal alveoli and the bases of the lungs. Air trapping causes a ventilation/perfusion (V/Q) mismatch with resultant hypoxemia. Even normal activities, such as walking and eating, can be exhausting to a patient with a chronic respiratory disorder. Nursing care for these patients includes teaching ways to reduce oxygen demand, such as:

- Pace activities with rest periods.
- Eat frequent, light meals to decrease metabolic demands and gastric fullness, which might press the diaphragm upward.
- Avoid holding the breath during activities, which will further diminish the P_{O_2} and increase dyspnea.

In the patient with chronic airflow limitation (CAL), the orthopnea position or tripod position may provide relief from dyspnea and enhance ventilation. This position involves the patient sitting at the bedside with a table in front of him or her, allowing for propping of the elbows on the table while compressing the lower chest.

If the patient is bedridden, he should be turned from side to side every 2 hours to allow improved chest expansion on the upward side and increased perfusion of the lung on the dependent side.

Patients with chronic respiratory disorders such as emphysema may have an impaired ability to oxygenate their blood and a decreased capacity to exert themselves.

- Avoid the Valsalva maneuver, which increases intrathoracic pressure and decreases blood return into the thorax, resulting in dizziness.
- Decrease temperature if febrile, as each degree (Fahrenheit) elevation results in a 7% increase in metabolic demand.
- Use energy conservation exercises such as performing the work part of an activity during exhalation and using pursed-lip breathing during exertion.

Preoperative teaching is important in providing patients with information regarding the risks of developing respiratory problems postoperatively. General anesthesia, postoperative pain, immobility, and pain medications can alter normal ventilation and put patients at risk for atelectasis, pneumonia, thrombophlebitis, and pulmonary embolism. Interventions to improve ventilation, oxygenation, and mobility postoperatively include the following:

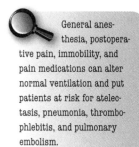

General anesthesia, postoperative pain, immobility, and pain medications can alter normal ventilation and put patients at risk for atelectasis, pneumonia, thrombophlebitis, and pulmonary embolism.

- Encourage breathing exercises and incentive spirometry every 1 to 2 hours to maximize lung expansion.
- Promote early ambulation and leg exercises to improve venous circulation.
- Maintain airway patency with coughing to clear secretions and, if necessary, suctioning.
- Administer pain medication prior to ambulation or chest physical therapy and use splinting to support surgical incisions.

 ## BREATHING EXERCISES

Breathing exercises may help patients control breathing, improve ventilation, decrease anxiety, and increase activity levels. Some exercises are more suited to patients with chronic airflow limitations (CAL), and others are more useful with anxious patients or those with postoperative pain.

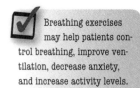

Breathing exercises may help patients control breathing, improve ventilation, decrease anxiety, and increase activity levels.

Diaphragmatic Breathing

Diaphragmatic breathing is indicated for patients with CAL or anxiety because it allows for slow, deep breaths. Slow deliberate breaths using the abdomen and chest muscles may slow the frequency of the ventilations and help the patient focus.

1. Place the patient in a sitting position on the side of the bed or in the semi- or high Fowler's position.

2. Have the patient place one hand on his or her chest and the other on his or her upper abdomen above the umbilicus. Another method that may be useful is to place a light object (e.g., tissue box) on the patient's abdomen so he or she can see abdominal movement during diaphragmatic breathing.

3. Teach the patient to inhale slowly through the nose, feeling the abdomen rise up under his hands but with little movement in the chest.

4. Instruct the patient to exhale through pursed lips using the abdominal muscles (see next section on pursed-lip breathing).

5. Assess the patient's response (e.g., dizziness and lightheadedness may indicate hyperventilation and necessitate slowing the frequency of the ventilations).

6. Repeat for three breaths and rest for 1 minute.

> Diaphragmatic breathing is indicated for patients with CAL or anxiety because it allows for slow, deep breaths.

Pursed-Lip Breathing

The **pursed-lip breathing** technique is especially useful in patients with diseases of chronic airway limitation because it slows the collapse of the small airways by maintaining a higher bronchiole pressure and prolonging expiration. It can also be used to control breathing in the dyspneic patient, to prevent holding the breath during activity (a common problem in patients with CAL), and to reduce air trapping in the alveoli.

1. Assist the patient into a sitting or high semi-Fowler's position.

2. Instruct the patient to purse his or her lips as if to whistle with lips slightly open.

3. Have the patient inhale through the nose to a count of two and slowly exhale through pursed lips to a count of four or until he or she has completely exhaled.

4. Repeat this technique for 10 minutes, increasing the frequency to four to five times a day.

The pursed-lip breathing technique is especially useful in patients with diseases of chronic airway limitation because it slows the collapse of the small airways by maintaining a higher bronchiole pressure and prolonging expiration.

Incentive Spirometry

Incentive spirometry or sustained maximal inspiration devices (SMI) are tools that help maximize ventilation by increasing lung volume, flow, and alveolar inflation. The device measures respiratory volume and provides a visual stimulus via a colored, plastic float to induce the patient to breath deeply. Incentive spirometry can be combined with breathing exercises to maximize ventilation.

Incentive spirometers are usually plastic, disposable units that patients may take home after discharge from a facility. They are useful in patients who have the diminished ability to breathe deeply and during the postoperative period, especially after thoracic or abdominal surgery when deep inhalation may be limited by pain. During the postoperative period, general anesthesia, incisional pain, and narcotic medications all diminish alveolar inflation. The incentive spirometer provides visual cues of preoperative functioning and postoperative goals. The preoperative levels are marked on the spirometer and can

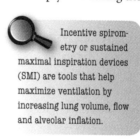

Incentive spirometry or sustained maximal inspiration devices (SMI) are tools that help maximize ventilation by increasing lung volume, flow and alveolar inflation.

be used to monitor recovery after surgery (see Figure 4-1). Flow incentive spirometers are useful for patients at low risk for developing postoperative atelectasis. Volume spirometers are useful with higher risk patients because they measure lung inflation more precisely.

MOBILIZING SECRETIONS

Clearing respiratory secretions promotes patent airways and easier ventilation of the lungs, and prevents mucus stasis. Secretions are easier to cough up if they are thin, rather than thick and tenacious. Therefore,

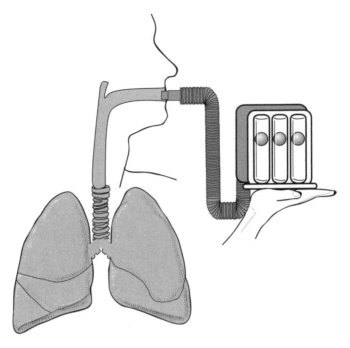

Figure 4-1 Incentive spirometer.

adequate fluid intake, humidification of inspired air, and possibly expectorant medication (e.g., guaifenesin) are important interventions in mobilizing secretions. Other medications that can be used before breathing exercises are inhaled bronchodilators such as albuterol or systemic bronchodilators such as theophylline (see Table 4-2). These medications allow the airways to relax and dilate so that the breathing and coughing exercises are more effective.

Patients with chronic respiratory disorders such as COPD and cystic fibrosis may require more aggressive interventions to remove mucous

Table 4-2 Instructions for Patients Taking Theophylline

1. Take theophylline with food to reduce nausea and vomiting.
2. Take it on a regular schedule to maintain steady blood levels of the drug.
3. Report signs and symptoms, such as dizziness, nausea, and vomiting.
4. Have theophylline blood levels measured periodically according to physician's protocol.

from the respiratory passages. A **mucus clearance device** or a *flutter* can help patients mobilize secretions. This handheld device has a ball valve that vibrates when the patient exhales, causing vibrations to be transmitted in the airways and loosen secretions. The device is held by the patient with the stem parallel to the floor. The patient exhales with flattened cheeks followed by huffing (see next section on coughing and huffing) to remove the secretions.

Coughing

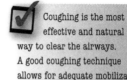

Coughing is the most effective and natural way to clear the airways. A good coughing technique allows for adequate mobilization and expulsion of pulmonary secretions. Normally a cough is an involuntary response, but it can be controlled consciously. In healthy patients, a cough begins with inhalation, followed by glottic closure, and then the rapid opening of the glottis and rapid expulsion of the air. Sometimes the air is expelled at speeds up to 100 miles per hour. In patients with some respiratory disorders, the normal cough reflex may be diminished or there may be excessive secretions. Three techniques that can be used to help patients clear secretions are cascade coughing, huff coughing (huffing), and quad coughing.

Cascade Coughing

Cascade coughing is a useful technique during the postoperative period with patients who have CAL or neuromuscular diseases or those who are bedridden. Cascade coughing allows the patient to increase chest expansion during inhalation and more forcefully expel secretions with coughing.

- Have the patient in an upright position such as sitting or semi-Fowler's position.
- Teach the patient to inhale and exhale slowly and deeply.
- Then, have the patient inhale deeply and exhale, closing his throat and using small coughs without inhaling again, pause, and then inhale again very slowly (to decrease the cough stimulus). If paroxysmal coughing starts, instruct the patient to use slow deep breaths or pursed-lip breathing until the coughing urge passes.
- Rest and repeat for a total of three cycles.

- Assess ability to expel secretions and/or auscultate the lungs.
- Try to set up a regular coughing schedule for patients with CAL to keep airways patent.

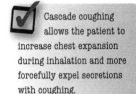
Cascade coughing allows the patient to increase chest expansion during inhalation and more forcefully expel secretions with coughing.

Huff or Open Glottis Coughing

Huff or open glottis coughing (**huffing**) is a useful technique in patients with chronic airway limitation such as COPD.

- Have the patient in the sitting or semi-Fowler's position with arms crossed below the rib cage (hugging a pillow may be more comfortable).
- Instruct the patient to inhale slowly, hold for 2 seconds, tighten the abdominal, leg, and gluteal muscles (to increase intrathoracic pressure), and then exhale in short huffs, actually saying the word *huff*.
- Repeat and try to cough on exhalation.
- Assess the patient's response and ability to expel secretions.
- Auscultate the lungs.

Quad Coughing

Quad coughing may assist patients with muscle weakness such as multiple sclerosis to expel secretions. Using a modified Heimlich maneuver, the patient places the heels of both hands between the umbilicus and the xiphoid process, pressing inward and upward during coughing or huffing to clear secretions.

Chest Physical Therapy

Outcomes of successful CPT include improved breath sounds, increased Pao2, expulsion of sputum, and improved airflow on spirometry.

Chest physical therapy (CPT) is another method to mobilize secretions and maintain airway patency and alveolar expansion. It may be combined with other interventions such as incentive spirometry, inhaled bronchodilators, and suctioning. Outcomes of successful CPT include improved breath sounds, increased Pao2, expulsion of sputum, and improved airflow on spirometry.

Chest physical therapy is composed of three techniques that may be used individually or in combination. These techniques—percussion, vibration, and postural drainage—are performed by respiratory therapists or nurses. **Percussion** is performed by applying cupped hands in a rhythmic sequence over a part or the entire lung. It is useful in patients with cystic fibrosis and bronchiectasis and may be com-

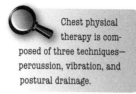

Chest physical therapy is composed of three techniques—percussion, vibration, and postural drainage.

bined with vibration. Using the percussion technique, a hollow sound is produced as the cupped hand creates an air pocket when applied to the chest wall. It is used to loosen secretions (see Figure 4-2). Percussion may be combined with postural drainage positions to optimize drainage of particular lung segments (see Figure 4-3). Percussion is contraindicated in patients with cardiac conditions, osteoporosis, pneumothorax, hemopneumothorax, or pleural effusion.

 Percussion is contraindicated in patients with cardiac conditions, osteoporosis, pneumothorax, hemopneumothorax, or pleural effusion.

Vibration is another technique of loosening secretions that usually follows percussion. It involves the placement of both hands pressing and vibrating the rib cage over the affected lung. The arm and shoulder muscles contract isometrically, producing a small vibration that is transmitted through the patient's chest wall and airways. This vibra-

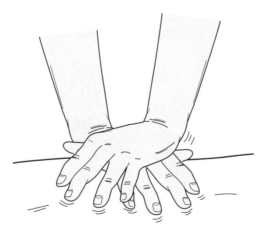

Figure 4-2 Hand position for vibration of the chest wall.

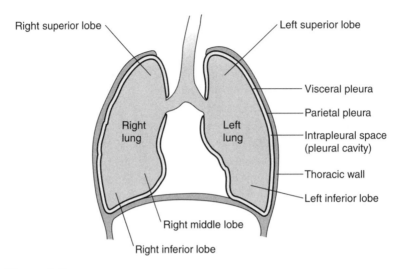

Figure 4-3 Lobes of the lungs.

tion is thought to increase the turbulence of the air in the lung and to loosen secretions. Vibration is useful in patients with cystic fibrosis and bronchiectasis.

Postural drainage involves positioning the patient in such a way as to allow gravity to drain particular segments of the lungs (see Figure 4-4). Several positions may not be tolerated by the patient because the head is lower than the torso. The positions can be adapted by raising the head of the bed so that the patient is comfortable and can breathe easily. Postural drainage may be contraindicated if the patient has cardiac conditions or

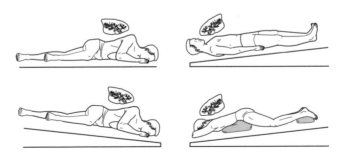

Figure 4-4 Postural drainage positions.

increased intracranial pressure. Particular positions can be combined with percussion and vibration to further mobilize secretions.

 Postural drainage may be contraindicated if the patient has cardiac conditions or increased intracranial pressure.

 ## MAINTAINING A PATENT AIRWAY

In all patients, maintaining a patent airway is the most important intervention to improve oxygenation. Airway patency is especially important if the patient is unconscious, anesthetized, or obtunded. In these conditions, the airways may collapse and secretions may accumulate, impeding the passage of air into the lungs. For example, patients who are semiconscious after anesthesia may not be able to maintain a patent airway because the tongue falls back and may occlude the posterior oropharynx. Artificial airways may be placed to maintain patency of the airway, allow for suctioning of secretions, and permit mechanical ventilation. The most common types of artificial airways are oral airways, nasopharyngeal airways, endotracheal tubes, and tracheostomy tubes.

 Patients who are semiconscious after anesthesia may not be able to maintain a patent airway because the tongue falls back and may occlude the posterior oropharynx.

Oral airways are rigid, plastic devices (see Figure 4-5 and Table 4-3) used to maintain the normal structure of the oropharynx. They are used for short-term airway maintenance, such as in postanesthesia units while the patient recovers from anesthetic agents. Oral airways are curved to follow the normal anatomy of the oropharynx from the lips, over the tongue, and into the posterior oropharynx. The opening allows for air passage through as well as around the airway and permits suctioning of secretions in the

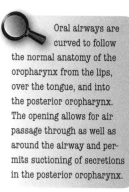 Oral airways are curved to follow the normal anatomy of the oropharynx from the lips, over the tongue, and into the posterior oropharynx. The opening allows for air passage through as well as around the airway and permits suctioning of secretions in the posterior oropharynx.

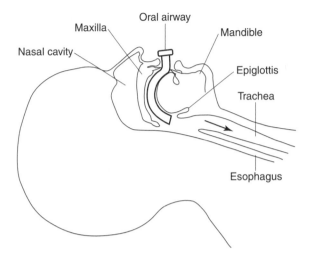

Figure 4-5 Oral airway.

Table 4-3 Insertion of an Oral Airway

1. Measure the oral airway along the patient's jaw with the open end of the curve facing the patient's neck to ensure that the airway is the correct size. The curve of the airway should follow the angle of the patient's jawline.
2. Check that dentures are removed and that there are no loose teeth before inserting the airway.
3. Place the patient in the supine position and open the mouth using the "cross-finger technique," using the thumb and forefinger on the upper and lower teeth to open the mouth.
4. Gently put the airway in upside down until past the teeth and then rotate it over the tongue to follow the curve of the oropharynx.
5. Tape the airway in place and position the patient on his side to prevent aspiration of secretions or vomitus.
6. Suction at least hourly to remove secretions.
7. Evaluate respiration and adequacy of the airway frequently.

posterior oropharynx. Once the patient is alert enough to maintain the airway and clear secretions, the oral airway is removed as it can be very irritating.

Nasal or **nasopharyngeal airways** are soft rubber or latex tubes that are placed through one nares into the pharynx. They are used for short-term airway maintenance if the oral route is not amenable due to surgery or loose teeth (see Table 4-4).

Endotracheal tubes (ET) are long tubes that are placed from the nose or mouth, past the glottis, and into the trachea. Endotracheal tubes are used in the following clinical situations:

- Oral or nasal airways cannot maintain a patent airway.
- Effective suctioning cannot be performed with other airways.
- There has been trauma to the upper airways.
- The patient needs assisted or mechanical ventilation.

Endotracheal tubes (ET) are long (240 to 360 mm in length) and 5 to 10 mm in internal diameter. Patients are intubated via the mouth or nose. Most ET tubes have a cuff at the distal end, which can be inflated with air via an external catheter to create a seal between the tube and the patient's trachea. The seal may be complete with "no leak" or incomplete with a "minimal leak" or "minimal occlusive pressure." The difference between these two depends on the patient's ventilatory requirements. The no-leak seal ensures that all air exchange takes place only through the tube. This is especially important when positive end-expiratory pressure (PEEP) is used in mechanical ventilation or if a feeding tube is in place (see Figure 4-6). The no-leak seal also prevents aspiration of secretions or gastric contents.

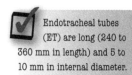

Endotracheal tubes (ET) are long (240 to 360 mm in length) and 5 to 10 mm in internal diameter.

Other conditions may allow for a minimal-leak seal to exist between the trachea and the cuff when the patient's condition does not require

Table 4-4 Insertion of a Nasal Airway

1. Measure the nasal airway following along the patient's cheek, starting at the nose and down the cheek past the jaw to ensure the tube is long enough to maintain an airway past the posterior oropharynx. The tube should be slightly wider than the patient's nares.
2. Using a water-soluble gel, lubricate the distal end of the airway.
3. Hyperextend the patient's neck, if allowable, and gently insert the airway in the nares. If any resistance is felt, stop and try the other nares.
4. Assess adequacy of respiration and air exchange and suction as necessary.
5. Examine the posterior oropharynx to ensure the tube is present and tape is in place.

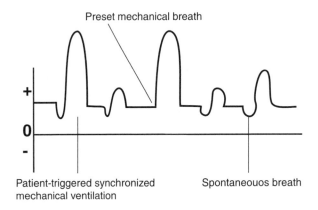

Figure 4-6 Positive end-expiratory pressure (PEEP).

complete ventilatory support. The minimal-leak seal also minimizes damage to the tracheal wall, such as irritation and necrosis, because microcirculation in the trachea is preserved. The cuff is inflated using a cufflator, and the pressure is measured. The nor-

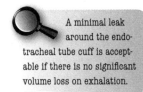

A minimal leak around the endotracheal tube cuff is acceptable if there is no significant volume loss on exhalation.

mal pressure in the cuff is approximately 25 mmHg. The amount of leak around the endotracheal tube cuff can also be auscultated by placing the stethoscope on the patient's trachea and slowly inflating the cuff or balloon with air. When there is no sound during the highest pressure phase of the ventilatory cycle, then there is no leak. When only a small rush of air is heard at peak inspiratory pressure, then there is a minimal leak. A minimal leak around the endotracheal tube cuff is acceptable if there is no significant volume loss on exhalation.

Patients with endotracheal tubes are cared for in the intensive care setting and require a great deal of nursing care. Because their ability to maintain an airway, mobilize secretions, and oxygenate adequately are all compromised, the team must work together to ensure the best outcome for the patient. Nurses, physicians, and respiratory therapists are all part of the team that plans the appropriate interventions for intubated patients.

Tracheostomy tubes, another type of airway, are placed through a surgically created opening in the trachea (see Figure 4-7). A **tracheostomy stoma** is created either electively or emergently between the third or fourth ring of the trachea. It is created after total laryngectomy for cancers of the vocal cords or larynx. It may also be created if the patient has a severe airway obstruction, difficulty expelling pulmonary secre-

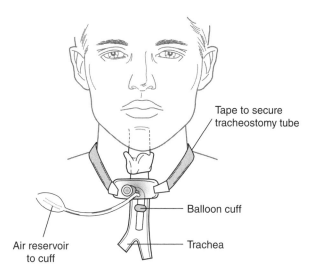

Tape to secure
tracheostomy tube

Balloon cuff

Trachea

Air reservoir
to cuff

Figure 4-7 Tracheostomy tube.

tions (as in some chronic airway diseases), as part of the care of a patient who requires long-term ventilation, or as a means of delivering oxygen to the distal tracheobronchial tree.

Tracheostomy tubes are inserted through the tracheostomy stoma and down into the trachea. They are made of two types of materials: plastic and metal. Metal tubes are used less frequently because the plastic has been found to be less irritating to the trachea. Metal tubes may be composed of an outer and inner cannula. The outer cannula is inserted into the trachea with a soft-ended guide called an obturator. The obturator is removed once the catheter is in place and an inner cannula is inserted. The inner cannula is removable for cleaning of dried secretions.

> A tracheostomy stoma is created either electively or emergently between the third or fourth ring of the trachea.

The tracheostomy tube may be either cuffed (having a balloon at the inner end, which may be inflated) or uncuffed (no balloon cuff or a metal cuff). The outer cannula of a metal tube or the outer portion of a plastic tube has a wider flange that allows the tube to be anchored and secured with sutures or taped around the neck. Fenestrated tracheostomy tubes have an opening in the outer cannula that when plugged allows the patient to phonate or speak. Otherwise, when a tracheostomy tube is in place, the patient cannot speak.

Tracheostomies require careful care to maintain the airway and prevent complications. Because the tube is a direct opening into the lower respiratory tract, all the protective mechanisms of the upper airways have been bypassed. Air is no longer filtered,

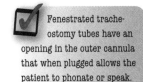

Fenestrated tracheostomy tubes have an opening in the outer cannula that when plugged allows the patient to phonate or speak.

warmed, or humidified. The ability to cough effectively is diminished because it is difficult to build up sufficient intrathoracic pressure with an opening in the trachea. Bacteria can easily access the lungs, and patients are at risk for infection.

Nursing Care of the Patient with a Tracheostomy

To maintain the airway in patients with tracheostomies, nursing care involves humidifying and warming the inspired air and suctioning the secretions (see Table 4-5). A tracheostomy collar is a specially designed oxygen delivery mask that fits over the tracheostomy to deliver humidified air or oxygen. Sterile water is always used when humidifying inspired air.

 The tracheostomy site and tube also require careful cleaning to prevent infection of the respiratory tract.

The tracheostomy site and tube also require careful cleaning to prevent infection of the respiratory tract. The tracheostomy stoma needs to be cleaned daily and more often if there are signs of infection (i.e., redness, drainage, or swelling). If an inner cannula is present, then it should be cleaned every 8 hours (see Table 4-6). Complications of tracheostomy tubes include both immediate problems and long-term risks. Postoperatively, patients with newly created tracheostomies are at risk for hemorrhage, **pneumomediastinum** (air in the mediastinum), **subcutaneous emphysema** (air in the tissues around the tracheostomy), and **tracheoesophageal (T-E) fistula**. T-E fistula can occur at any time after tracheostomy creation. Tracheoesophageal fistulas may develop because of necrosis of the posterior wall of the larynx from prolonged pressure (from the cuff) or malposition of the tube. Long-term problems include dislodgment of the tube, expelled tubes, and infection. Patients with permanent tracheostomies need to observe for signs of infection (fever, painful cough, increased sputum, and chest pain) and notify their healthcare providers.

Table 4-5 Suctioning a Tracheostomy Tube

1. Assess the patient's breath sounds and breathing patterns. Loud, noisy respiration, an increased respiratory rate, crackles, wheezes, or rhonchi on auscultation may indicate the need for suctioning or the patient himself may request it.
2. Prepare the needed equipment and always have suctioning equipment in the room of a patient with a tracheostomy (some prepackaged suctioning kits are available):
   - Sterile and nonsterile gloves
   - Sterile saline or water and a container for it
   - Manual resuscitation bag
   - Suction catheters
   - Syringe (5 mL)
   - Suction machine (at 60 to 80 mm suction) or wall suction
3. Wash your hands.
4. Explain the procedure to the patient. Be calm and reassuring because the patient may be concerned about choking and being unable to communicate.
5. Ventilate the patient with 100% oxygen using the manual resuscitation bag for five breaths. If there are superficial secretions, suction them first before manually inflating the lungs.
6. Fill the container with saline or sterile water.
7. Place a sterile glove on the dominant hand that will hold the sterile catheter and a nonsterile glove on the nondominant hand that will control the suction.
8. Insert the sterile catheter into the tracheostomy and down into the bronchus about 6 to 12 inches or until resistance is felt. (Do not use suction during insertion.)
9. Withdraw the catheter slowly, rotating it and applying suction only intermittently so as not to damage the airway walls. (Suction for no more than 10 seconds.)
10. Return the tracheostomy collar (oxygen), and assess the patient's status. If the patient requires more suctioning, wait at least 2 minutes before performing it again.
11. Clear the suction catheter when finished by suctioning with sterile water or saline from the container until the tubing is clear. Discard the suction catheter.
12. Document the color, type, amount, consistency, and any odor of the secretions.

Table 4-6 Care of the Tracheostomy Site

1. Gather the needed equipment or a prepackaged kit. Supplies include:
   - Sterile hydrogen peroxide
   - Sterile saline
   - Sterile plastic forceps or swabs
   - Sterile tracheostomy dressing
   - Sterile bowl for soaking inner cannula if present
2. Explain to the patient what you are going to do.
3. Suction the patient as described in Table 4-5 before removing the cannula.
4. Use gloves to remove and discard the old tracheostomy dressing. Assess the drainage on the dressing and the site.
5. Pour sterile saline into one bowl and sterile hydrogen peroxide into the other bowl.
6. Put on sterile gloves.
7. Hold the tracheostomy tube with one hand to keep it from moving (which could stimulate coughing) and use the other hand to gently clean around the tube with sterile saline (or half-strength saline and peroxide depending on the institution's guidelines).
8. Soak the inner cannula, if present, in the peroxide for 1 minute and rinse it in the saline. Allow it to drip dry on the sterile field or gauze.
9. If you are changing the tapes that anchor the tube (usually done every 48 hours or more often if soiled), have another nurse help you keep the tube secure while changing them. Check the tension on the ties frequently to make sure that they are not too tight. They should be snug enough to prevent slippage but loose enough to allow circulation.
10. Keep a spare tracheostomy tube with its obturator of the patient's size taped over his bed at all times in case the tube should become dislodged during cleaning.

Tracheoesophageal fistulas may develop because of necrosis of the posterior wall of the larynx from prolonged pressure (from the cuff) or malposition of the tube.

CLOSED CHEST DRAINAGE

Many disease processes and surgeries can result in the accumulation of air and fluid in the pleural space. Irritation of the pleural lining from malignancy or infection can produce fluid. For example, a thoracotomy for lung cancer may produce excess fluid accumulation in the pleural cavity, preventing lung re-expansion.

The pleural space is a potential space where the pressure is subatmospheric (lower than atmospheric pressure), allowing the lungs to remain expanded. When the pleural space is opened, air rushes into the pleural space and the lung collapses. Increased pressure in the pleural space can result in complete collapse of the lung on the affected side and shifting of the mediastinal contents to the opposite side of the chest. This dangerous and life-threatening condition, a mediastinal shift, may kink the great vessels in the thoracic cavity, compromising cardiac and respiratory function and requiring immediate treatment.

 A mediastinal shift, may kink the great vessels in the thoracic cavity, compromising cardiac and respiratory function and requiring immediate treatment.

Closed chest drainage (i.e., chest drainage that is closed to atmospheric pressure) allows a system for drainage of fluid and air from the pleural space and re-expansion of the lung. Closed chest drainage systems were historically made of three glass bottles: one to collect drainage, one to maintain a seal to atmospheric pressure, and one for suction control. Now, disposable single unit systems are used in most healthcare facilities (see Figure 4-8).

The closed chest drainage system is used to accomplish the following:

- Collect drainage and evacuate air from the pleural space.
- Re-establish negative intrapleural pressure to promote lung re-expansion.
- Equalize pressure in the thoracic cavity to prevent mediastinal shift.

Each component of the chest drainage system must be frequently assessed to ensure proper functioning. The chest tubes that run from the patient to the unit must be free of kinks and clots. The unit itself must always be lower than the patient to allow gravity to assist in draining fluid from the chest. The unit usually has hooks for hanging on the end of the bed or feet to permit standing it on the floor. It should always be upright. If the chest drainage system tips over, the entire unit must be replaced. The amount of drainage should be marked on the container every hour

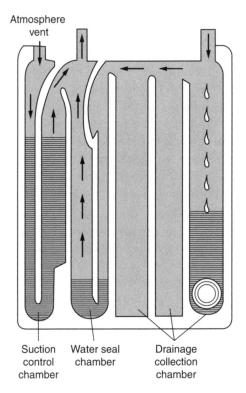

Figure 4-8 Closed chest drainage.

immediately postoperatively to assess the flow rate and the amount of blood loss. The surgeon should be notified if the drainage exceeds specific parameters.

 If the chest drainage system tips over, the entire unit must be replaced.

The closed chest drainage system is used to collect drainage and evacuate air from the pleural space, re-establish negative intrapleural pressure to promote lung re-expansion, and equalize pressure in the thoracic cavity to prevent mediastinal shift.

The water seal compartment allows for a one-way valve between the intrapleural space and atmospheric pressure. Air and fluid can leave the cavity but atmospheric air can not enter the pleural cavity. The air bubbles out of the water seal chamber and the fluid drains into the drainage compartment. An air vent at the top of the water seal chamber allows the air to escape the unit. Intermittent bubbling in the water seal chamber is normal and indicates that air is leaking into the pleural space and out into the unit. Continuous bubbling means that there is an air leak in the system and it needs to be found and corrected. The water level in this chamber fluctuates (tidaling) during inspiration and expiration.

Suction allows for rapid evacuation of air and drainage. The suction chamber permits suction to be applied to the intrapleural space in a regulated manner. Depending on the amount of sterile water instilled in the chamber, the suction may be 10 to 20 cm H_2O. The more water in the chamber means that there is more suction. Continuous bubbling in the suction chamber indicates that

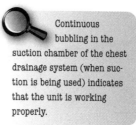

Intermittent bubbling in the water seal chamber of the chest drainage system is normal and indicates that air is leaking from the pleural space and out into the unit.

Continuous bubbling in the suction chamber of the chest drainage system (when suction is being used) indicates that the unit is working properly.

the unit is working properly. Newer systems apply "dry" suction, using a spring or dial mechanism in place of a water column.

Nursing Care of the Patient with Closed Chest Drainage

Nursing care of the patient with a closed chest drainage system involves frequent assessment of the patient's status and the functioning of the unit.

1. Keep the chest tubes free of kinks or bends. Patients may compress the tubes if they are lying on them, so follow positioning orders carefully. Clots may block the tubes postoperatively, and "milking" the tube may be necessary to clear the clots (see Figure 4-9). Be aware, milking is a controversial practice because it greatly increases the suction into the pleural space, so check the surgeon's orders before performing this technique.

2. Place the chest drainage unit lower than the patient and always in the upright position.

3. Check the suction chamber to make sure that it is bubbling continuously when suction is applied to the system.

4. Encourage the patient to cough and deep breathe not only to clear secretions but to help re-expand the lung.

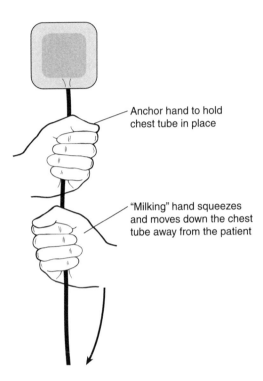

Figure 4-9 Milking (or "stripping") chest tubes to remove blood clots.

5. Check the water seal chamber for tidaling during breathing. Lack of fluctuation in the water seal chamber may indicate a blocked tube or the lung has reexpanded.

6. Never clamp a chest tube without a physician's order. When necessary, this may be done to assess lung expansion and pleural leaks.

7. Medicate the patient 30 minutes before chest tube removal, as it is a moderately painful procedure.

 Never clamp a chest tube without a physician's order.

Preoperative Care of the Patient Undergoing Surgery

A special note needs to be made about the patient undergoing surgery. Preoperatively, every patient needs thorough assessment and comprehensive teaching about the operative experience. The preoperative assessment should identify patients at risk for problems with oxygenation (e.g., smokers, those with pre-existing lung disease such as COPD or asthma, the elderly, and those with circulatory problems such as varicose veins). Varicosities can predispose patients to venous stasis in the extremities with the potential for the development of deep vein phlebitis and pulmonary embolus. Some of the most common postoperative complica-

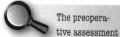

The preoperative assessment should identify patients at risk for problems with oxygenation (e.g., smokers, those with pre-existing lung disease such as COPD or asthma, the elderly, and those with circulatory problems such as varicose veins).

tions are atelectasis, pneumonia, deep vein thrombosis, and pulmonary emboli.

Preoperative teaching about the operative experience is an important part of nursing care. It involves teaching the patient about what to expect during the perioperative period and what the patient can do to facilitate his recovery from the anesthesia and surgery (see Table 4-7). Preoperative teaching not only allays anxiety in the patient but it also shortens the recovery time and prevents complications. Use handouts such as the one seen in Table 4-7 to enlist the patient as a partner in the recovery process.

Table 4-7 What You Can Do to Help Your Recovery

1. Take deep breaths every few minutes or when the nurses remind you. Inhale, filling the lower chest, then the midchest, and finally the upper chest, holding for 5 seconds and then slowly exhaling for 6 to 8 seconds.
2. Cough every 1 to 2 hours if you have secretions. Remember to splint the incision with a pillow or your hands to decrease the pain.
3. Use your incentive spirometer as directed or every 1 to 2 hours. Remember that slow breaths and holding the deep breath for 2 to 5 seconds help open the airways.
4. Ask for pain medication when you start to get uncomfortable. Do not wait until the pain is severe.
5. Remember to move from side to side if your surgeon approves this to allow your lungs to expand.
6. Start ambulating with assistance as soon as your surgeon says that it is all right. Take pain medication before you start walking.
7. Perform leg exercises as allowed by the surgeon to facilitate blood flow in the legs.
8. Remember that the staff is here to help your recovery—call them if you are having any problems or questions.

OXYGEN THERAPY

The purpose of oxygen therapy is to deliver more oxygen than is present in room air (21%). It is the most common treatment for patients with respiratory problems, such as chronic bronchitis, emphysema, arterial hypoxemia, and adult respiratory distress syndrome. The goals of oxygen therapy are the prevention or treatment of hypoxemia. Although it does not cure any diseases, it can reduce the cardiac workload and decrease tissue hypoxia. The correction of hypoxemia will decrease the work of breathing and facilitate myocardial and tissue oxygen supply.

Oxygen is prescribed by a physician with orders specifying the technique, amount, and route. The prescription for oxygen is written in liters per minute (L/min) or the Fio_2, the fraction of inspired oxygen (e.g., 40% or 0.4). The safest way to administer oxygen is to titrate it to achieve a particular So_2 or Pao_2. In patients without chronic respiratory diseases, a Pao_2 of 70 to 100 mmHg would be acceptable. But in those with chronic respiratory disease, whose stimulus to breathe may be their hypoxic drive, the goal of oxygen therapy can be 55 to 60 mmHg. The order for oxygen has to be customized for each patient and his or her condition.

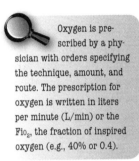

Oxygen is prescribed by a physician with orders specifying the technique, amount, and route. The prescription for oxygen is written in liters per minute (L/min) or the Fio_2, the fraction of inspired oxygen (e.g., 40% or 0.4).

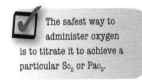

The safest way to administer oxygen is to titrate it to achieve a particular So_2 or Pao_2.

Oxygen can be delivered by several routes depending on the patient's age, respiratory disorder, and the desired fraction of inspired oxygen (Fio_2). All oxygen delivery systems consist of an oxygen source: cylinder or piped-in wall; valve handles to open the cylinder/system; flow meter to regulate the control of oxygen flow in L/min; tubing that connects the oxygen supply source to the patient's oxygen administration device; and a humidifier to counteract the drying effects of oxygen flowing over mucus membranes (some institutions do not use humidifiers with very low-flow oxygen systems unless requested by the patient).

Oxygen is available in canisters (green is the universal color for oxygen-carrying containers) or in wall sockets in healthcare facilities. The least invasive method to deliver oxygen is the nasal cannula or prongs into the patient's nostrils (see Figure 4-10). Patients may still speak and clear secretions while wearing nasal prongs. Oxygen may also be delivered by a variety of masks such as the Venturi (Venti) mask, where oxygen flows into the mask via a port at the bottom of the mask and exits via holes in the side of the mask. **Partial rebreathing** and **nonrebreathing masks** have a reservoir bag at the bottom of the mask. A portion of exhaled air (approximately one third) remains in the reservoir bag and the remainder exits the mask via the holes in the mask. The nonrebreathing mask has a one-way inspiratory valve to allow the greatest concentration of oxygen delivery short of mechanical ventilation.

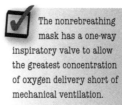

The nonrebreathing mask has a one-way inspiratory valve to allow the greatest concentration of oxygen delivery short of mechanical ventilation.

Newer routes include the **transtracheal catheter**, where oxygen is delivered via an implanted tracheal catheter to allow greater mobility, less oxygen, and more discretion.

Green is the universal color for oxygen-carrying containers.

Hyperbaric oxygen is the use of higher percentages of oxygen at pressures greater than atmospheric pressure to increase the amount of oxygen dissolved in the blood. It is useful in healing skin grafts and ischemic or gangrene tissue, and treating carbon monoxide poisoning. Hyperbaric oxygen chambers may hold the entire body (see Table 4-8).

Tubing connects to oxygen source

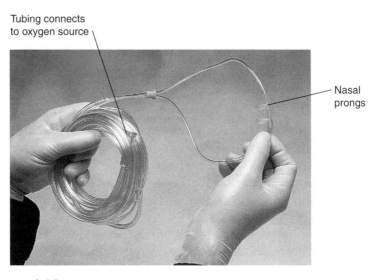

Nasal prongs

Figure 4-10 Nasal cannula (prongs).

Table 4-8 Oxygen Delivery Systems (FiO$_2$)

Delivery System	% FiO$_2$
Nasal cannula	1–6 L/min (1 L = 3% FiO$_2$)
Venturi mask	24, 28, 31, 35, 40, 50
Face mask	35–60
Partial rebreathing mask	60–90
Partial nonrebreathing mask	90–100
Trach collar	24, 28, 31, 35, 40, 50

Hazards of Oxygen Therapy

Oxygen should be viewed as a drug with concerns about potential complications. Obviously oxygen therapy is a highly beneficial treatment; however, it is not without risks. The number one hazard associated with oxygen delivery is that it is extremely flammable. Patients and family members should be aware of the dangers associated with smoking and oxygen therapy, and nurses need to teach the appropriate precautions.

> The number one hazard associated with oxygen delivery is that it is extremely flammable. Patients and family members should be aware of the dangers associated with smoking and oxygen therapy, and nurses need to teach the appropriate precautions.

Physiologic adverse effects to oxygen therapy occur when treatment has been prolonged or when the FiO$_2$ has been greater than 50%. Adverse effects include pulmonary oxygen toxicity and hypoventilation. Pulmonary oxygen toxicity is a result of higher than normal amounts of oxygen in the lower airways for a prolonged time period such as an FiO$_2$ greater than 50–70% for longer than 48–72 hours. This prolonged exposure may lead to ciliary dysfunction, impaired mucus removal, fibrosis of the alveolar capillary membrane, and respiratory distress syndrome. Early signs and symptoms of oxygen toxicity include increased respiratory rate, dyspnea, coughing, fatigue, lethargy, malaise, restlessness, paresthesias in the extremities, nausea, vomiting, and anorexia. Later symptoms include cyanosis, severe dyspnea, use of accessory muscles during respiration, and asphyxia. Hypoventilation may occur during oxygen therapy in patients with COPD who need a hypoxic drive to stimulate breathing. As the Pao$_2$ increases with supplemental oxygen, the stimulus for respiration can be blunted or eliminated. This could result in hypoventilation and possibly respiratory arrest. Signs and symptoms of hypoventilation include a decrease in the rate and depth of respiration and a decreasing level of consciousness.

 Hypoventilation may occur during oxygen therapy in patients who need a hypoxic drive to stimulate breathing.

The most common side effect of oxygen therapy is drying of the mucus membranes. Normally, inspired air passes over the nasal mucosa where it is humidified before it reaches the lower respiratory tract. When supplemental oxygen is delivered at greater than 4 L/min, it should be humidified. This is accomplished by passing the oxygen through a container of sterile water before it enters the patient.

 Pulmonary oxygen toxicity is a result of higher than normal amounts of oxygen in the lower airways for a prolonged time period such as an Fio_2 greater than 50–70% for longer than 48–72 hours.

Oxygen Delivery Systems

 Oxygen via nasal cannula is prescribed in liters per minute (L/min).

Nasal Cannula

Nasal cannulas are utilized when the patient requires low to medium concentrations of oxygen. Because the cannula is a low-flow system, a large part of the tidal volume inspired by the patient will be ambient (room) air (see Table 4-9). Therefore, the inspired oxygen concentration is dependent on the flow of oxygen through the unit, the patient's respiratory rate, and the patient's own tidal volume. Dyspneic patients with high respiratory rates and tidal volumes entrain a high volume of room air, which results in a lower Fio_2 delivery.

Oxygen via nasal cannula is prescribed in liters per minute (L/min). With each increase of 1 liter of oxygen, the inspired oxygen concentration increases by approximately 3%. The normal range of prescribed flow rate is 1 to 6 L/min. This oxygen flow rate in a patient with a normal respiratory rate and tidal volume deliver an Fio_2 of approximately 24% to 44%. Flow rates greater than 6 L/min via nasal cannula may result in irritation to the nasal and pharyngeal mucosa and possibly contribute to air swallowing. Humidification at a 1 to 6 L/min flow rate is not required but is frequently utilized to prevent mucosal drying. Mouth breathing does not affect the concentration of delivered oxygen unless there is complete obstruction of

Table 4-9 Low-Flow Systems

Device	Flow Rate (L/min)	FiO$_2$ (%)*
Nasal cannula	1	22–24
	2	26–28
	3	28–32
	4	32–36
	5	36–40
	6	40–44
Simple mask	5–6	40
	6–7	50
	7–8	60
Partial rebreathing mask	7	65
	8–15	70–80
	12–15	85–100
Nonrebreathing	Set to prevent collapse of oxygen reservoir	

*FiO$_2$ will vary with respiratory pattern, rate, and tidal volume.

the nares because oxygen will be inhaled from the anatomic reservoirs, the oropharynx and nasopharynx.

There are multiple advantages of the nasal cannula system. Nasal cannulas are comfortable, well-tolerated, and relatively inexpensive. They also allow the patient to communicate, eat, drink, and cough without disrupting oxygen flow. A disadvantage of the nasal cannula system is the variability of oxygen delivery with changing respiratory rates and tidal volumes. Nasal cannulas (see Figure 4-10) are utilized when the patient requires low to medium concentrations of oxygen. Because the cannula is a low-flow system, a large part of the tidal volume inspired by the patient will be ambient (room) air. Cannula systems may also cause pressure sores around the nose and ears. Care of the patient using the nasal cannula includes close assessment of skin for signs of breakdown around the ears, cheeks, and nares, lubrication of the nares if humidification is not being utilized, and cleaning of the equipment as needed.

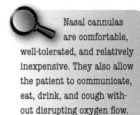

Nasal cannulas are comfortable, well-tolerated, and relatively inexpensive. They also allow the patient to communicate, eat, drink, and cough without disrupting oxygen flow.

Oropharyngeal Catheter

The **oro- or nasopharyngeal catheter** is rarely utilized because of the need to move the catheter daily to minimize pharyngeal damage. A possible scenario in which it may be used is the short-term delivery of oxygen in low to moderate concentrations. As with the nasal cannula, oxygen delivery varies with respiratory rate, oxygen flow rate, and tidal volume.

Simple Face Mask

Face masks for oxygen delivery are generally well-tolerated by adults (see Figure 4-11). Openings cut into both sides of the mask stop a possible accumulation and rebreathing of expired air, which is high in CO_2. Oxygen flow rates in a simple face mask should exceed

> ✓ The recommended flow rate through a simple face mask is 5 to 8 L/min. At this flow, the simple face mask can provide oxygen concentrations between 40% and 60%.

5 L/min. This rate facilitates flushing out of expired air. The recommended flow rate through a simple face mask is 5 to 8 L/min. At this flow rate, the simple face mask can provide oxygen concentrations between 40% and 60%. However, as noted with the nasal cannula, the FiO_2 in a simple face mask is diluted by room air and can be affected by respiratory rate and tidal volume.

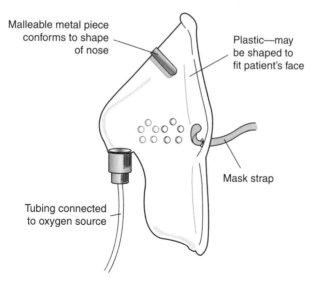

Malleable metal piece conforms to shape of nose

Plastic—may be shaped to fit patient's face

Mask strap

Tubing connected to oxygen source

Figure 4-11 Simple face mask.

Care of patients being treated with oxygen therapy via a simple mask includes recognition of the risk for aspiration of vomitus, assessment of facial skin and ears for irritation or breakdown, maintaining oxygen flow rate at greater than 5 L/min, maintaining adequate water in the system for humidification, emptying connecting tubing of condensed water, and cleaning the masks when necessary.

Face Mask with an Oxygen Reservoir

Face masks with an oxygen reservoir bag are divided into two types: partial rebreathing and nonrebreathing (see Figure 4-12). These systems provide a constant flow of oxygen into an attached reservoir bag. The design of the **partial rebreathing mask** is similar to that of the simple face mask. The difference between the two is that the partial rebreathing mask has an oxygen reservoir bag attached. The purpose of the partial rebreathing mask is to

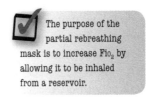

The purpose of the partial rebreathing mask is to increase Fio₂ by allowing it to be inhaled from a reservoir.

increase Fio_2 by allowing it to be inhaled from a reservoir. Exhaled air also enters the reservoir bag, allowing some rebreathing of CO_2.

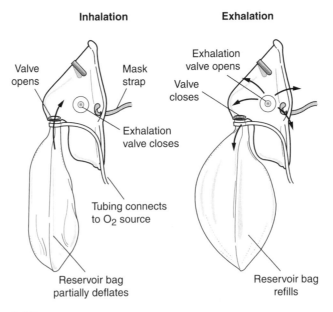

Inhalation

Valve opens

Mask strap

Exhalation valve closes

Tubing connects to O₂ source

Reservoir bag partially deflates

Exhalation

Exhalation valve opens

Valve closes

Reservoir bag refills

Figure 4-12 Rebreathing and nonrebreathing masks.

In order to achieve an FiO_2 greater than 60%, a **nonrebreathing mask** must be used. A nonrebreathing mask consists of a face mask with an attached reservoir bag and a one-way valve between the reservoir bag and the mask. The one-way valve between the reservoir bag and the mask prevents exhaled air from re-entering the reservoir bag and diluting the FiO_2. At a flow of 6 L/min, an FiO_2 of approximately 60% can be achieved. Each additional liter per minute of oxygen flow will increase the FiO_2 by approximately 10%. This system can deliver the highest oxygen concentration in spontaneously breathing patients. At flow rates of 12 to 15 L/min, and a one-way valve between the reservoir and the mask and one-way valves covering both ports in the mask's sides preventing inhalation of room air, this system can deliver almost a 100% oxygen concentration. However, because a tight fit is seldom achieved with these masks, room air may be pulled in around the mask, diluting the FiO_2 to 80% to 90%.

Care of patients being treated with oxygen therapy via a partial or nonrebreathing mask mirror that of a patient using a simple mask but also includes monitoring of the reservoir bag to assure continuous inflation and adjustment of the mask to minimize leaks.

 A nonrebreathing mask consists of a face mask with an attached reservoir bag and a one-way valve between the reservoir bag and the mask.

Venturi Mask

The **Venturi (Venti) mask** delivers oxygen under pressure through various-sized orifices in the mask (see Figure 4-13). As the oxygen exits the orifice, it creates a subatmospheric pressure, which entrains room air into the system. The size of the orifice and the oxygen flow rate dictate the oxygen concentration. The Venturi mask can be adjusted to deliver the following fractions of inspired oxygen: 24, 28, 35, 40, and 60 (see Table 4-10). This system is used frequently in patients with chronic hypercapnia who rely on an hypoxic drive for respiration and are at high risk of respiratory depression caused by sudden increases in PaO_2 because it offers a more precise inspired oxygen fraction.

 The Venturi mask can be adjusted to deliver the following fractions of inspired oxygen: 24, 28, 35, 40, and 60.

 In the Venturi (Venti) mask, oxygen under pressure is forced through various-sized orifices in the mask. As the oxygen exits the orifice, it creates a subatmospheric pressure, which entrains room air into the system. The size of the orifice and the oxygen flow rate dictate the oxygen concentration.

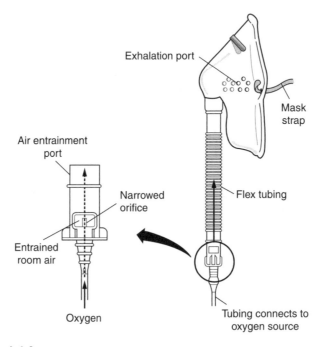

Figure 4-13 Venturi mask.

Table 4-10 Venturi Devices

Flow Rate (L/min)	FiO$_2$ (%)*
2	24
4	28
6	35
8	40
12	60

*Color-coded adapters exist for each desired FiO$_2$.

Oxygen therapy via a Venturi mask at an FiO$_2$ of 24% is usually used initially. The patient's response to this dose of oxygen is then evaluated and the mask adjusted to the desired level of SaO$_2$ or PaO$_2$. Care of patients treated with oxygen therapy via the Venturi mask is the same as patients being treated via a simple mask.

Transtracheal Catheter

The transtracheal catheter is a small catheter inserted into the trachea percutaneously between the second and third tracheal cartilage. This option may be used for patients who require home oxygen therapy. The advantages of this oxygenation technique are that they are cosmetically more appealing, and the catheter may be concealed by clothing. These catheters do not interfere with eating, drinking, or talking. Patients with these catheters report an improved sense of taste and smell and an improved appetite. The disadvantages of transtracheal catheters include the risk of infection, the need for meticulous care of the site, a possibly difficult insertion technique, and the possibility of subcutaneous emphysema should the catheter be dislodged before a mature tract is formed. Care of patients with transtracheal catheters includes teaching patients how to recognize and report evidence of infection: fever, warmth, erythema, edema at insertion site; a change in the color, consistency, and/or amount of secretions; and assessment of their catheters for patency.

Continuous Positive Airway Pressure and Bilevel Positive Airway Pressure Mask (CPAP)

Continuous positive airway pressure (**CPAP**) is continuous positive pressure above atmospheric pressure at the airway opening throughout a spontaneous breathing cycle. CPAP systems deliver oxygen via a nasal or facial mask while applying CPAP. CPAP improves oxygenation by enhancing the transport of oxygen across the pulmonary capillary membrane and reducing the shunt created by collapsed alveoli. The **positive end-expiratory pressure** (**PEEP**) helps to prevent alveolar collapse. A CPAP device is used by alert patients whose oxygen requirements can not be met despite the delivery of maximum supplemental oxygen. A CPAP device is also used to maintain a patent airway, as in the case of obstructive sleep apnea.

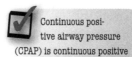

Continuous positive airway pressure (CPAP) is continuous positive pressure above atmospheric pressure at the airway opening throughout a spontaneous breathing cycle.

CPAP systems consist of a face or nasal mask with an inflatable cushion and head strap to hold the mask tightly in place; a PEEP valve is incorporated into the exhalation port to maintain positive expiratory pressure, and in the face mask version, a port exists through which nasogastric suction may be accomplished. **Bilevel positive airway pressure (BIPAP)** provides pressure-supported ventilation by assisting inhalation, increasing tidal volume, and creating positive end-expiratory pressure (PEEP). BIPAP is delivered via nasal or facial mask. Patients using CPAP or BIPAP must be alert enough to protect their airway.

 Patients using CPAP or BIPAP must be alert enough to protect their airway.

The advantage of using CPAP or BIPAP devices is improved oxygenation with lower levels of inspired oxygen. Disadvantages of utilizing CPAP or BIPAP include oral and nasal dryness, burning, bleeding, eye irritation, and interference with talking, eating, and expectorating sputum. These devices also put the patient at high risk for aerophagia, aspiration, the development of pressure sores, and decubitus ulcers under the perimeter of the mask. The care of patients being treated with these devices includes vigilant skin assessment, possible treatment with nasogastric tubes for decompression, antigas medications, and hydration measures for the oropharynx and nasopharynx.

MECHANICAL VENTILATION

Case Study

Mrs. P, a 76-year-old female with a history of COPD secondary to cigarette smoking (50 pack-years) and hypertension (HTN), transient ischemia attack (TIA), and coronary artery disease (CAD), presents to the emergency room with complaints of increasing shortness of breath (SOB) and chest pressure. She states this began approximately 5 hours ago when she returned from a shopping trip with her friend. She has taken three nitroglycerin tablets without relief of her chest pain and has used her Ventolin inhaler five to six times without any change in her SOB. Physical exam reveals an anxious, elderly, obese female who is pale, cool, diaphoretic, and using accessory muscles to breathe. Vital signs: temperature—96.5°F, AP—143 and irregular, BP—194/102 mmHg on the right and 198/104 mmHg on the left, RR—40 breaths per min and labored, Sao_2 is 84 on 100% oxygen via nonrebreathing mask. Lung sounds: inspiratory and expiratory crackles; posterior: T3 (thoracic vertebrae) down bilaterally; anteriorly: fourth intercostal space down bilaterally. The quality of the crackles does not change with deep breathing and coughing. Jugular venous distention is noted bilaterally with the patient sitting at a 75° angle. A systolic murmur and an S3 heart sound are heard on auscultation. The EKG reveals 4 mm ST segment elevation across the precordium (anterior septal leads). The results of the arterial blood gas (ABG) are: pH—7.16, Pco_2—74, Po_2—47, Sao_2—84. A diagnosis of anterior septal myocardial infarction (MI) and pulmonary edema with resulting respiratory failure is made. The ER physician orders nitroglycerin IV and titrate up until relief of chest pain, maintaining a systolic blood pressure (SBP) of greater than 90 mmHg, furosemide 60 mg IVP, 2 mg MSO_4 IV every 3 minutes until relief of chest pain, and directs the respiratory therapist to prepare for endotracheal intubation and mechanical ventilation.

Mechanical ventilation is indicated when a patient's lungs are incapable of delivering an adequate amount of oxygen to the tissues and/or removing a sufficient amount of carbon dioxide. This condition can be the result of a myriad of diseases or injury processes, such as drug overdose, COPD, asthma, pneumonia, inhalation injury, multiple trauma, neuromuscular disease, shock, multisystem failure, and postoperative states where anesthesia is not reversed or the integrity of the muscles of breathing are compromised.

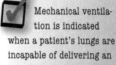 Mechanical ventilation is indicated when a patient's lungs are incapable of delivering an adequate amount of oxygen to the tissues and/or removing a sufficient amount of carbon dioxide.

Endotracheal Intubation

A patient who can no longer maintain adequate gas exchange or a patent airway and requires intervention with mechanical ventilation must have an artificial airway inserted. This artificial airway can be either an **endotracheal tube (ETT)** or a **tracheostomy tube**. The rationale for use of a tracheostomy tube as the initial artificial airway is described earlier in this chapter. The most common artificial airway utilized for short-term airway management and ventilatory support is the ETT. The ETT is a polyvinylchloride tube that is passed via either the nares or mouth through the vocal cords into the trachea with the tip positioned approximately 2 to 3 cm above the carina.

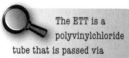 The ETT is a polyvinylchloride tube that is passed via either the nares or mouth through the vocal cords into the trachea with the tip positioned approximately 2 to 3 cm above the carina.

The ETT design is standardized with a 15 mm outside diameter on the connector that facilitates connection to standard ventilatory equipment, ventilator circuitry, manual resuscitator bag (MRB), or anesthesia devices. The ETT body has a radiopaque stripe that runs the length of the tube to facilitate tube location on chest X-ray. The body also has centimeter markings that allow for the determination of the depth of insertion. This distal tip of the ETT is beveled to allow easier passage. At the distal tip is a cuff that when inflated produces a seal in the trachea, allowing for the application of positive pressure ventilation and minimizing aspiration of secretions and gastric contents. When the cuff is inflated, no air can pass through the vocal cords from the lungs to the nose and mouth, therefore the patient cannot speak. The inflating system for the cuff consists of a small bore tube that is fused to the body of the ETT with a pilot balloon at the proximal end. This pilot balloon has a spring-loaded, one-way valve that is activated by the insertion of a syringe. Air can be inserted or withdrawn from the cuff through this valve.

 Adult women are commonly intubated with a 7 to 8 mm tube; men with an 8 to 9 mm tube.

ETTs are available in a variety of sizes. Adult sizes range from 5 to 10 mm in diameter. The tube size is determined by its internal diameter and marked on the connector/adapter and/or tube body. Adult women are commonly intubated with a 7 to 8 mm tube; men with an 8 to 9 mm tube.

Intubation is usually performed by an experienced professional, trained in the technique (i.e., an anesthesiologist, pulmonologist, nurse anesthetist, or specially trained RN or RCP). After the ETT is inserted, its position is assessed by auscultation with a stethoscope over both lung fields and abdomen. Many institutions now use a **capnography** device to aid in the assessment of proper positioning of the ETT by measuring carbon dioxide in expired air. The gold standard of assessment for ETT position is the chest X-ray. Once the tube is determined to be in proper position, it is stabilized by either taping it to the face or with a variety of stabilizing devices. The depth of the tube at the teeth, lip, or nares opening should be documented in the patient's medical record.

The goals of mechanical ventilation are to accomplish the following:

* Provide an adequate amount of oxygen delivery to the lung.
* Maintain alveolar ventilation and the elimination of carbon dioxide.
* Reduce the work of breathing.

Mechanical ventilation does not cure diseased lungs, but it may be used to correct impaired ventilation and oxygenation. It is used as adjunctive therapy to support the patient through a period where lung function is inadequate as demonstrated by hypercapnia, hypoxia, and symptoms of respiratory distress. Therapy during mechanical ventilation is aimed at correcting the underlying disease process and preventing the possible complications of mechanical ventilation. Once the patient is capable of maintaining adequate tissue oxygenation and alveolar ventilation (removal of CO_2), ventilatory support can be withdrawn.

Classification of Ventilators

The main classifications of mechanical ventilators are: negative pressure, positive pressure, or high frequency ventilators. **Negative pressure ventilators**, such as the Drinker respirator tank (iron lung), chest cuirass (tortoise shell), and the body wrap (pneumowrap) are rarely utilized now in the treatment of acute respiratory failure (see Figures 4-14 and 4-15). They are most commonly used as home nighttime ventilatory support by patients who cannot generate adequate inspiratory pressures, such

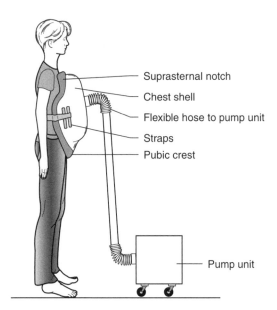

Figure 4-14 Negative pressure ventilator—chest shell.

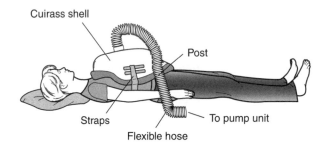

Cuirass shell

Post

Straps

To pump unit

Flexible hose

Figure 4-15 Negative pressure ventilator—cuirass shell.

as polio survivors and persons with neuro-muscular disease, CNS disorders, COPD, or spinal cord injuries. Negative pressure ventilators do not require intubation. They are airtight devices that enclose either the chest wall cavity (tortoise shell, pneumowrap) or the entire body (iron lung), leaving the head exposed (see Figures 4-16 and 4-17). They function by creating negative pressure around the thoracic cavity during inspiration, promoting air entry into the lungs, and then negative pressure is stopped, allowing air to flow passively out of the lungs. These devices are used with patients who have compliant lungs and the ability to clear their own secretions.

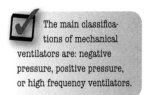

The main classifications of mechanical ventilators are: negative pressure, positive pressure, or high frequency ventilators.

Positive pressure ventilators are the type most commonly used in the acute care setting and can be volume-cycled, pressure-cycled, or set by time parameters. Positive pressure ventilators force gas into the lungs under positive pressure via an artificial airway (endotracheal tube or tracheostomy tube) during inspiration. Expiration occurs passively when the flow of gas from the mechanical ventilator ceases.

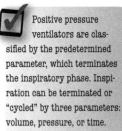

Positive pressure ventilators are classified by the predetermined parameter, which terminates the inspiratory phase. Inspiration can be terminated or "cycled" by three parameters: volume, pressure, or time.

High-frequency ventilation systems deliver high ventilation rates synchronized to the patient's inspiratory efforts. The peak airway pressures are low during ventilations.

Positive pressure ventilators are classified by the predetermined parameter, which terminates the inspiratory phase. Inspiration can be terminated or "cycled" by three parameters: volume, pressure, or time. **Volume-cycled ventilators** deliver gas to a preset volume. When the preset volume is reached, gas delivery is terminated, inspiration ends,

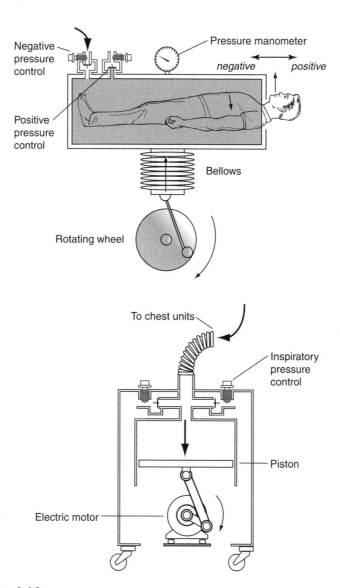

Figure 4-16 Negative pressure ventilator—inspiration.

and passive expiration begins. Puritan Bennett MA-1, MA-2, and 7200 A, and the Bourns Bear I- V are examples of volume-cycled ventilators.

Pressure-cycled ventilators deliver gas until a preset pressure in the airway is attained, terminating inspiration and allowing passive expiration. The volume of gas delivered is affected by any variable that alters

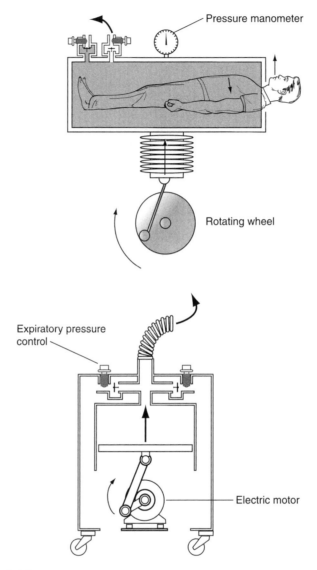

Figure 4-17 Negative pressure ventilator—exhalation.

airway resistance or chest wall/lung compliance. If airway resistance increases or lung/chest wall compliance decreases, the volume of gas decreases. If airway resistance decreases or lung/chest wall compliance increases, the volume of gas increases.

Time-cycled ventilators deliver gas for a preset amount of time. The volume of gas delivered is determined by the flow rate of the gas and a preset time internal. Changes in airway resistance or chest wall/lung compliance also affect the volume of gas delivered by a time-cycled ventilator. This type of ventilation is used more commonly in neonatal and pediatric populations. Many microprocessor-driven ventilators are capable of functioning in a variety of inspiratory flow patterns. The majority of positive pressure ventilators have built-in safety features with alarm functions to prevent the delivery of excessively high pressures, rates, or volumes to the patient being treated with mechanical ventilation (see Figure 4-18).

Ventilator Settings and Controls

The volume-cycled ventilator is currently the most commonly used ventilator in acute care. Each ventilator has a number of parameters prescribed by the physician and set or adjusted by the nurse caring for the

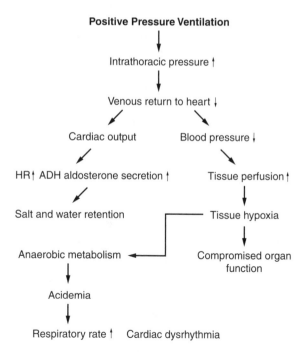

Figure 4-18 Physiologic sequelae to positive pressure ventilation.

patient receiving mechanical ventilation. The parameters requiring physician prescription and which are universal to most ventilators include the following:

- **Respiratory rate (RR), breaths per minute (BPM), frequency (f)**—These terms are the number of breaths the ventilator delivers every minute. The patient's respiratory rate equals the number of breaths delivered by the ventilator plus the patient's own spontaneous breaths.
- **Tidal volume (Vt)**—Volume of gas delivered with each breath. This is usually set between 5 to 15 cc/kg.
- **Fraction of inspired oxygen (FiO_2)**—The percent of oxygen being delivered with each breath. It is recommended that the lowest FiO_2 possible to meet the patient's needs be used.
- **Positive end-expiratory pressure (PEEP)**—Amount of pressure, measured in cm of H_2O, exerted by the ventilator during the expiratory phase of ventilation. PEEP improves oxygenation by enhancing gas exchange and preventing atelectasis. PEEP set at 3 to 5 cm H_2O is considered physiologic. Persistent hypoxemia despite high FiO_2s may be treated by increasing the amount of PEEP. PEEP, by increasing intrathoracic pressure, may decrease venous return to the heart, thereby possibly decreasing BP and cardiac output.
- **Continuous positive airway pressure (CPAP)**—Application of positive airway pressure throughout the entire ventilatory cycle, inspiration and expiration, in spontaneously breathing patients. CPAP aids in alveolar recruitment during inspiration and prevents alveolar collapse during expiration. CPAP is indicated for the treatment of sleep apnea and is also used as a method to wean patients from ventilatory support.
- **I:E**—Determined by the preset volume being delivered and the rate of inspiratory flow. Normal I:E ratio is 1:2.
- **Sensitivity**—The amount of negative pressure the patient must generate to trigger the ventilator to respond. Sensitivity is adjusted to require minimal patient effort, usually around 2 cm H_2O.
- **Sighs**—Volumes of air that are 1.5 to 2 times the preset Vt delivered 6 to 10 times an hour. Sighs are used to prevent atelectasis in certain circumstances.
- **Pressure limits**—Settings used to limit the pressure the ventilator can use to deliver a specified volume. The pressure limit is usually set 10 to 15 cm H_2O greater than the pressure it takes

to deliver a normal breath to a patient. Once a preset pressure limit is reached, the ventilator stops delivering volume, even if the preset Vt is not obtained, to protect the patient against barotrauma. This is accompanied by an alarm system.

◆ **Alarm systems**—Visual and audible warning that alerts caretakers that certain conditions exist (e.g., low or high pressures, low volumes, disconnection, inappropriate I:E ratio or Fio_2). Various tones are utilized for specific conditions, allowing the RN or RCP to expedite their trouble shooting when specific alarm conditions exist.

Parameters such as inspiration to expiration ratio (I:E ratio), sensitivity, sighs, pressure limits, flow rate, flow wave patterns, pressure and/or flow triggers, and alarms may be dictated by the type of ventilatory mode utilized or may be adjusted by the nurse responsible for ventilator management.

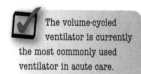

The volume-cycled ventilator is currently the most commonly used ventilator in acute care.

Modes of Ventilation

The mode of ventilation (see Figures 4-19 and 4-20) describes the pattern by which the ventilator delivers breaths to the patient. There are five basic modes of **ventilatory support:** controlled mechanical ventilation (CMV), assist/control ventilation (A/C), synchronized intermittent mandatory

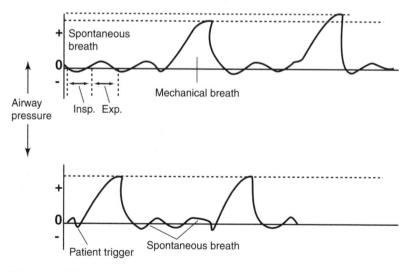

Figure 4-19 Modes of ventilation (I).

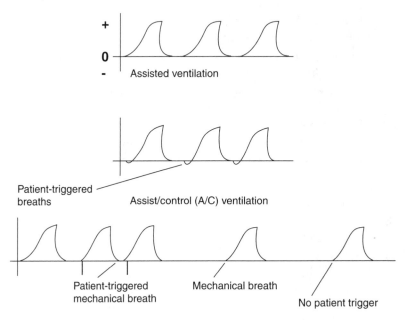

Figure 4-20 Modes of ventilation (II).

ventilation (SIMV), pressure support ventilation (PSV), and pressure control ventilation (PCV).

Controlled Mechanical Ventilation

Controlled mechanical ventilation (CMV) is the least frequently used mode of ventilation. During CMV, the patient receives a preset Fio_2, rate, and tidal volume. No spontaneous breaths are allowed. This mode is only utilized in patients who are not capable of spontaneous respiratory effort (i.e., patients who are totally anesthetized or paralyzed).

Assist/Control Ventilation

In **assist/control ventilation (A/C)**, a preset tidal volume is delivered at a preset rate (control), but the patient may also initiate breaths (assist). The ventilator delivers the preset volume each time it "senses" the patient initiating a breath. Therefore, every breath the patient receives is at the preset tidal volume. In this mode, the work of breathing may be significantly decreased. A/C mode also allows for complete rest for the muscles of respiration. A/C is the most commonly used mode for the treatment of acute respiratory failure.

Synchronized Intermittent Mandatory Ventilation

Synchronized intermittent mandatory ventilation (**SIMV**) mode is similar to the A/C mode in that a preset rate, tidal volume, and FiO_2 are programmed into the ventilator. However, in the SIMV mode, the ventilator synchronizes its delivery of the preset volume breath to coincide with a patient's spontaneous effort within a specified time. It accomplishes this by having a control algorithm that has the ventilator wait a specified period of time to sense a spontaneous inspiratory effort. For example, if the preset rate is 6, the ventilator will wait for 10 seconds (if the rate were 4, the ventilator would wait for 15 seconds) to sense an inspiratory effort. If one is sensed, then the preset tidal volume is delivered with the patient's effort. Any additional breaths initiated by the patient within that time frame have a volume dependent on the patient's inspiratory effort. If no inspiratory effort is sensed in that time frame, the ventilator delivers a breath at the end of the prescribed time period. This mode allows the patient to breathe spontaneously at variable volumes between ventilator breaths. It also assures that a minimum ventilatory pattern is maintained. The FiO_2 is constant for both ventilator and patient-initiated breaths.

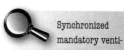

Synchronized mandatory ventilation (SIMV) mode is similar to the A/C mode in that a preset rate, tidal volume, and FiO_2 are programmed into the ventilator.

Pressure Support Ventilation

In **pressure support ventilation (PSV)**, the patient's spontaneous inspiratory effort is augmented by the delivery of a preset level of positive inspiratory pressure. When the patient initiates inspiration, the preset amount of pressure support is delivered and held constant throughout inspiration, facilitating the flow of gas into the lungs. In the PSV mode, the tidal volume is variable, dependent on patient effort, and the amount of pressure support selected. PSV is used to assist the patient in overcoming the increased resistance and work of breathing imposed by a disease process, as well as the implements of mechanical ventilation (e.g., endotracheal tubes, inspiratory valves, and tubing).

In pressure support ventilation (PSV), the patient's spontaneous inspiratory effort is augmented by the delivery of a preset level of positive inspiratory pressure.

Pressure Control Ventilation

In **pressure control ventilation (PCV)**, a preset number of breaths per minute is augmented by a preset amount of inspiratory pressure. When the preselected pressure is reached, the flow of gas is stopped, allowing passive expiration. In PCV, there is no preset tidal volume (Vt). The Vt the patient receives is determined by the set inspiratory pressure, the inspiratory time, the patient's lung compliance, and the resistance of both

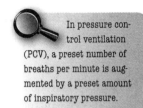

In pressure control ventilation (PCV), a preset number of breaths per minute is augmented by a preset amount of inspiratory pressure.

the patient's airways and the ventilator circuit. The nurse and respiratory therapist must carefully monitor Vt and minute ventilation because any factor that increases resistance or decreases compliance negatively impacts Vt and minute ventilation. Conversely, any situation that decreases resistance or improves compliance may result in an increase in Vt and subsequent overdistention and excessive ventilation.

Management of Patients Requiring Mechanical Ventilation

Patients requiring mechanical ventilation need a multidisciplinary approach to successfully manage their care. This team usually consists of a nurse, physician, respiratory therapist (RT), nutritionist, occupational and/or physical therapist, speech therapist (ST), social worker, pharmacist, and pastoral care provider. If possible, a team meeting involving the patient and family prior to the initiation of mechanical ventilation could help allay some fear and anxiety. The team should explain, in understandable language, the reason(s) for mechanical ventilation, frequently reported sensations and experiences, possible duration of treatment, risks and benefits, strategies employed to facilitate weaning from mechanical ventilation, and what rights and responsibilities the patient and family have during this experience.

However, patients are often intubated and placed on mechanical ventilation during an emergency situation. The nurse, in this scenario, plays the invaluable role of patient advocate and educator. The nurse is the ventilated patient's vital link to the health delivery system, acting as a direct caregiver and coordinator of essential services. It is imperative that the nurse understand the underlying pathology that resulted in the patient's need for mechanical ventilation. Understanding the disease process can guide the nurse in the provision and coordination of care. For example, a patient who is ventilated for respiratory failure secondary to pneumonia has different needs than a patient ventilated for respiratory failure secondary to cardiogenic shock. There are, however, many collaborative diagnoses common to patients requiring mechanical ventilation. By successfully managing these issues, nurses have an enormous impact on the experience of the intubated, ventilated patients and their families.

The nurse's primary goal is to monitor and evaluate the patient's response to mechanical ventilation. Physiologic parameters that must be closely monitored include vital signs, heart rate, blood pressure, respiratory rate and effort, oxygen saturation, breath sounds, breathing pattern, and arterial blood gases. The nurse is the person at the bedside who understands the patient's response to mechanical ventilation, and collaborates and coordinates the expertise of the other disciplines involved in the patient's care.

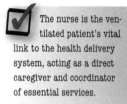
The nurse is the ventilated patient's vital link to the health delivery system, acting as a direct caregiver and coordinator of essential services.

Care of the Mechanically Ventilated Patient

When patients are mechanically ventilated, they require coordinated care from multiple disciplines. Careful and frequent assessment is necessary to detect potential problems as they develop and begin early interventions to minimize the adverse effects of mechanical ventilation on patients. Potential collaborative problems and diagnoses include the following:

- High risk for inadequate gas exchange or ineffective breathing pattern
- Ineffective airway clearance
- Impaired communication
- Fear and anxiety
- Powerlessness
- Isolation and sensory deprivation
- Altered nutritional intake
- Altered bowel functioning
- Disuse syndrome

High Risk for Inadequate Gas Exchange or Ineffective Breathing Pattern

Patients on ventilators may experience inadequate gas exchange and/or ineffective breathing patterns due to a variety of factors, such as occluded or partially occluded endotracheal tube or tracheostomy tube, dysynchrony due to "fighting" or "bucking" the ventilator, hemothorax, pneumothorax, pulmonary embolus, exhaustion, and any other condition that would increase airway resistance (asthma) or decrease lung compliance (ARDS). The nurse must carefully assess the mechanically ventilated patient for increased work of breathing; increased use of accessory muscles; fear, agitation, and confusion; any factors that indicate fatigue and increased respiratory rate; and dysynchronous respiratory pattern. The nurse must watch for decreases in tidal volumes, increased heart rate and blood pressure, decreased oxygen saturation, adventitious breath sounds, increased airway pressures, and decreased lung compliance. The ventilator function must also be carefully assessed to rule out any possible mechanical failures. Ventilator settings must be evaluated to ensure they are appropriate for the patient's current condition. The underlying problem must be discovered and appropriate interventions undertaken to facilitate the patient's return to normal respiratory functioning.

The nurse must carefully assess the mechanically ventilated patient for increased work of breathing; increased use of accessory muscles; fear, agitation, and confusion; any factors that indicate fatigue and increased respiratory rate; and dysynchronous respiratory pattern.

Ineffective Airway Clearance

The ability of the patient to expectorate his or her own secretions can be affected by multiple factors: length and diameter of the endotracheal tube, muscle strength, viscosity of the secretions, and level of sedation. If the patient cannot clear the airway, it is the responsibility of the nurse or respiratory therapist to suction the airway.

Over the past 10 years, there has been excellent research done in the area of suctioning for the management of secretions in mechanically ventilated patients. Suctioning should only be performed if indicated by coughing, visible secretions, increased work of breathing, decrease in Sao_2, high peak inspiratory pressures, and/or breath sounds revealing coarse wheezing or crackles.

Deep endotracheal or tracheostomy suctioning in the healthcare facility is a sterile procedure. The patient should be well-oxygenated with 100% oxygen either through the ventilator circuit or via manual resuscitation bag prior to the initiation of the procedure. It has been well-supported that the ritual of instillation of normal saline prior to suctioning does not liquefy or break up secretions, but it may stimulate the cough response. It also may introduce bacteria present on the distal end of the ETT or TT into the lower respiratory tract, increasing the risk of nosocomial pneumonia. Instead of the instillation of normal saline, the cough response can be

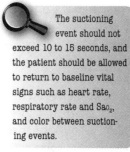

The suctioning event should not exceed 10 to 15 seconds, and the patient should be allowed to return to baseline vital signs such as heart rate, respiratory rate and Sao_2, and color between suctioning events.

stimulated during suctioning using the "sigh" setting on the ventilator or by using a manual resuscitation bag. Wall suction should be regulated not to exceed a maximum of 120 mmHg. The suctioning event should not exceed 10 to 15 seconds, and the patient should be allowed to return to baseline vital signs such as heart rate, respiratory rate and Sao_2, and color between suctioning events. The nurse must be cognizant of the possible complications of suctioning including hypoxemia, hypoxia, tissue trauma to the tracheal and/or bronchial mucosa, cardiac dysrhythmias or arrest, bronchospasm, pulmonary bleeding, hemorrhage, infection, hyper- or hypotension, and be prepared to intervene if they should occur.

> The nurse must be cognizant of the possible complications of ETT suctioning: hypoxemia, hypoxia, tissue trauma to the tracheal and/or bronchial mucosa, cardiac dysrhythmias or arrest, bronchospasm, pulmonary bleeding, hemorrhage, infection, and hyper- or hypotension.

Impaired Communication

Any patient being mechanically ventilated either by endotracheal (ET) or tracheostomy (T) tube is unable to speak. Endotracheal tubes pass directly through the vocal cords. A tracheostomy tube is situated below the vocal cords but with the cuff inflated (required for positive pressure ventilation) air does not pass through the vocal cords. Many of these patients have manual dexterity and/or visual impairments that limit their ability to communicate via the written word. Patients with dentures and ETTs will have had dentures removed; altering the musculature in the face. The ETT will be taped to their mouths or faces, making even lip-reading almost impossible.

The nurse, working with the respiratory therapist and speech therapist, must establish a form of communication to handle at least the patient's basic needs (i.e., pain, toileting, and thirst). The inability to communicate creates anxiety in the patient, and anxiety can play a major role in a patient's ability to tolerate mechanical ventilation. Inability to communicate also produces feelings of isolation. By establishing a communication system, the nurse can assist the patient to regain some control over the environment. There are valves on the market that can be utilized with mechanically ventilated patients to facilitate speaking. These valves require intense manipulation and monitoring of ventilatory parameters and are commonly only used for very short periods of time.

 Any patient being mechanically ventilated either by endotracheal (ET) or tracheostomy (T) tube is unable to speak. By establishing a communication system, the nurse can assist the patient to regain some control over the environment.

Fear and Anxiety

Many patients report fear as a dominant experience during mechanical ventilation. Ventilators have many alarms that often sound for benign problems (e.g., high pressure secondary to a cough or hiccup). However, the patient experiences the alarms as something seriously wrong and possibly life-threatening. They may experience extreme dyspnea as a result of a "disconnect" from the ventilator and they are unable to call for help. It is of utmost importance for the nurse to provide support to these patients, assure them of their safety, and educate them as to the response time of the staff.

Powerlessness

All patients requiring mechanical ventilation are tethered to a machine. This condition limits their ability to communicate, toilet themselves, and even change position. Many mechanically ventilated patients are receiving drugs that alter their sensorium and judgment requiring measures to ensure their safety, including wrist restraints, bite blocks, and side rails. Bite blocks are used to prevent biting down on the ETT as this may interrupt gas flow and possibly damage the

 Many mechanically ventilated patients are receiving drugs that alter their sensorium and judgment and may require measures to ensure their safety, including wrist restraints, bite blocks, and side rails.

conduit to the cuff. These safety measures may also engender powerlessness. The nurse can mitigate some sources of powerlessness by offering choices during routine care such as treatment scheduling, rest periods, and positioning. The nurse also needs to elicit the patient's desires and needs and incorporate these into the plan of care.

Isolation and Sensory Deprivation

Mechanically ventilated patients are unable to communicate easily, limited in their physical activity, and often in a single room. These conditions can contribute to sensory deprivation and loneliness. Nurses have an enormous impact on the patient's experience. Interview the patient and family to discover this patient's interests and incorporate them into the plan of care. Watching baseball on TV, listening to show tunes, affixing a bird feeder to the window, or arranging for family, friends, and volunteers (or nurses if time permits) to read or play cards with the patient will go a long way toward lifting spirits. Complementary therapies such as massage, guided imagery, healing touch, therapeutic touch, and acupressure can be employed to help allay fear and feelings of isolation.

Altered Nutritional Intake

All patients on mechanical ventilation are unable to eat normally. The ETT bypasses the protective reflex of epiglottis closure, making normal eating impossible. The tracheostomy tube cuff impinges into the esophageal space, possibly compromising the ability to swallow. Malnutrition is a common problem in this population. Malnutrition leads to a loss of muscle mass and strength. The diaphragm, the major muscle of ventilation, is weakened early on by malnutrition. This weakening of the diaphragm can produce an ineffective breathing pattern. This causes fatigue, further compromising the patient's ability to wean from the venti-

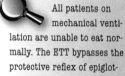

All patients on mechanical ventilation are unable to eat normally. The ETT bypasses the protective reflex of epiglottis closure, making normal eating impossible.

lator. The nurse needs to consult with the dietitian to formulate a plan for the institution and monitoring of nutritional support. Enteral feedings are the preferred method if the patient can tolerate this. Electrolytes must be monitored closely. Adequate amounts of calcium, magnesium, and phosphorous are essential for respiratory muscle contraction.

The inability to take anything by mouth intensifies the patient's need for excellent oral hygiene. Most intubated patients have their mouths

partially kept open by the ETT, exposing
the mucus membranes to dehydration. Oral
secretions contain numerous bacteria that
can be introduced into the lower respiratory
tract during routine care, increasing the risk
for nosocomial infection in mechanically
ventilated patients. Also, many patients are
dehydrated from medication such as diuret
ics for their underlying medical problems.
Many products exist to cleanse and hydrate the oral cavity. Oral care is a
task easily taught to family members and may provide patients and their
family members with much comfort and relief as they are more involved
in the patients' care.

Oral secretions contain numerous bacteria that can be introduced into the lower respiratory tract during routine care, increasing the risk for nosocomial infection in mechanically ventilated patients.

Altered Bowel Functioning

Patients on mechanical ventilation may have a variety of elimination
problems related to medications, altered nutritional intake, and inactivity. As a result of the necessity of enteral tube feeding, many ventilated
patients suffer from diarrhea. Research at this time does not support the
use of one feeding method, bolus or continuous, over another. The nurse
must provide for adequate toileting, skin protection, and medication to
alleviate diarrhea. Electrolyte levels, especially potassium, need to be
closely monitored in patients experiencing diarrhea.

Many patients who require mechanical ventilation are receiving high
doses of analgesic and anxiolytic medications. These medications, especially when coupled with inactivity and low-fiber enteral feedings, decrease bowel motility and can lead to constipation and an ileus. Patients
receiving enteral feedings must have comprehensive abdominal assessments, which include observation of the
size of the abdomen, auscultation of bowel
sounds, palpation to detect firmness or pain,
careful monitoring for the frequency and
quality of bowel movements, and quantity of
residual tube feedings in the stomach after a
predetermined time. The nurse should col-
laborate with the physician around the use
of a promotility agent to help prevent the
development of an ileus. The use of stool
softeners and laxatives to maintain adequate

Many patients who require mechanical ventilation are receiving high doses of analgesic and anxiolytic medications. These medications, especially when coupled with inactivity and low-fiber enteral feedings, decrease bowel motility and can lead to constipation and an ileus.

bowel function is frequently necessary because of inadequate fiber in commercially prepared enteral feeding formulas, medications that slow bowel function, and relative lack of physical activity.

Disuse Syndrome

Many ventilated patients are initially confined to bed by their underlying medical problem and confined to a limited geographic area as a result of being tethered to a ventilator. The lack of mobility imposed by mechanical ventilation results in "disuse syndrome," a degradation of muscle tissue

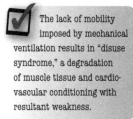

The lack of mobility imposed by mechanical ventilation results in "disuse syndrome," a degradation of muscle tissue and cardiovascular conditioning with resultant weakness.

and cardiovascular conditioning with resultant weakness. As soon as the patient is stable, the nurse, OT/PT, and the patient should formulate a conditioning program. Physical exercise improves overall muscle tone and strength, facilitates gas exchange, promoting oxygen delivery to the tissues, and improves mood. Improved muscle strength enhances a patient's ability to wean from ventilatory support. Family members can also be encouraged to participate in training by being taught the regimen and acting as coaches for the patient.

Complications of Mechanical Ventilation

Intubation and mechanical ventilation may produce many adverse sequelae (see Table 4-11). A manual resuscitation bag with an oxygen source must be readily available in case of equipment failure or malfunction or loss of electrical power. Many ventilators do not have backup battery systems.

Positive pressure ventilation can cause serious physiologic complications. Pulmonary **barotrauma** related to overdistention of the alveolar units may result in pneumothorax, pneumomediastinum, and subcutaneous emphysema. Positive pressure ventilation increases intrathoracic pressure, thereby decreasing venous return to the heart. This may result in decreased cardiac output that may cause a compensatory increase in HR. Decreased cardiac output also may decrease blood pressure, thereby decreasing blood and oxygen delivery to the tissues.

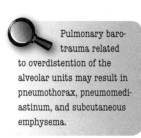

Pulmonary barotrauma related to overdistention of the alveolar units may result in pneumothorax, pneumomediastinum, and subcutaneous emphysema.

Table 4-11 Complications of Mechanical Ventilation

Mechanical
1. Failure in ventilator function or alarm system
2. Loss of electrical power
3. Inadequate humidification
4. Overheating of inspired air leading to mild hyperthermia
5. Volume overload due to humidification of inspired air

Physiologic
1. Barotrauma: pneumothorax, pneumomediastinum, subcutaneous emphysema
2. Cardiac dysrhythmias
3. Decreased cardiac output: tachycardia, hypotension, tissue hypoxia, water and salt retention
4. Oxygen toxicity
5. Tracheal or laryngeal damage
6. Stress ulcer or gastritis
7. Aspiration of gastric contents
8. Nosocomial pulmonary infection

Decreased oxygen to the tissues can result in tissue hypoxia and possible anaerobic metabolism, leading to acidemia. Decreased cardiac output may also trigger a compensatory increase in the secretion of antidiuretic hormone (ADH) and aldosterone that leads

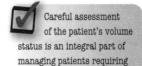

Careful assessment of the patient's volume status is an integral part of managing patients requiring mechanical ventilation.

to salt and water retention. Recognize, report, and intervene quickly to prevent long-term effects from positive pressure ventilation. For example, the prescribing physician may decide it is appropriate to treat cardiac dysrhythmias by increasing the FiO_2. Signs and symptoms of decreased cardiac output may be treated by decreasing the amount of PEEP or tidal volume. Careful assessment of the patient's volume status is an integral part of managing patients requiring mechanical ventilation.

To utilize positive pressure ventilation, the endotracheal tubes must have a cuff that seals the trachea during ventilation. This cuff exerts pressure. If the pressure in the cuff of the endotracheal tube exceeds capillary arterial perfusion pressure, approximately 30 to 32 cm H_2O in a patient with normal hemodynamics, then blood flow to the tracheal tissues will be compromised. Because venous and lymphatic flow occurs at even lower pressures, ideally the cuff pressure should be maintained at

25 cm H_2O. Higher pressures result in a decreased blood flow and subsequently impair oxygen delivery to the tracheal tissue. This in turn may cause tissue erosion and ischemic damage leading to the development of **tracheomalacia** and possible tracheoesophageal fistula. To prevent this, cuff pressure should be measured at least every 24 hours. Pressures in the cuff may be measured with a standard sphygmomanometer or aneroid cuff pressure manometer, such as the cufflator. If pressure exceeds 25 cm H_2O, the physician should be notified and steps taken to remedy the situation. These steps may include administering sedative agents to reduce tracheal muscle tone or possibly changing the endotracheal tube to one with a smaller diameter.

If the pressure in the cuff of the endotracheal tube exceeds capillary arterial perfusion pressure, approximately 30 to 32 cm H_2O in a patient with normal hemodynamics, then blood flow to the tracheal tissues will be compromised.

The ETT can move for a variety of reasons, resulting in a cuff that does not totally occlude the trachea. If the cuff does not occlude the trachea, the patient may aspirate oral secretions or gastric contents into the lungs. Endotracheal and tracheostomy tubes bypass the normal lines of defense for the lung, putting patients at higher risk for acquiring nosocomial and aspiration pneumonias.

Research has demonstrated that patients being treated with mechanical ventilation are at very high risk of developing stress ulcers or gastritis. Monitor the patient for complaints of gastric discomfort or the presence of blood in the gastric aspirate or stool. Most physicians prescribe medications (i.e., a hydrogen ion blocker or proton pump inhibitor) for stress ulcer prophylaxis for mechanically ventilated patients.

The use of mechanical ventilation places enormous responsibility on all the disciplines caring for these patients. Coordinated care and good communication are necessary to provide frequent assessments, early interventions, and safe and effective treatments.

Weaning from Mechanical Ventilation

No simple parameters exist that indicate when weaning or liberation from mechanical ventilation should be attempted. The underlying condition that precipitated the institution of mechanical ventilation should be resolved or at least improving. Weaning is usually not attempted until the Fio_2 is less than 50%, PEEP is less than 10 cm H_2O, and the patient is hemodynamically stable and possesses intact protective (cough, gag) reflexes. Research demonstrates that if a patient cannot generate a negative inspiratory force when coughing (NIF: the amount of negative pressure the patient can generate when inhaling against a closed valve) of greater than -20 cm H_2O and a vital capacity (quantity of gas exhaled after the deepest possible inhalation) of greater than 10 to 15 cc/kg, then the probability of successful weaning is very low. A variety of methodologies and ventilatory modes are employed to wean patients from ventilatory support. These techniques include the use of a T-piece, CPAP, IMV, and PSV.

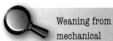 Weaning from mechanical ventilation is usually not attempted until the Fio_2 is less than 50%, PEEP is less than 10 cm H_2O, and the patient is hemodynamically stable and possesses intact protective (cough, gag) reflexes.

The collaborative team should begin to prepare patients and families for the experience of weaning as soon as it is appropriate to do so. The process of weaning must be carefully explained to patients and families to avoid fear and undue anxiety. The patient must be reassured that he or she will not be alone during the weaning process and struggling for breath, and that a team member will be closely monitoring the condition and progress. Team members and family can provide emotional support and act as coaches and cheerleaders.

 The patient must be reassured that he or she will not be alone during the weaning process and struggling for breath, and that a team member will be closely monitoring the condition and progress.

The patient should be placed in a position that will facilitate diaphragmatic movement. Sitting or semirecumbent positions are usually the best tolerated. The airway should be cleared of any secretions. The use of complementary therapies, such as music therapy, guided imagery, and biofeedback, should be explored with the patient to decrease anxiety during the weaning process.

Common practice is to attempt **extubation**, removal of the ETT, if the patient meets the following criteria:

- Intact protective reflexes (cough and gag)
- Capable of generating a Vt of 5 cc/kg, a VC of 10 cc/kg

- NIF greater than -20 cm H_2O
- Minute volume of 6 to 10 L/minute
- Sao_2 greater than 92%
- RR, HR, and BP within 10% to 20% of baseline

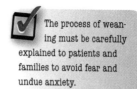
The process of weaning must be carefully explained to patients and families to avoid fear and undue anxiety.

If these criteria are met, then extubation can be attempted. If these criteria are unable to be met, then depending on the wishes of the patient, family, and durable power of attorney, the option of either a tracheostomy (see tracheostomy section) or terminal wean will be pursued.

Nursing Care for the Patient During Weaning from Mechanical Ventilation

1. Prepare patients and families for the experience of weaning and reassure them that they will not be alone and struggling for breath and that a team member will be closely monitoring their condition and progress.

2. Place patient in a sitting or semirecumbent position to allow for the most diaphragmatic movement.

3. Clear the airway of any secretions.

4. Establish patient possesses intact cough and gag reflexes.

5. Ensure that the patient requires an Fio_2 of less than 50% to maintain an Sao_2 greater than 92%.

6. PEEP is less than 10 cm H_2O.

7. Vital capacity (quantity of gas exhaled after the deepest possible inhalation) of greater than 10 to 15 cc/kg and a tidal volume of 5 cc/kg

8. Minute volume of 6 to 10 L/min

9. Respiratory rate, heart rate, and blood pressure within 10–20% of baseline

10. Patient can generate a negative inspiratory force (NIF) of greater than -20 cm H_2O when coughing.

11. Assess patient's vital signs frequently, and monitor for signs of respiratory distress.

12. Continue supplemental oxygen as ordered to maintain Sao_2 greater than 92%.

Extubation

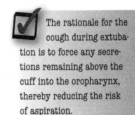

The rationale for the cough during extubation is to force any secretions remaining above the cuff into the oropharynx, thereby reducing the risk of aspiration.

If a patient has been successfully weaned from the ventilator, either the physician, nurse, or respiratory therapist will remove the ETT. Explain the procedure to the patient. Usually patients who have been intubated require supplemental oxygen after extubation; therefore, this should be set up and ready for use prior to extubation. Then, with the patient in an upright or semirecumbent position, the ETT and mouth are suctioned. The tape is removed, the patient is instructed to take a deep breath, and the cuff is deflated via aspiration of the pilot balloon. The patient is told to cough while the tube is swiftly removed. The rationale for the cough during extubation is to force any secretions remaining above the cuff into the oropharynx, thereby reducing the risk of aspiration. Supplemental oxygen, if prescribed, should be administered at this point and titrated to maintain prescribed Sao_2.

The patient should be asked to speak and cough. Patients need to be closely monitored postextubation for the development of upper airway obstruction due to vocal cord or laryngeal edema. In this case, the patient will become stridorous and dyspneic. This is an emergency, and the physician should be contacted immediately. Cool mist and/or nebulized racemic epinephrine may be utilized to reduce edema. If these treatments are unsuccessful and the patient's airway is compromised, immediate intubation or tracheostomy is indicated. Many patients postextubation experience hoarseness and difficulty swallowing. Food and fluids are usually withheld for a period of hours postextubation. Ice chips are normally allowed. When fluids are begun, water is first given so that the nurse can assess the patient's ability to swallow.

Patients need to be closely monitored postextubation for the development of upper airway obstruction caused by vocal cord or laryngeal edema.

Nursing Care During Extubation

1. Explain the procedure to the patient.

2. Set up supplemental oxygen for use prior to extubation.

3. Place the patient in an upright or semirecumbent position.

4. Suction the ETT and mouth.

5. Remove the tape.

6. Instruct the patient to take a deep breath.

7. Deflate the cuff via aspiration of the pilot balloon.

8. Instruct the patient to cough while the tube is swiftly removed.

9. Give supplemental oxygen as ordered.

10. Ask the patient to cough and speak.

11. Monitor vital signs frequently and report signs of respiratory distress.

Tracheostomy

A **tracheotomy** is a surgical incision into the trachea in the area of the second, third, and fourth tracheal rings (see Figure 4-7). A **tracheostomy** is the resulting opening, or stoma, that is made during a tracheotomy procedure. A tracheostomy tube is inserted into the stoma. A tracheostomy is used for a variety of reasons; however, use of a tracheostomy tube implies that an artificial airway will be necessary for a prolonged period of time. A tracheostomy is performed when a patient has been unsuccessful at weaning from ventilatory support. This usually occurs between 2 weeks and 4 weeks after the initial intubation.

Indications for tracheostomy include the following:

1. Long-term secretion management

2. Airway protection from aspiration

3. Acute upper airway obstruction from trauma or burns

4. Prophylaxis against airway obstruction: radical neck, neurological surgeries, laryngectomy

5. Prolonged intubation and mechanical ventilation are necessary to maintain oxygenation.

Tracheostomy tubes are generally better tolerated than endotracheal intubation. They create less airflow resistance, allowing for improved oral care and intake, and may permit talking, depending on the patient condition and tube design. Tracheostomy tubes are available in a number of materials, sizes, and designs: cuffed or uncuffed, plastic, nylon or metal, single or double lumen, and fenestrated or nonfenestrated.

 Tracheostomy tubes create less airflow resistance, allowing for improved oral care and intake, and may permit talking, depending on the patient condition and tube design.

Generally, tracheostomy tubes consist of a neck flange, which rests flush against the skin on the neck. The flange has openings at both sides through which cloth or Velcro ties are inserted for securing the airway. The flange should be secured against the skin of the patient's neck to prevent movement of the tube in the stoma, minimizing airway trauma. The tube itself usually has a 15 mm adaptor on the proximal end, allowing easy interface with ventilatory devices. Most plastic tracheostomy tubes have a radiopaque stripe for radiologic position identification. On the proximal end of cuffed tubes is a cuff whose design and function mirror that of an ETT (see section on endotracheal intubation). An **obturator** (a device to block the opening of the tube) is included with the tracheostomy tube. When inserted into the tube, the obturator's smooth, rounded tip slightly protrudes from the body of the tube. The function of the obturator is to prevent injury to the tracheal wall during insertion of the tracheostomy tube. After insertion, it must be removed to allow air to pass through the tube. The obturator is usually kept at the bedside should emergency reinsertion of the tube be necessary.

Tracheostomy care (see Table 4-12) is necessary to keep the tracheostomy tube and stoma clean, dry, and free from secretions and mucus, thereby preventing infection and maintaining a patent airway. In acute care, the tracheostomy tube is suctioned prior to the onset of tracheostomy care to remove

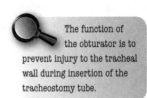 The function of the obturator is to prevent injury to the tracheal wall during insertion of the tracheostomy tube.

any excess secretions. The nurse must assure that the tracheostomy tube is secure at all times to prevent accidental dislodgment. Tracheostomy ties are usually changed every 24 hours or when necessary. Velcro or other manufactured devices are changed as needed. A properly applied tracheostomy-securing device allows space for one finger to be placed between the tie and the neck.

Table 4-12 Tracheostomy Care (in the Acute Setting)

1. Assemble the following equipment
   - Goggles
   - Sterile gloves
   - Scissors (if tracheostomy ties are in place)
   - Sterile normal saline
   - Suctioning equipment
   - Tracheostomy care components or kit:
     - H_2O_2
     - Sterile, precut tracheostomy dressing (precut, sewn-edge dressings necessary to prevent threads from falling into the stoma and lung)
     - Tracheostomy securing devices: ties, Velcro holder
     - Pipe cleaners, brush cleaner, cotton-tipped swabs
     - Forceps
     - 4 x 4 sterile gauze pads, two sterile bowls
     - Sterile inner cannula (if indicated)
2. Wash hands.
3. Explain procedure to patient.
4. Place patient in position of comfort (this allows nurse easier access to tracheostomy).
5. Suction the tracheostomy tube.
6. Remove soiled dressing and discard in appropriate receptacle.
7. Pour half-strength H_2O_2 into one bowl and plain normal saline into other.
8. Wear sterile gloves.
9. Remove inner cannula and either discard or cleanse it (according to institutional policy):
   - Immerse inner cannula in half-strength H_2O_2.
   - Use brush and pipe cleaners to remove secretions.
   - Immerse cannula in N/S, and remove excess solution with sterile gauze.
   - Reinsert cannula, assuring it is locked in place. If patient is ventilator dependent or outer cannula diameter is not correct size, attach an adapter or spare inner cannula to ventilator to assure uninterrupted ventilation.
   - Wet sterile gauze or cotton-tipped swabs with sterile N/S, and clean peristomal skin.
   - Change tracheostomy ties.

The type of tracheostomy care varies depending on the type of tube. If the tracheostomy tube is a single lumen, only stoma care is required. If it is a double lumen, the inner cannula may need to be changed or cleaned. If the inner cannula is disposable, current recommendations allow for its replacement every 24 hours. If the inner cannula is not disposable, it is recommended that it be cleansed every 8 hours and whenever necessary with half-strength hydrogen peroxide. Tracheostomy dressings should be changed whenever they are wet or soiled. Wetness irritates the skin and provides an excellent medium for

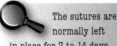
The sutures are normally left in place for 7 to 14 days, allowing for a tracheostomy tract to form.

the growth of bacteria. Some tracheostomies are sutured into place to prevent dislodgment. The sutures are normally left in place for 7 to 14 days, allowing for a tracheostomy tract to form. Care must be taken to assess what effect the sutures have on the peristomal skin and note any breakdown.

Decannulation

If the indications for tracheostomy have been resolved and the patient is stable, then the physician will make the decision to proceed with removal of the tracheostomy tube (**decannulation**). This process may either be immediate or gradual. In immediate decannulation, the tracheostomy tube is removed and the stoma covered by a sterile, nonocclusive dressing. If air loss is a problem, then the stoma may be covered with petroleum-impregnated gauze and covered by dry gauze. The patient will immediately need to use his or her natural airway for ventilation and secretion removal.

There are multiple techniques for gradual decannulation. The tracheostomy tube may be replaced at prescribed intervals by a tube of a smaller size—downsizing. This allows for gradual closing of the stoma. The tracheostomy tube may also be plugged for a prescribed period of time and the patient assessed for the tolerance to this procedure. If it is well-tolerated, immediate decannulation may ensue. A tracheostomy button may be placed in the tracheal stoma after decannulation. The tracheostomy button prevents the stoma from closing, thereby allowing for immediate access should that be necessary. With the button in place, the patient must use his or her natural airway for ventilation and secretion removal.

Tracheostomy care may be done with two people; one person securing the tube while the other removes the ties and performs the care. If the nurse performs tracheostomy care alone, the old ties must remain intact until the new ties are secured.

The tracheostomy button prevents the stoma from closing, thereby allowing for immediate access should that be necessary.

Changing tracheostomy ties involves the following steps:

1. Manufacturer's devices should be changed according to their instruction.

2. If using cloth ties:
   • Assure skin on the neck is clean, dry, and without breakdown. If breakdown is present, treat according to institutional guidelines.
   • Cut hole 3/4 of an inch from end of tape.
   • Pass cut end through the hole in flange of tracheostomy tube.
   • Thread noncut end through hole and pull tightly. Do this on both sides.
   • Bring ties to side of neck and tie with a square knot. Knot must be secured so only one finger can be placed between tie and neck.

3. Place new tracheostomy dressing around the tube.

CHAPTER 4 MULTIPLE-CHOICE QUESTIONS

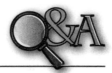

1. When Mr. J is receiving oxygen via nasal prongs, the nurse understands that this method of oxygen administration does all of the following except:
   a. Delivers a set concentration of oxygen
   b. Does not require humidification
   c. Is traumatic to the respiratory tract
   d. Allows the patient to speak

2. If Mr. J's O_2 saturation does not respond to oxygen delivered by nasal prongs, then a facial mask with a reservoir bag may be needed. The risks of higher inspired oxygen (FiO_2) include all of the following except:
   a. Dryness of the mucus membranes
   b. Risk of hypoventilation
   c. Potential for oxygen toxicity
   d. Excessive, watery pulmonary secretions

3. After a chest X-ray, a diagnosis of left lower lobe pneumonia is made. Chest physical therapy and an incentive spirometer are ordered. All the following actions show that the patient understands how to use the spirometer except:
   a. The patient holds the spirometer in the upright position.
   b. The patient places the spirometer in his mouth and completely exhales.
   c. The patient places the spirometer in his mouth, takes a deep breath, and holds it for 2 to 5 seconds before removing the mouthpiece and exhaling.
   d. The patient tries to cough after using the spirometer.

4. Mr. J's fever has resolved, and he is being discharged with theophylline, as well as with clarithromycin, an antibiotic. Your teaching about theophylline would include all of the following except:
a. Take theophylline on an empty stomach.
b. Report signs of theophylline toxicity such as nausea, dizziness, rapid heart rate, or muscle twitching to the healthcare provider.
c. Decrease caffeine and chocolate intake as theophylline has similar effects.
d. Take theophylline at regular intervals.

5. Which type of mechanical ventilation supplies all ventilation to the patient?
a. Pressure control ventilation
b. Pressure support ventilation
c. Synchronized intermittent mandatory ventilation
d. Controlled mechanical ventilation

CHAPTER 4 ANSWERS AND RATIONALES

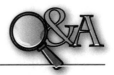

1. c.

   Rationale: Nasal prongs or cannula are the least traumatic oxygen delivery system.

2. d.

   Rationale: Higher levels of Fio_2 do not produce increased pulmonary secretions but are usually more drying.

3. b.

   Rationale: Most incentive spirometers are used to improve inspiratory capacity and are used during inhalation.

4. a.

   Rationale: Theophylline should be taken on a full stomach because of the risk of stomach upset.

5. d.

   Rationale: Controlled mechanical ventilation is used to fully support patient breathing in patients who are not breathing spontaneously.

The cardiovascular and respiratory systems are both integral to oxygenation. The cardiovascular system provides oxygen to the tissues and removes carbon dioxide and waste products. In this chapter, we will review the following:

- Anatomy of the cardiovascular system

- Processes of circulation and perfusion

- Relationships between resistance, pressure, viscosity, and blood flow

- Components of blood pressure

5

Anatomy and Physiology of the Cardiovascular System

TERMS
- ☐ perfusion
- ☐ myocardium
- ☐ pulmonic circuit
- ☐ systemic circuit
- ☐ blood pressure
- ☐ resistance
- ☐ cardiac output
- ☐ sinoatrial node
- ☐ diastole
- ☐ systole

CASE STUDY

Mr. M is a 76-year-old man with newly diagnosed coronary artery disease. In the past, he has had chest pain after overexerting himself. When this happens, he usually stops what he is doing, sits down, and the pain subsides in a few minutes. Today, he wants to know why he still has chest pain even after sitting down for an hour.

INTRODUCTION

Although the respiratory system provides oxygen to the body, it is the cardiovascular system that moves the oxygen to the cells and removes carbon dioxide. The heart works as a pump to move oxygenated blood throughout the arterial system and returns deoxygenated blood to the heart and lungs via the venous system. This process of pumping and circulating is called **perfusion**, and without it the other processes—ventilation and diffusion—would not provide oxygen to the cells.

The cardiovascular system is composed of two parts: a heart that pumps the blood and the vascular network through which blood is channeled. The vascular network consists of **arteries** and **veins.** The arteries carry blood away from the heart, and the veins return blood to the heart. In this chapter, the heart and the components of the vascular network will be discussed as they pertain to the process of oxygenation.

THE HEART

The heart is an amazing organ and the cardiovascular system could not function without it. Although the heart is small, about the size of a clenched fist in an adult, it can pump 100,000 times a day. The heart rate can change depending on the needs of the body. The heart rate and cardiac output are finely regulated by neural and hormonal mechanisms to ensure oxygenation of the tissues.

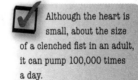
Although the heart is small, about the size of a clenched fist in an adult, it can pump 100,000 times a day.

The heart is a muscular organ, lying near the center of the thoracic cavity (see Figure 5-1). It is somewhat anterior in the chest and situated directly behind the sternum. The heart lies within a pericardial cavity, which is lined by a thin, serous membrane called the **pericardium**. A membrane called the **epicardium** surrounds the heart itself. Pericardial fluid is the lubricant between the pericardium and the epicardium. There is only about 10 cc of pericardial fluid, but it reduces friction between the surfaces of the two membranes.

The heart is composed of three layers: the epicardium, the **myocardium** or cardiac muscle, and the endocardium. The epicardium is one of three layers of the heart that is part of the serous pericardium. The myocardium contracts rhythmically to move blood through the heart, into the pulmonary vasculature, and out again into the systemic vasculature. The **endocardium** is the lining of the inner surfaces of the heart's chambers.

The heart is divided into four chambers: the **right atrium**, the **right ventricle**, the **left atrium**, and the **left ventricle** (see Figure 5-2). The atria serve to collect blood as it returns to the heart, draining it into the ventricles to be pumped into circulation. The atria contract at the end of diastole, providing the "**atrial kick**"—a 30% increase in blood return to the ventricle that is particularly useful in increasing cardiac output during exertion.

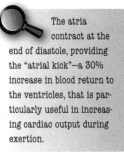 The atria contract at the end of diastole, providing the "atrial kick"—a 30% increase in blood return to the ventricles, that is particularly useful in increasing cardiac output during exertion.

The two cycles of the heart are referred to as diastole and systole. During **diastole**, the chambers of the heart fill with blood. **Systole** is the contraction of the heart muscle, expelling blood from the heart into the aorta and

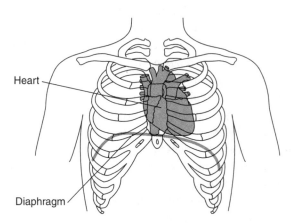

Heart

Diaphragm

Figure 5-1 Position of the heart in the thoracic cavity.

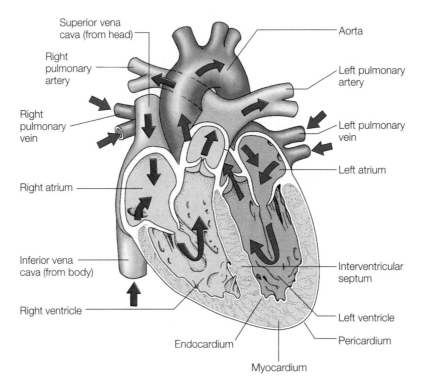

Superior vena cava (from head)
Right pulmonary artery
Right pulmonary vein
Right atrium
Inferior vena cava (from body)
Right ventricle
Endocardium
Myocardium
Aorta
Left pulmonary artery
Left pulmonary vein
Left atrium
Interventricular septum
Left ventricle
Pericardium

Figure 5-2 The chambers and the layers of the heart.

pulmonary artery. Venous blood enters the right atrium from the superior and inferior vena cavae. It flows into the right ventricle and then leaves the right side of the heart via the pulmonary artery. Blood passes through the pulmonary vasculature in the lungs, where gas exchange takes place at the alveolar membrane. Reoxygenated blood returns to the left side of the heart at the left atrium via the pulmonary vein. It moves into the left ventricle and is pushed into the aorta by the contraction of the myocardium, where it begins its journey through the systemic vasculature.

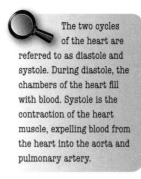

The two cycles of the heart are referred to as diastole and systole. During diastole, the chambers of the heart fill with blood. Systole is the contraction of the heart muscle, expelling blood from the heart into the aorta and pulmonary artery.

Valves control the flow of blood between the atria and ventricles of the heart and some of the blood vessels that are connected to the heart (see Figure 5-3). The valves of the heart alternately open and close to ensure one-way blood flow through the heart. There are four valves in

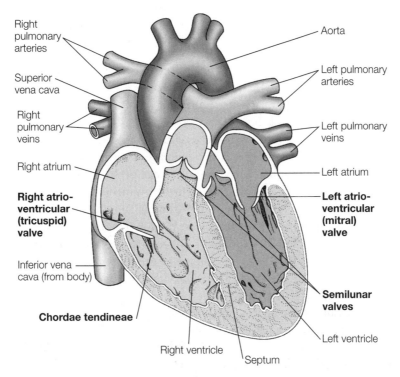

Right pulmonary arteries

Superior vena cava

Right pulmonary veins

Right atrium

Right atrio-ventricular (tricuspid) valve

Inferior vena cava (from body)

Chordae tendineae

Right ventricle

Aorta

Left pulmonary arteries

Left pulmonary veins

Left atrium

Left atrio-ventricular (mitral) valve

Semilunar valves

Left ventricle

Septum

Figure 5-3 The heart valves. A cross section of the heart showing the four chambers and the location of the major vessels and valves.

the heart: the **aortic**, **pulmonic**, **mitral**, and **tricuspid** valves. There are no valves where the large vessels drain into the atria.

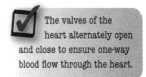

The valves of the heart alternately open and close to ensure one-way blood flow through the heart.

Circulation through the heart valves flows in an orderly sequence when the valves are working properly. Blood drains from the superior and inferior vena cavae into the right atrium. It passes the tricuspid valve lying between the right atrium and right ventricle. During systole, the pulmonic valve opens and blood flows from the right ventricle into the pulmonary artery. After a trip through the pulmonary vasculature, reoxygenated blood flows through the pulmonary vein and into the left atrium. It passes through the mitral valve between the left atrium and left ventricle. The final valve that blood passes through as it leaves the heart is the **aortic valve**, which lies where the left ventricle connects to the aorta. The closing of the heart valves can be heard as heart sounds (the assessment of heart sounds will be reviewed in Chapter 6).

Blood flows from an area of higher pressure to an area of lower pressure. As blood moves from the heart through the circulatory system, it slowly loses pressure. The blood pressure in the aorta is approximately 120/80 mmHg: 120 mmHg being the systolic blood pressure and 80 being the diastolic blood pressure. The **mean arterial pressure** is the arithmetic mean of the blood pressure in the arterial circulation (between 70 to 100 mmHg). **Mean capillary pressure**, the arithmetic mean of the blood pressure in the capillary circulation, is approximately 40 mmHg. As blood travels in the venous circulation, the mean pressure is 10 mmHg, and when it reaches the right atrium the pressure is only 2 to 5 mmHg.

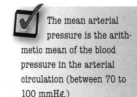

The mean arterial pressure is the arithmetic mean of the blood pressure in the arterial circulation (between 70 to 100 mmHg.)

The heart muscles work continuously, requiring oxygen and nutrients just like other tissues. The muscles of the heart are supplied with oxygen by the coronary circulation. The **coronary arteries** begin at the ascending aorta just past the aortic valve where blood pressure is the highest in the systemic circulation. They branch into smaller arteries to supply different parts of the heart muscle. When coronary arteries are blocked by atherosclerosis or clots, hypoxia occurs in the heart muscle distal to the blockage (see Figure 5-4). Patients with hypoxic cardiac tissues may experience chest pain or angina, especially during exertion. If hypoxia continues and the heart muscle does not receive enough oxygen, part of the myocardium dies. This is called a "heart attack" or **myocardial infarction**. This part of the heart muscle no longer functions properly. Depending on the location and extent of the tissue death, a myocardial infarction may make the heart incapable of maintaining adequate blood flow and output or impair the conduction system, both potentially life-threatening complications.

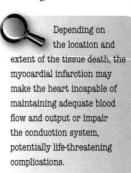

Depending on the location and extent of the tissue death, the myocardial infarction may make the heart incapable of maintaining adequate blood flow and output or impair the conduction system, potentially life-threatening complications.

Patients with hypoxic cardiac tissues may experience chest pain or angina, especially during exertion. If hypoxia continues and the heart muscle does not receive enough oxygen, part of the myocardium dies.

The myocardium contracts due to an electrical conduction system contained within the muscle walls (see Figure 5-5). This electrical sys-

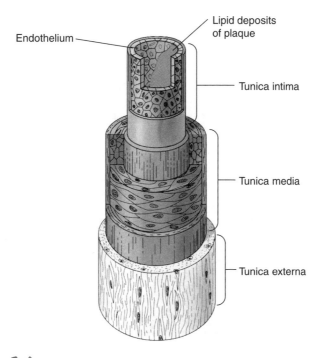

Endothelium

Lipid deposits of plaque

Tunica intima

Tunica media

Tunica externa

Figure 5-4 Cross section of arteriosclerotic plaque in an arterial wall.

tem stimulates the specialized muscle fibers of the heart to contract. The atria fill and contract first followed by the filling and contraction of the ventricles. In this rhythmic pattern the heart fills and then pushes blood out into the pulmonic and systemic circulation. The conduction system originates in the sinoatrial node in the right atrium. The **sinoatrial node (SA node)** is considered the "pacemaker of the heart." The electrical impulse travels down the fibers to the **atrioventricular node (AV node)** at the base of the right atrium. At least four smaller branches, including **Bachmann's bundle**, travel from the right atrium to the left atrium, allowing for synchronized contraction of both atria. At the AV node, the conduction pathway branches into the right and left bundle branches, innervating the ventricles of the heart. Special cells called **Purkinje fibers** carry the impulses to the myocardial cells of the ventricles. The electrical activity in the heart can be recorded on an **electrocardiogram (EKG)**. The EKG is used to represent

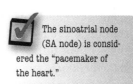

The sinoatrial node (SA node) is considered the "pacemaker of the heart."

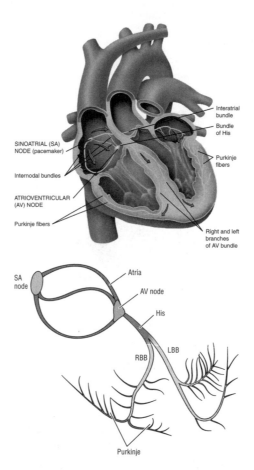

Interatrial bundle

Bundle of His

SINOATRIAL (SA) NODE (pacemaker)

Purkinje fibers

Internodal bundles

ATRIOVENTRICULAR (AV) NODE

Purkinje fibers

Right and left branches of AV bundle

SA node

Atria

AV node

His

LBB

RBB

Purkinje

Figure 5-5 The conduction system of the heart.

the mechanical activity of the heart during the cardiac cycle (the use of the EKG in the assessment of the heart will be reviewed in Chapter 6).

THE VASCULAR NETWORK

The miles and miles of blood vessels that distribute oxygen and nutrients to the cells and remove waste products make up the vascular network. This network can be further divided into two main circuits: the systemic circuit and the pulmonic circuit (see Figure 5-6). The **systemic circuit** supplies

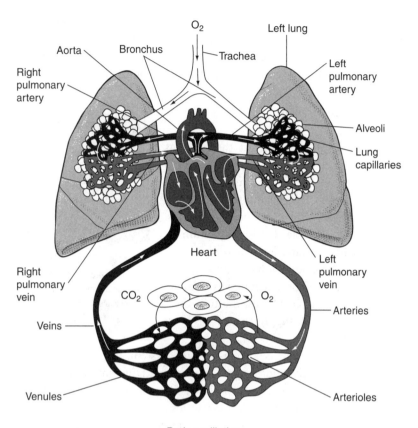

O_2

Left lung

Aorta

Bronchus

Trachea

Right pulmonary artery

Left pulmonary artery

Alveoli

Lung capillaries

Right pulmonary vein

Heart

Left pulmonary vein

CO_2

O_2

Arteries

Veins

Venules

Arterioles

Body capillaries

Figure 5-6 The vascular circuits: pulmonic and systemic.

all the body's tissues, except the lungs, with blood. The lungs are provided with blood via the **pulmonic circuit**. Both circuits are made up of a central pump (the heart), and arteries, veins, and capillaries. The pump for the pulmonic system is the right ventricle of the heart, and the pump for the systemic circuit is the left ventricle. Both circuits are connected and dependent on the adequate and equal functioning of the other. The circulatory system is a closed, pressurized system; if

There are two main circuits of circulation: the systemic circuit and the pulmonic circuit. The systemic circuit supplies all the body's tissues, except the lungs, with blood. The lungs are provided with blood via the pulmonic circuit. The pump for the pulmonic system is the right ventricle of the heart, and the pump for the systemic circuit is the left ventricle.

one side of the heart fails, then the other side is affected. For example, if a patient is in a right-sided heart failure, then blood backs up in the venous vasculature. Or, in the case of left-sided heart failure, blood will accumulate in the pulmonary vasculature with resulting pulmonary edema.

The Arterial System

The arterial system begins at the heart as the aorta leaves the left ventricle. The **aorta** is a large vessel, about 2.5 cm in diameter. The aorta begins to branch into smaller and smaller arteries and then into **arterioles**. Arteries and arterioles have a large number of elastic fibers that allow them to stretch and recoil with changing blood pressures of the cardiac cycle. Blood then moves from the arterioles into the capillaries, the tiny, thin-walled vessels that supply the tissues with oxygenated blood.

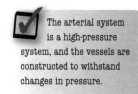

The arterial system is a high-pressure system, and the vessels are constructed to withstand changes in pressure.

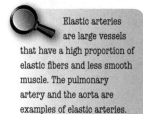

Elastic arteries are large vessels that have a high proportion of elastic fibers and less smooth muscle. The pulmonary artery and the aorta are examples of elastic arteries.

The arterial system is a high-pressure system, and the vessels are constructed to withstand changes in pressure. Different types of arteries have different proportions of elastic fibers and smooth muscle depending on their function. Elastic arteries are large vessels that have a high proportion of elastic fibers and less smooth muscle. The **pulmonary artery** and the aorta are examples of elastic arteries. They are very resilient and stretch during changes in blood pressure. Muscular arteries are medium-size arteries that distribute blood to the organs. These arteries have proportionately more smooth muscle, allowing the vessels to change diameter and blood flow to distal tissues. The carotid arteries are an example of muscular arteries.

The Capillaries

Capillaries, are the tiniest vessels in the circulatory system and the only ones that permit the exchange of gases and nutrients between the tissues and the circulating blood. Their thin walls are composed of a single layer of endothelial cells. Gaps between the endothelial cells and the specialized basement membrane allow diffusion of oxygen and carbon dioxide, as well as nutrients and cellular waste products. The average diameter of a capillary is only 8 μm. Blood flow also slows in the capillaries, allowing adequate time for diffusion. The capillaries form a network of communicating vessels called a **capillary bed** or plexus. The entrance to each capillary is guarded by a band of smooth muscle called a **precapillary sphincter** (see Figure 5-7). This sphincter controls the flow of blood into the capillary and is influenced by neural and hormonal impulses. Capillary walls are also involved in the secretion and removal of vasoactive substances in the circulation.

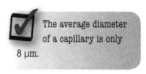

The average diameter of a capillary is only 8 μm.

The Venous System

The venous system begins when capillaries in the tissues drain deoxygenated blood back into small vessels called **venules**. The return trip to the heart and lungs is the reverse of the arterial system, with small venules merging with others to create larger and larger veins. Veins continually join together on the return path to the heart until they reach the right side of the heart as the two largest veins: the inferior and superior vena cavae.

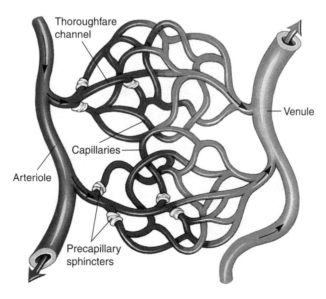

Figure 5-7 Structure of capillary bed with precapillary sphincters.

Veins are structured differently from arteries because the venous system is a low-pressure system. The blood pressure in the veins is only 10% of that in the ascending aorta, the beginning of the arterial system. The walls of veins are thinner and more elastic because they have less smooth muscle (see Figure 5-8). Veins do not have to withstand wide pressure changes like arteries, but they do have to compete with the force of gravity. A system of valves is needed to prevent backflow of blood in the smaller veins (see Figure 5-9). Large veins like the vena cavae do not have valves.

> A system of valves is needed to prevent backflow of blood in the smaller veins.

In addition to valves, the muscles of the extremities and the thoracoabdominal pump assist in returning venous blood to the heart. The skeletal muscles in the extremities push blood through the venous system as they contract and relax during activity. The **thoracoabdominal pump** refers to the pressure changes in the chest during breathing that facilitate venous blood return to the heart. On inhalation, the negative pressure in the chest pulls venous blood into the thoracic cavity and back to the right side of the heart.

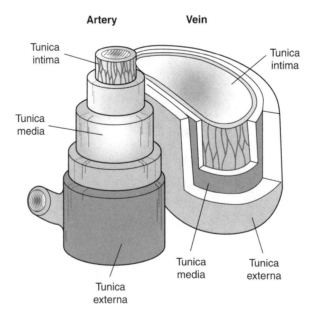

Figure 5-8 Structure of arteries versus veins.

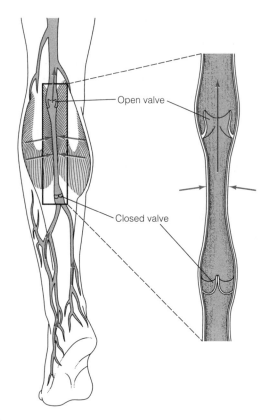

Open valve

Closed valve

Figure 5-9 Valves of the venous system preventing backflow of blood.

The Pulmonic Circuit

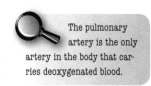

The pulmonary artery is the only artery in the body that carries deoxygenated blood.

The pulmonic circuit, as previously discussed in this chapter, is separate from the systemic vasculature. It delivers the blood from the right side of the heart to the lungs for removal of carbon dioxide from the blood followed by reoxygenation, and return of blood to the left side of the heart for delivery into the systemic circuit (see Figure 5-6). Blood leaves the right side of the heart for delivery to the lungs via the pulmonary artery. The pulmonary artery is the only artery in the body that carries deoxygenated blood. This artery branches into smaller arteries in the lungs and then into capillaries surrounding the alveoli. The walls of the alveoli are very thin, allowing for diffusion of gases. Carbon dioxide diffuses across the capillary membrane and alveolar wall into the alveoli to be exhaled. Oxygen in the alveolar air crosses over the alveolar wall into the blood. The reoxygenated blood begins its return trip to the heart via the pulmonary venules and then the larger veins. The blood returns from the lungs to the left atrium via the pulmonary vein. It is the only vein in the body that carries oxygenated blood.

The pulmonic circuit is shorter than the systemic circuit, and the vessels are much shorter. The heart and lungs are only centimeters apart. The pressure required to pump blood from the right side of the heart (**pulmonary artery pressure**) through the pulmonic circuit and back to the left side of the heart is only about 15 mmHg. This is much less than the pressure that must be generated by the left side of the heart for the systemic circuit (about 120 mmHg.)

The Structure of Arteries and Veins

Arteries and veins are hollow pipes composed of three cellular layers (see Figure 5-10). The exterior of the vessels is called the **tunica externa**. It is a connective tissue sheath that protects and supports the vessel. The middle layer of a blood vessel, the **tunica media**, is made of concentric

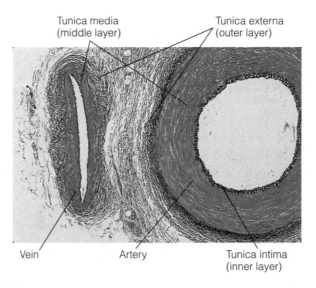

Figure 5-10 Layers of blood vessels. *Source:* © Cabisco/Visuals Unlimited.

layers of smooth muscle within a matrix of collagen and elastic fibers. The smooth muscle constricts to control the diameter of the blood vessel and regulate blood flow. The **tunica intima** is the innermost layer that lines the inside of the vessel. It is composed of a smooth layer of endothelial cells that promotes blood flow and, when functioning properly, prevents platelet adherence and clotting.

> The tunica intima is the innermost layer that lines the inside of the vessel. It is composed of a smooth layer of endothelial cells that promotes blood flow and, when functioning properly, prevents platelet adherence and clotting.

Distribution of Blood in the Vasculature

The total blood volume is not divided equally between the arterial and venous vasculature (see Figure 5-11). The arterial system (i.e., the heart, arteries, and capillaries) holds only 30% to 35% (about 1.5 L) of the total volume of blood. The remaining 65% to 70% is in the venous system (about 3.5 L). The

> The arterial system (i.e., the heart, arteries, and capillaries) holds only 30% to 35% (about 1.5 L) of the total volume of blood. The remaining 65% to 70% is in the venous system (about 3.5 L).

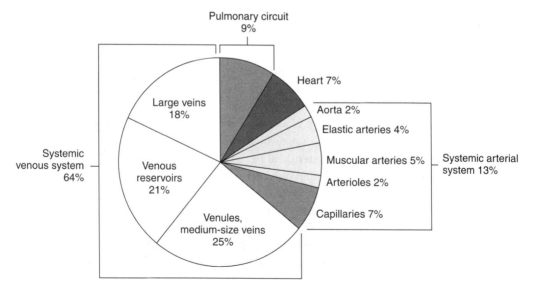

Figure 5-11 Distribution of blood in the circulatory system.

veins are thinner-walled and more elastic than the arteries and can stretch eight times more than an artery. The venous system can act as a reservoir of blood for the body. This reservoir, or **venous reserve**, can be called upon to increase arterial blood flow

 Veins are thinner-walled and more elastic than the arteries and can stretch eight times more than an artery.

if needed. For example, if severe hemorrhaging occurs, the medulla activates the smooth muscles around the veins. The veins contract and blood leaves the venous system and contributes to the general circulation to increase the blood pressure in the arterial system.

THE PHYSIOLOGY OF THE CIRCULATORY SYSTEM

The main function of the cardiovascular system is to maintain an adequate blood flow. As simple as this may sound, it takes a complex system of checks and balances to keep pace with the changing needs of different tissues in the body. Normally, blood flow is equal to the cardiac output, the volume of blood expelled by the ventricles of the heart during systole. But there are two factors that affect the flow of blood: pressure and resistance.

Pressure

Fluids flow from areas of high pressure to areas of lower pressure. Flow is proportional to the difference in pressure. **Blood pressure** is the force needed to move blood through the arterial system into the relatively lower pressures of the venous system and back to the heart. The pressure difference between the aorta, where the arterial system begins,

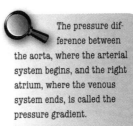 The pressure difference between the aorta, where the arterial system begins, and the right atrium, where the venous system ends, is called the pressure gradient.

and the right atrium, where the venous system ends, is called the **pressure gradient**. Blood flow through the capillaries at the cellular level is directly proportional to the arterial blood pressure. Blood pressure must be kept relatively high because of the force working against it: namely resistance.

Resistance

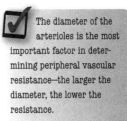

The diameter of the arterioles is the most important factor in determining peripheral vascular resistance—the larger the diameter, the lower the resistance.

Resistance is the force that opposes movement. The relationship between blood flow and resistance is inversely proportional: the greater the resistance, the lower the blood flow. **Total peripheral resistance** (**TPR**) or **systemic vascular resistance** (**SVR**) is the resistance of the entire circulatory system to blood flow. Because the greatest pressures are in the arterial system, the term **peripheral vascular resistance** refers to the resistance of the arterial system. For perfusion to occur, the circulatory pressure must be greater than the peripheral resistance. The diameter of the arterioles is the most important factor in determining peripheral vascular resistance—the larger the diameter, the lower the resistance.

Sources of resistance include vascular resistance, viscosity, and turbulence. **Vascular resistance** is the friction caused by blood moving along the vessel wall. Any decrease in the diameter of the blood vessel, particularly of the arterioles, will decrease the blood flow. The wider the diameter of the blood vessel, the more quickly the blood flows through it.

Viscosity refers to the resistance to flow caused by the friction of molecules in a liquid. The number of molecules or particles suspended in the liquid interacts to make fluids more or less viscous. A thin liquid, like water, has a low viscosity and can be moved at low pressures. A thicker liquid such as corn syrup flows at relatively higher pressures. Whole blood is about five times more viscous than water. Blood viscosity remains relatively stable except in pathological states such as dehydration or **polycythemia** (a high percentage of red blood cells in whole blood), that can change the viscosity of blood and the peripheral vascular resistance.

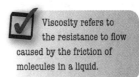

Viscosity refers to the resistance to flow caused by the friction of molecules in a liquid.

Turbulence occurs in areas of high flow, in areas of changing surfaces, and in areas of changing diameters. An example of turbulence found in nature would be the water flow over rocks in a river, causing rapids. Normally, blood flow is relatively smooth, but it becomes more turbulent when it flows through the chambers of the heart and the large vessels. Increasing turbulence slows blood flow. Turbulence through incompetent valves in the heart may be heard as murmurs through a stethoscope.

Atherosclerotic plaques can cause turbulence in larger vessels like the carotid arteries, producing sounds called **bruits**.

Atherosclerotic plaques can cause turbulence in larger vessels like the carotid arteries, producing sounds called bruits.

Blood Pressure

Blood pressure is actually three different pressures: arterial, venous, and capillary. As was previously reviewed, the rate of blood flow is dependent on the pressure and the diameter of the blood vessel. The pressure is highest at the beginning of the arterial system where the blood in the aorta leaves the left ventricle (about 120 mmHg). As blood travels away from the heart, the blood vessels become narrower and resistance increases. Blood pressure decreases continually until it reaches

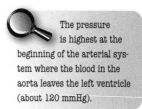

The pressure is highest at the beginning of the arterial system where the blood in the aorta leaves the left ventricle (about 120 mmHg).

the capillaries where the pressure is very low and the blood moves very slowly, allowing for diffusion across the capillary membrane. The lower pressure in the capillaries also protects the thin walls of the vessels in the capillary beds from damage. As the blood leaves the capillary beds and enters the venous system, the vessel diameters begin to increase, thus decreasing resistance. Flow increases even though the pressures are low.

The venous blood pressure is one tenth of the arterial system, but the system of valves, the muscular pump, and the thoracoabdominal pump all assist in returning venous blood to the heart. The blood pressure is lowest as blood enters the right atrium at the end of the venous system. In the pulmonic circuit, pressures are quite low when compared to the systemic circuit because the system is much shorter and the vessels are more elastic, providing less resistance.

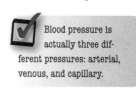

Blood pressure is actually three different pressures: arterial, venous, and capillary.

Blood pressure fluctuates depending on the cardiac cycle. It is highest when both ventricles are contracting (**systolic pressure**) and lowest when the ventricles are filling (**diastolic pressure**). Blood pressure can be measured because it not only pushes blood through the circulatory system; it also pushes outward against the vessel walls. Blood pressure can be measured using a **sphygmomanometer**. This is an inflatable cuff used to exert pressure over a muscular artery to the point that blood flow can be obstructed and then the pressure lowered so that the pressure at which blood flow returns can be heard by a stethoscope and measured.

Different arterial pulse points in the body can be palpated and used to measure the blood pressure against the vessel walls with or without a stethoscope (see Figure 5-12). Palpated blood pressures can provide a rapid systolic reading without a stethoscope.

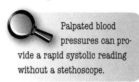

Palpated blood pressures can provide a rapid systolic reading without a stethoscope.

Blood pressure is measured in millimeters of mercury (mmHg) with systolic pressure listed over the diastolic pressure. The difference between the systolic and diastolic pressures is referred to as the **pulse pressure**:

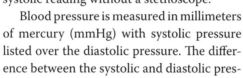

Systolic pressure – diastolic pressure = pulse pressure

* Systolic pressure/diastolic pressure: 120/80 mmHg
* Systolic pressure – diastolic pressure = pulse pressure
* If BP is 120/80, then 120 – 80 = 40 mmHg (pulse pressure)

If only a single value is used to record the blood pressure, it is referred to as the mean arterial pressure (MAP). A mean arterial pressure (MAP) is about 90 to 100 mmHg. The formula for the MAP is:

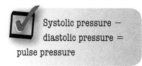

1/3 pulse pressure + diastolic pressure = mean arterial pressure

* 1/3 pulse pressure + diastolic pressure = mean arterial pressure
* If BP = 120/90 then PP = 30, so 1/3 (30) + 90 = 100

Blood pressure varies depending on the cardiac output, the peripheral vascular resistance, and the blood volume. Cardiac output and blood pressure can increase or decrease depending on the heart rate, stroke volume, and venous return to the heart. Peripheral vascular resistance can be increased by vasoconstriction and decreased by vasodilation. Changes in resistance change the blood flow and pressure. Changes in blood volume will affect the venous return to the heart. For example, if a patient is hemorrhaging, less blood will return to the heart, and the cardiac output and blood pressure will drop. How the body alters blood pressure and blood flow to compensate for the changing needs of the tissues will be reviewed in the next section.

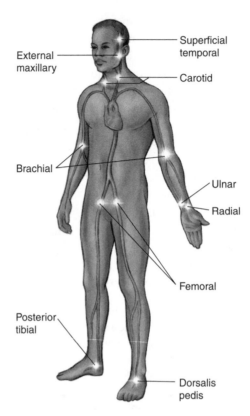

Figure 5-12 Arterial pulses.

 # REGULATION OF THE CARDIOVASCULAR SYSTEM

Many mechanisms are involved in maintaining adequate perfusion of the tissues. All cells require oxygen and nutrients to function and waste products need to be removed. Whether blood reaches the cellular level depends on the cardiac output, the blood pressure, and the peripheral resistance (see Figure 5-13).

Cardiac output (CO) is the volume of blood pumped every minute into the systemic circulation by the heart. It is normally equal to peripheral blood flow. Cardiac output is affected by the heart rate, the stroke volume, and the peripheral resistance (see Figure 5-14). The formula for calculating the cardiac output is:

Cardiac output (CO) = stroke volume (SV) × heart rate (HR)

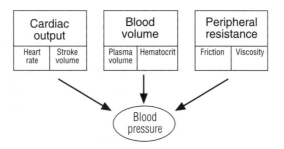

Figure 5-13 Factors influencing blood pressure.

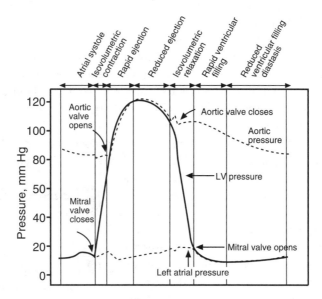

Figure 5-14 Pressure wave.

For example:

$$SV\ (80\ mL) \times HR\ (60\ bpm) = CO\ (4800\ mL\ or\ 4.8\ L/min)$$

A discussion of each factor influencing the cardiac output, heart rate, stroke volume, and peripheral vascular resistance will clarify how important the heart's pumping action is to the oxygenation of the tissues.

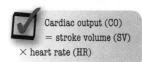

Cardiac output (CO)
= stroke volume (SV)
× heart rate (HR)

Heart Rate

The heart rate is influenced by local, neural, and hormonal factors. The SA node of the heart is the pacemaker of the heart and sets the heart rate, which is normally 60 to 100 beats per minute. This intrinsic rate can be altered by the autonomic nervous system (ANS). The cardiac centers for the ANS are located in the medulla and receive input from the hypothalamus and the peripheral chemoreceptors and barore-ceptors. The chemoreceptors in the aortic arch and carotid bodies provide information about the oxygen and carbon dioxide lev-els in the blood. The baroreceptors provide information about the blood pressure. All this information is coordinated to adjust the functioning of the cardio-vascular system. For example, if the oxygen levels or the blood pressure fall or the carbon dioxide levels rise, then the heart rate (and cardiac output) are increased to ensure that the vital organs and tissues receive adequate circulation.

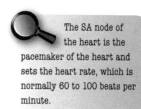

The SA node of the heart is the pacemaker of the heart and sets the heart rate, which is normally 60 to 100 beats per minute.

The autonomic nervous system ANS provides sympathetic and para-sympathetic innervation of the heart (see Figure 5-15). The sympathetic nervous system increases the heart rate and cardiac contractility. The parasympathetic nervous system decreases the heart rate via the vagus nerve. The heart can vary its rate by 2.5 times. As the heart rate increases, the cardiac output increases. However, at higher heart rates, less time of the cardiac cycle is spent in filling the ventricles (diastole), and the cardiac output can actually decrease.

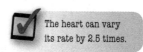

The heart can vary its rate by 2.5 times.

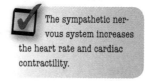

The sympathetic ner-vous system increases the heart rate and cardiac contractility.

The hormones epinephrine and norepi-nephrine are produced by the sympathetic neurons in the heart and by the adrenal glands. These hormones can also increase the heart rate, cardiac contractility, and car-diac output. The so-called "fight or flight"

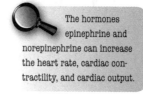

The hormones epinephrine and norepinephrine can increase the heart rate, cardiac con-tractility, and cardiac output.

mechanism can be triggered in times of stress or physical exertion, in-creasing the heart rate and cardiac output to increase circulation and performance.

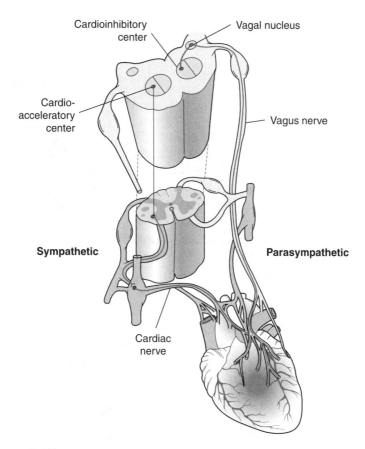

Cardioinhibitory
center

Vagal nucleus

Cardio-
acceleratory
center

Vagus nerve

Sympathetic

Parasympathetic

Cardiac
nerve

Figure 5-15 Regulation of heart rate by the autonomic nervous system.

The autonomic nervous system allows the circulatory system to respond to a variety of stresses in daily life. When a patient moves from the lying to the standing position, 20% of the blood in the heart and lungs is redistributed to the legs. Venous return to the heart drops and the blood pressure falls. The baroreceptors are stimulated, and the sympathetic nervous system increases the heart rate and peripheral vascular resistance. These mechanisms increase the blood pressure and compensate for the postural redistribution of the blood volume. Decreased responsiveness of the sympathetic nervous system to postural changes can cause a significant drop in blood

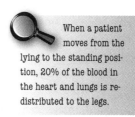

When a patient moves from the lying to the standing position, 20% of the blood in the heart and lungs is redistributed to the legs.

pressure when changing position called **postural hypotension**. During exercise, the skeletal muscle pump also contributes to the venous return to the heart.

Stroke Volume

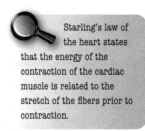

The stroke volume is the amount of blood ejected from the ventricle during systole and is normally 55 to 100 mL per beat.

The **stroke volume** is the amount of blood ejected from the ventricle during systole. It is normally 55 to 100 mL per beat. Because both sides of the heart must function equally, if the left ventricle pumps out 80 mL, then the right atrium must also receive 80 mL. When the ventricles contract, they do not eject every millimeter of blood. This residual volume of blood after systole, the **end-systolic volume**, is the amount of blood remaining in the ventricles after systole.

The specialized muscle cells of the myocardium contract more forcefully when they are stretched. The greater the venous return to the heart, the more the myocardium is stretched and the more strongly it will contract. This general rule of "more in = more out" is named Starling's law of the heart, after the physiologist who discovered it. **Starling's law of the heart** states that the energy of the contraction of the cardiac muscle is related to the stretch of the fibers prior to contraction. The filling of the ventricles at the end of diastole just prior to contraction produces a pressure on the walls of the ventricles called **preload**. Starling's mechanism works best if the cardiac muscle fibers are stretched to 2.5 times their resting length. If the stretch is excessive, then the strength of the contraction may decrease.

Starling's law of the heart states that the energy of the contraction of the cardiac muscle is related to the stretch of the fibers prior to contraction.

Resistance

When the preload pressure has been reached, the ventricle begins to contract. On the left side of the heart, the aortic valve opens when the left ventricular pressure overcomes diastolic pressure (see Figure 5-16). As the left ventricle continues to contract, systolic pressure is achieved as it pushes against resistance in the arterial system. **Afterload** is the pressure created in the ventricular wall to achieve systolic pressure. **Systemic vascular resistance (SVR)** is the clinical measure of the left ventricular afterload. The principles of preload and afterload also apply to the right

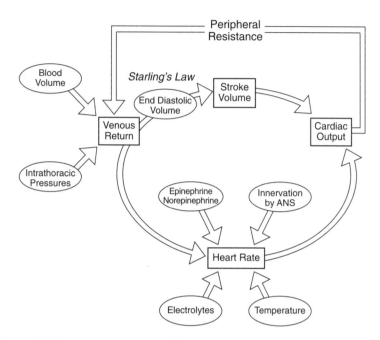

Figure 5-16 Regulation of blood flow.

side of the heart. **Pulmonic vascular resistance** (**PVR**) is the clinical measure of the right ventricular afterload.

Systemic vascular resistance (SVR) can be increased and decreased by the arterioles and the capillaries. The capillaries can regulate their blood flow through the precapillary sphincters. Local, hormonal, and neural impulses can dilate or contract the sphincters, altering the blood flow in the capillary beds. Local tissue factors that dilate the sphincters and increase circulation to the tissues are released. For example, during exercise, the precapillary sphincters respond to the needs of the tissues and dilate to allow greater blood flow to the muscles. Conversely, if the patient is hemorrhaging, then the sphincters can contract in response to sympathetic hormones such as epinephrine. This shunts more blood into the systemic circulation to maintain blood pressure and blood flow to vital organs such as the heart and brain.

In summary, the cardiovascular system is a well-tuned machine, consisting of a pump and blood vessels. The pump (the heart) is well-suited for pushing blood throughout the systemic and pulmonary circulation. The arteries, veins, and capillaries are each constructed to serve their individual functions. Many neural and hormonal mechanisms allow regulation of the system to provide oxygen and nutrients to the tissues. Oxygen and nutrients must be delivered to every cell in the body, and the cellular waste products and carbon dioxide need to be removed. The cardiovascular system ensures the perfusion of the tissues with oxygen.

CHAPTER 5 MULTIPLE-CHOICE QUESTIONS

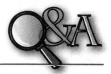

1. The main function of the atria of the heart is to:
   a. Contract and push blood into the systemic circulation
   b. Collect blood from the pulmonary and systemic circuits
   c. Be the pacemaker of the heart
   d. Sense changes in the carbon dioxide and oxygen levels

2. Arteries and veins are structured differently because:
   a. The veins need to withstand higher pressures.
   b. The arterial system is a low-pressure system.
   c. Arteries need valves to help push the blood to the tissues.
   d. Veins operate at one-tenth of the pressure of the arteries.

3. In general, the contraction of the myocardium is regulated by the:
   a. Sinoatrial node in the left ventricle
   b. Purkinje fibers in the ventricles
   c. SA node in the right atrium
   d. Bachmann's bundle

4. The relationship between resistance and blood flow could be summarized as:
   a. The lower the resistance, the more pressure is needed to make blood flow.
   b. The higher the resistance, the faster the flow.
   c. The lower the resistance, the faster the flow.
   d. The higher the resistance, the less pressure is needed to make blood flow.

5. Both diastole and systole are important in the cardiac cycle because:
   a. The chambers of the heart fill with blood during diastole.
   b. The ventricles contract during diastole to move blood throughout the circulatory system.
   c. The atria and ventricles fill during systole.
   d. When ventricles stretch less during diastole, they expel more blood during systole.

CHAPTER 5 ANSWERS AND RATIONALES

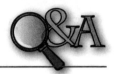

1. **b.**

    Rationale: The right and left atria collect blood from the systemic and pulmonary venous systems.

2. **d.**

    Rationale: The venous system is a low-pressure system with thinner-walled vessels.

3. **c.**

    Rationale: The SA or sinoatrial node in the right ventricle is known as the "pacemaker of the heart."

4. **c.**

    Rationale: Resistance and blood flow are inversely related—the lower the resistance, the faster the flow.

5. **a.**

    Rationale: The chambers of the heart fill during diastole, allowing the forceful contraction of the blood-filled chambers during systole.

QUICK LOOK AT THE CHAPTER AHEAD

This chapter reviews the assessment of the cardio-vascular system as it pertains to tissue perfusion and cell oxygenation, including:

* General health assessment

* Physical assessment of the cardiovascular system

* Heart sounds

* Diagnostic testing

* Hemodynamic monitoring

6

Assessment of the Cardiovascular System

CASE STUDY

Mr. H has a long-standing history of chronic obstructive lung disease and high blood pressure, and is 60 pounds overweight. He has continued to smoke despite urgings from his physician to quit. He called the office this morning because his chest felt tight and he could not catch his breath. When the nurse asked him what he did to help the pain, he said that he laid down an hour ago but the pain did not go away. Suspecting that his pain could be cardiac in origin, the nurse asked if his son was available to take him to the hospital or if he could call an ambulance. This scares Mr. H, but the nurse reassured him that this is the best place for him because they can get to the root of his pain and make him feel better. The nurse reminded him not to smoke any more cigarettes. Vital signs, an EKG, blood work, and pulse oximetry were done on Mr. H's arrival in the emergency department. His vital signs were as follows: HR—108 bpm, RR—32, and BP—176/94 mmHg. His Sao_2 was 89%. The nurse started oxygen via nasal cannula at 2 L/min and gave him aspirin per the protocol. His EKG showed ST segment elevations and his chest pain was not fully relieved by sublingual nitroglycerine, so a cardiac catheterization was ordered.

Important Questions to Ask

- How would you explain the purpose of the cardiac catheterization to Mr. H?
- What allergies would you ask Mr. H about prior to the procedure?
- What feelings should Mr. H report to the nurses during the procedure?
- Why is bed rest important after the catheterization?

Assessment of the cardiovascular system involves evaluating the adequacy of the heart's ability to pump blood and perfuse tissues. The **perfusion** process is similar to a plumbing system: the heart acts as the pump to deliver oxygenated blood to the cells, and the vascular network functions as the pipes. Perfusion through the cardiovascular network is a closed system that responds to changes in pressure. Unlike plumbing, the cardiovascular system is also responsive to changes in the

 Perfusion through the cardiovascular network is a closed system that responds to changes in pressure.

tissue demands and can alter flow to meet the demands of the body. This chapter will review the assessment of the cardiovascular system as it pertains to tissue perfusion and cell oxygenation.

GENERAL ASSESSMENT

A general overview of the patient's health provides clues to the overall functioning and the efficiency of the cardiovascular system. Examine the patient and estimate his apparent age. A comparison of his apparent and stated age may reveal that the patient looks older because of smoking, sun exposure, or poor health. Notice any cyanosis around the mouth and nose or in the extremities as seen in clubbing of the nails. Central cyanosis could indicate poor oxygenation or circulation. Assess the patient's facial expression, posture, and body language. These may allude to problems with breathing, pain, or anxiety. Pallor may indicate anemia or low cardiac output. Diaphoresis may suggest hypotension or myocardial infarction. Note the patient's respiratory patterns during activity. Increased breathlessness during a mild activity like disrobing may indicate problems with the respiratory or cardiovascular systems. While these are only general clues, they can direct a more detailed assessment of the heart and circulatory system.

ASSESSMENT OF THE CARDIOVASCULAR SYSTEM

An assessment of the cardiovascular system begins with questions about the patient's family health history. Any history of heart disease in the patient's family is important in understanding the patient's health risks. Family history would include congenital heart disease, angina, myocardial infarction, elevated cholesterol levels (dyslipidemia), high blood pressure, and strokes. Other diseases associated with heart problems include a family history of diabetes, hypertension, and thyroid disease.

Ask about the patient's health history, including the following:

- Heart disease—Acute, chronic, or congenital heart problems, hypertension, diabetes, dyslipidemia, heart murmurs, rheumatic fever, or varicose veins
- Lifestyle—Occupation, hobbies, sleep habits, stressors, exercise, smoking, and alcohol intake

- Medications—Cardiac medications, antihypertensives, over-the-counter medications, oral contraceptives, herbal remedies, and nutritional supplements
- Nutritional habits—Caloric intake, fat, salt, and caffeine consumption

The patient's health history should include questions about the presenting problem plus nonspecific symptoms. Ask the patient about what brought him to seek a healthcare provider and use follow-up questions to determine the timing of the symptom(s), alleviating factors, and how they affect the patient's functioning. Nonspecific symptoms might include fatigue, cough (refer to Chapter 2), dizziness, palpitations, or problems with sleep including snoring and sleep apnea. Some common signs and symptoms of patients with cardiovascular disorders include the following:

- Chest pain—Including arm, shoulder, and neck pain, and epigastric discomfort, as well as timing of the pain to activities
- Pain in the extremities on exertion—**Intermittent claudication** is relieved by rest, and heaviness in the extremities caused by varicose veins is relieved by rest and elevation.
- Dyspnea on exertion or with ordinary activities—Note the timing, the precipitating activity, and the alleviating factors.
- Orthopnea or difficulty breathing when recumbent—Note the timing of the orthopnea, including paroxysmal nocturnal dyspnea (PND). Ask about the number of pillows the patient uses when sleeping.
- Palpitations (awareness of heart beating)—Note any precipitating factors like caffeine, nicotine, alcohol, sugar, or stress. Also ask about awareness of skipped beats.
- Edema of the extremities—Note location of unilateral or bilateral swelling, any discoloration of the extremities, presence of ulcerations, and time during the day when the edema is noticeable.
- Episodes of dizziness or fainting— These may indicate cardiac arrhythmias, postural hypotension, or a vasovagal response.

> Ask the patient about what brought him or her to seek a healthcare provider and use follow-up questions to determine the timing of the symptom(s), alleviating factors, and how they affect the patient's functioning.

To begin an examination of the cardiovascular system, have the patient disrobe. The examining room should be warm, well-lit, and quiet. Start by assessing the skin and mucus membranes: color, lesions, ulcers, pigmentation changes, temperature, and hair distribution on the extremities. Patients with venous insufficiency may have brownish pigmentation or ulcers on the lower extremities. Those with arterial insufficiency may present with reddened, cool, or swollen extremities that are hairless. Check the nail beds for clubbing, a symptom of central cyanosis.

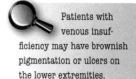

Patients with venous insufficiency may have brownish pigmentation or ulcers on the lower extremities.

Pulses

Assess the adequacy of arterial perfusion by palpating the peripheral pulses (see Figure 6-1). The pulses that are palpable include the temporal, carotid, brachial, radial, femoral, popliteal, dorsalis pedis, and posterior tibial pulses. Using the pads of the index and middle fingers, gently palpate over the pulse and grade it on a scale of 0 to 4 (see the section on grading pulses). Too much pressure can obliterate the pulse during assessment. Assessing and grading the pulses allows the nurse to evaluate perfusion by documenting the patient's baseline status, monitoring changes in circulation, and comparing the corresponding pulses on the opposite side of the body. Compare findings with the medical record and document the present findings.

 Too much pressure can obliterate the pulse during assessment.

Sometimes the pulses are difficult to palpate, especially when there is arterial insufficiency of the lower extremities. A **Doppler ultrasound (DUS)** may be used to listen for the presence of a pulse. The DUS apparatus has a special stethoscope with a transducer and an audio unit. The transducer is applied to the skin, and ultrasound waves detect the movement of red blood cells in the blood vessels. The pressure wave of increased blood flow after the heart contracts is detectable by the transducer as a pulse. A water-soluble gel is used on the skin to enhance the transmission of the sounds. The pulse sites may be marked with a waterproof marker so that they are easier to locate during subsequent assessments.

With arterial insufficiency, the pulses may be weak or absent in the extremities. Capillary filling may be slow (return to normal color greater

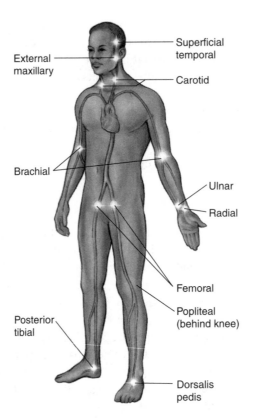

External maxillary

Superficial temporal

Carotid

Brachial

Ulnar

Radial

Femoral

Popliteal (behind knee)

Posterior tibial

Dorsalis pedis

Figure 6-1 Sites for palpating arterial pulses.

than 1 second after tissue compression), and the affected extremity starts to blanch when elevated above the heart for 1 to 2 minutes. When patients have venous insufficiency of the extremities, the pulses are present but may be difficult to palpate due to peripheral edema.

Pulse Rate

Using the patient's radial pulse on the wrist, count the pulsation for a full minute to get a sense of the heart rate and regularity. Use the finger pads of the middle fingers pressed lightly over the pulse. If the pulse is regular, count the pulsation for 30 seconds and multiply by 2 to get the 1-minute pulse rate. If the pulse is irregular, count the pulsation for a full minute.

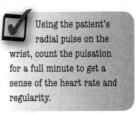

Using the patient's radial pulse on the wrist, count the pulsation for a full minute to get a sense of the heart rate and regularity.

The most accurate method for obtaining the heart rate, especially when the pulse is irregular, is by listening to the apical pulse with a stethoscope for a full minute (see Cardiac Assessment section later in this chapter.) An irregular heart rate can represent premature beats that might not be palpable peripherally at the radial pulse because left ventricular filling was incomplete prior to systole. When a pulse is irregular, note the type of irregularity: regularly irregular (e.g., beat, beat, pause, beat, beat, pause), irregular with respiration (e.g., an increasing rate with inspiration and decreasing rate with expiration), or totally irregular. Alternately, take a radial and apical pulse rate and note any discrepancies as they may vary with cardiac output.

When a pulse is irregular, note the type of irregularity: regularly irregular (e.g., beat, beat, pause, beat, beat, pause), irregular with respiration (e.g., an increasing rate with inspiration and decreasing rate with expiration), or totally irregular.

Blood Pressure

The blood pressure is an important determinant of cardiovascular functioning. As the heart relaxes and contracts, it sends a pressure wave of blood through the circulatory system. The pressure wave produces the impulse detected as an arterial pulse and the **Korotkoff sounds** that are heard when auscultating a blood pressure with a stethoscope. Normally, the blood pressure is finely controlled by neural and hormonal influences that maintain adequate tissue perfusion. Measuring the blood pressure can assess the adequacy of the circulation and the regulatory mechanisms.

Blood pressure can be measured either directly or indirectly. Direct measurement requires the insertion of a catheter into an artery (see Figure 6-2). Indirect blood pressure readings are done with a blood pressure cuff and auscultation of **Korotkoff sounds** or Doppler reading of the pressure wave. Using a **sphygmomanometer** (a blood pressure cuff attached to a manometer) and a stethoscope, the blood pressure is usually taken on the upper arm. A mercury sphygmomanometer aneroid instrument may be used to take a blood pressure (see Table 6-1).

The blood pressure measurement should be taken on both arms.

When hypertension is suspected, the blood pressure should be repeated on three separate occasions.

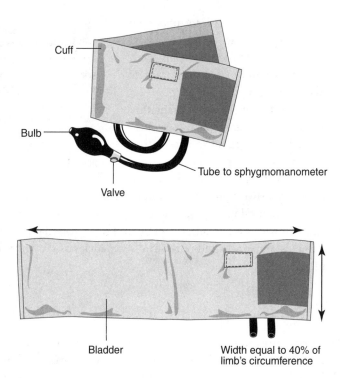

Figure 6-2 Blood pressure cuff-appropriate size for accurate mesurement.

The blood pressure measurement should be taken on both arms. When hypertension is suspected, the blood pressure should be repeated on three separate occasions. The patient should refrain from smoking cigarettes or drinking caffeine for 30 minutes before the blood pressure measurements. In patients with symptoms of dizziness and syncope, the blood pressure should be taken in the reclined, sitting, and standing positions to assess for orthostatic hypotension. Changing from the reclined to the standing position does not normally change the systolic pressure and may only slightly increase the diastolic pressure. But a decrease in the systolic blood pressure of more than 20 mmHg when changing from the sitting to standing positions may indicate **orthostatic hypotension**. Dehydration, hypovolemia, and certain antihypertensive medications are common causes of postural hypotension.

Dehydration, hypovolemia, and certain antihypertensive medications are common causes of postural hypotension.

Table 6-1 Measuring Blood Pressure

1. Choose a cuff of the appropriate size; the width should be 40% of the upper arm circumference (about 12 to 14 cm) (Figure 6-2). The bladder should be 80% of the circumference. A cuff that is too small may give an abnormally high reading.
2. Have the patient uncross his or her legs. Palpate the brachial pulse and position the arm at the level of the patient's heart with the palm facing up.
3. Wrap the cuff around the upper arm and brachial artery so that the bottom of the cuff is about 2.5 cm above the brachial pulse. It is best to have no clothing on the arm when taking a blood pressure.
4. To know how high to inflate the cuff, first take a palpable systolic reading. Palpate the radial pulse and rapidly inflate the cuff until the radial pulse disappears. Then, while deflating the cuff, palpate the return of the radial pulse. This is the palpable systolic pressure. Add 30 to this number, and use this as the highest pressure to which the cuff is to be inflated.
5. Place the stethoscope over the brachial pulse. The bell of the stethoscope picks up the low-pitched sounds (Korotkoff sounds) better than the diaphragm.
6. Inflate the cuff to the predetermined number (30 above the palpable systolic pressure), and slowly deflate the cuff (2 to 3 mmHg per second), listening for two consecutive sounds. Note this number as the systolic pressure. Continue deflating the cuff until the sounds become muffled and disappear. This is the diastolic pressure. The point of disappearance gives the best measure of diastolic pressure.

Paradoxical blood pressure is a decrease of greater than 10 mmHg in the systolic pressure during inspiration. This change is sometimes called **pulsus paradoxus.** It can be assessed by taking the blood pressure twice, once during inspiration and again at rest. First, palpate the systolic pressure while the patient stops breathing for a moment. Then, auscultate the blood pressure during inspiration and note when the sounds are first heard. Subtract the second number from the first and note any discrepancy between the two systolic pressures. Causes of pulsus paradoxus include pericardial tamponade, pulmonary hypertension, and restrictive pericarditis.

Causes of pulsus paradoxus include pericardial tamponade, pulmonary hypertension, and restrictive pericarditis.

Blood pressure ranges for normal and high blood pressure have been labeled by the Joint National Committee on Detection, Evaluation, and Treatment of High Blood Pressure in the United States. Values for normal and abnormal blood pressures are seen in Table 6-2.

High blood pressure can be categorized in different ways. If both the systolic and diastolic pressures are elevated, the highest pressure determines the category of hypertension. When only the systolic or diastolic pressure is elevated, it is called isolated systolic or isolated diastolic hypertension.

Examination of the Chest

The examination of the chest allows assessment of the structure and functioning of the cardiovascular system as well as the respiratory system. To review, the landmarks for both cardiac and respiratory assessments are established by the anatomy of the thorax: the midsternal line, the midclavicular line, the sternal notch, the midscapular line, the midaxillary line, and the intercostal spaces between the ribs (see Figure 6-3). Several key landmarks are used in cardiac assessment as they approximate the location of cardiac structures within the bony thorax (see Figure 6-4). These cardiac landmarks are used during palpation of the chest wall and auscultation of the heart.

The landmarks for both cardiac and respiratory assessments are established by the anatomy of the thorax: the midsternal line, the midclavicular line, the sternal notch, the midscapular line, the midaxillary line, and the intercostal spaces between the ribs. The examination of the chest follows three steps: **inspection**, **palpation**, and **auscultation**.

Table 6-2 Normal and Abnormal Blood Pressures

Category	Systolic	Diastolic
Normal	< 130	< 85
High normal	130–139	85–89
Mild hypertension	140–159	90–99
Moderate hypertension	160–179	100–109
Severe hypertension	180–209	110–119

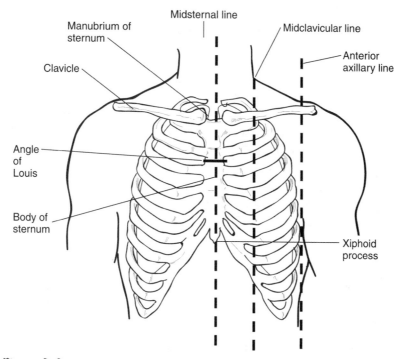

Figure 6-3 Thoracic landmarks.

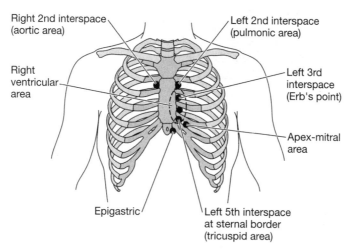

Figure 6-4 Cardiac landmarks.

Inspection

Start examining the patient by looking at the anterior chest while the patient is sitting. Take care to drape female patients as much as possible while allowing for adequate visualization of the thorax. Notice any pulsation, retractions, or movements of the chest wall. Inspect the large vessels of the neck: the carotid arteries and jugular veins. Note their location and how high up the neck the pulsations are visible. The jugular veins may also be used to estimate the venous pressure and the pressure in the right atrium of the heart. A noninvasive method of estimating venous pressure is to observe the jugular vein in the neck.

Take care to drape female patients as much as possible while allowing for adequate visualization of the thorax during assessment.

Assess the jugular venous distention using the following steps:

1. Position the patient in a supine position with the head of the bed at a 30° angle and turn the patient's head slightly away from the side being inspected.

2. Use oblique lighting and observe the neck for the pulsation of the jugular vein on either side of the neck. It is usually above the sternal notch or just posterior to the sternocleidomastoid muscle.

3. Find the highest point up the neck where the jugular venous pulsation is visible.

4. Measure from the sternal angle (the connection of the second ribs to the sternum and manubrium) to this level using a vertical ruler and a horizontal reference point to the highest point of jugular venous pulsation (see Figure 6-5).

5. Measurements greater than 3 to 4 cm above the sternal angle may indicate elevated venous pressure. Central venous pressure can also be measured using central lines and electronic equipment.

Palpation

After inspecting the thorax and the neck veins, continue the examination by palpating the chest wall. The patient can remain in the supine position with the head of the bed at a 30° angle with the examiner on the patient's right side. Using the cardiac landmarks in Figure 6-4 (aortic, pulmonic,

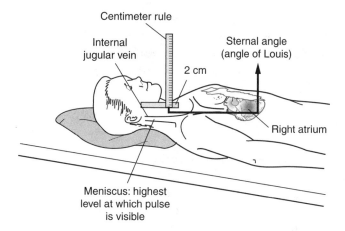

Figure 6-5 Measuring jugular vein distention.

tricuspid, and mitral areas), palpate with the finger pads along the chest wall, noting any thrills or vibrations. **Thrills** are palpable vibrations that may accompany loud, rumbling heart murmurs. (Heart murmurs are addressed more specifically in a later section). Vibrations may accompany murmurs or extra heart sounds. Locate the **apical pulse** by palpating along the fourth and fifth intercostal spaces and slightly medial to the midclavicular line. Remember that the inter-costal spaces are labeled by the rib above them (e.g., the second inter-costal space is just below the second rib). In female patients with large breasts, move the breast gently upward or ask the patient to do this. This will allow better palpation of the chest wall. Note the location, amplitude, and regularity of the apical pulse.

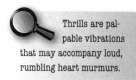

Thrills are palpable vibrations that may accompany loud, rumbling heart murmurs.

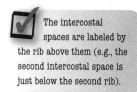

The intercostal spaces are labeled by the rib above them (e.g., the second intercostal space is just below the second rib).

Auscultation

Auscultation is one of the most frequently used techniques for assessing cardiac functioning and one which requires practice in order to become proficient. Clean and warm the stethoscope prior to applying it to the patient. With the patient in the supine position with the head of the bed at a 30° angle, begin listening to the heart using the bell of the stethoscope and then repeat the same steps using the diaphragm. Begin listening at the same cardiac landmarks that were used for palpation of the chest wall. Start at the base of the heart (the aortic and pulmonic sites) and progress to the apex of the heart (the tricuspid and mitral sites). Do not forget to listen at **Erb's point** (the third intercostal space at the left sternal border), as extra heart sounds and murmurs are often heard there.

Do not forget to auscultate heart sounds at Erb's point (the third intercostal space at the left sternal border), as extra heart sounds and murmurs are often heard there.

The first heart sounds the nurse should listen for are the "lub" and "dup" sounds of the heartbeat, or S1 and S2. Each "lub-dup" or S1 and S2, equals one heartbeat. Identifying the two sounds takes some practice and knowledge about the physiologic basis for the sounds. Heart sounds are caused by the closing of valves and the rapid distension of the chambers of the heart with blood. It is easiest to think about heart sounds as the

Heart sounds are caused by the closing of valves and the rapid distending of the chambers of the heart with blood.

valves closing during the cardiac cycle. "Lub" or S1 is the sound that accompanies the closing of the **atrioventricular valves** (tricuspid and mitral valves) just before contraction of the ventricles (systole). "Dup" or S2 is the sound that accompanies the closing of the aortic and pulmonic valves after the ventricles have emptied and the heart enters the filling phase of the cardiac cycle (diastole). Using the first letter of each valve to represent each valve closing, think about the heart sounds and the cardiac cycle using Table 6-3. The opposite pair of valves is open during each heart sound, allowing blood to fill the chambers. For example, when S1 is heard, the tricuspid and mitral valves are closing to allow blood to

Table 6-3 Cardiac Cycle

	One heartbeat		One heartbeat	
	Lub	Dup	Lub	Dup
Heart sound	S1	S2	S1	S2
Valves closing	T-M	A-P	T-M	A-P
	Systole	Diastole	Systole	Diastole

Note: T = tricuspid valve; Diastole = ventricular filling; M = mitral valve; Systole = ventricular contraction; P = pulmonic valve; A = aortic valve.

fill the atria. At the same time, the aortic and pulmonic valves are open-ing as the ventricles contract and are pushing blood into the systemic and pulmonic circulation.

Using the cardiac landmarks (see Figure 6-4 for the aortic, pulmonic, tricuspid, and mitral areas) listen for S1 and S2 at each site. S2 is loudest at the base of the heart at the aortic and pulmonic sites. S1 is loudest at the apex of the heart, the tricuspid, and mitral sites. To identify S1, gently palpate the carotid pulse while listening to the heart sounds. The carotid pulse will immediately follow S1. Sometimes it is easier to identify each heart sound by tapping with the first and second fingers with the "lub" and "dup" sounds to get the rhythm of the heart beat.

Occasionally, in healthy, young adults, the second heart sound, S2, is split into two parts. Each part represents a valve closing—first the aortic and then the pulmonic valve because they are not closing simultaneously. When the second heart sound is split on inspiration but the split disap-pears on expiration, this is called **normal** or **physiologic splitting**.

While listening to the heart sounds, assess the rate, rhythm, and qual-ity of the heartbeat. As with assessing the pulse, label the rate as normal, bradycardia (less than 60 beats/min), or tachycardia (greater than 100 beats/min). Note whether the rate is regular or irregular. While auscul-tating, listen for the intensity of the heart sounds during each beat and note whether they sound of the same strength or vary-ing strengths with each beat. Take an apical pulse by listening to the apex of the heart for a full minute. Remember that the api-cal pulse is usually at the left fourth or fifth intercostal space at the midclavicular line. If the apical pulse has been located on palpation first, it is much easier to locate it when auscultating the apical pulse. Always compare the findings to the patient's baseline data by reviewing the chart.

 The apical pulse is usually at the left fourth or fifth intercostal space at the midclavicular line.

 S3 may be one of the first signs of congestive heart failure.

Extra heart sounds are heard when the heart is not functioning prop-erly. Extra sounds include S3, S4, heart murmurs, opening snaps, and friction rubs. Both S3 and S4 are diastolic sounds. S3, or a **ventricular gallop**, signals decreased ventricular compliance (stiffness). It may be one of the first signs of congestive heart failure. It is best heard with the bell of the stethoscope because it is a low-frequency sound. Listening at the tricuspid area at the lower-left sternal border, S3 is heard immediately after S2 and the heart beat sounds like *Tennessee:*

S1	S2 S3	S1	S2 S3

The fourth heart sound, S4, is sometimes called a **presystolic** or **atrial gallop** and is heard with decreased ventricular compliance. It is also heard with the bell of the stethoscope at the apex of the heart. The heart beat sounds like *Kentucky:*

S4 S1	S2	S4 S1	S2

Opening snaps are made when a stenotic mitral valve opens. It is an early, diastolic sound and heard best with the diaphragm of the stethoscope.

Heart Murmurs

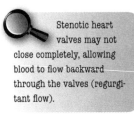

Stenotic heart valves may not close completely, allowing blood to flow backward through the valves (regurgitant flow).

Heart murmurs are extra heart sounds that signal valvular dysfunction. Valves can become incompetent because they do not open and close properly. Stenotic heart valves may not close completely, allowing blood to flow backward through the valves (**regurgitant flow**). They also may not open fully, causing turbulent forward flow. The abnormal blood flow produces sounds that can be heard with a stethoscope and sometimes palpated as thrills.

Heart murmurs are described by their timing during the cardiac cycle, their location, the presence of radiation, the intensity, the pitch, and quality of the sound. Murmurs are first differentiated by whether they are systolic (occurring between S1 and S2) or diastolic (occurring between S2 and S1). The timing of the murmur during the cardiac cycle is important because it can help identify which valve is incompetent. Murmurs occur only during a particular point during the cardiac cycle (e.g., pansystolic), during the whole systolic component of the cycle, or across the whole cycle (i.e., continuous murmur). The location of the maximal intensity and the presence of radiation of the sound to other locations such as the neck or axilla should also be noted (see Table 6-4).

The intensity of the murmur may vary during the cycle. The varying intensity or configuration of a heart murmur may be described

Table 6-4 Murmur Intensity Scale

Grade 1—Very faint
Grade 2—Quiet but immediately heard with a stethoscope
Grade 3—Moderately loud
Grade 4—Loud
Grade 5—Very loud, may be heard with stethoscope partly off the chest wall
Grade 6—Can be heard with a stethoscope off the chest wall

as increasing during the cycle (crescendo) or decreasing in intensity (decrescendo).

Pitch refers to whether the murmur is of high, medium, or low pitch. The stethoscope can help differentiate the pitch. The bell picks up low-pitched sounds and the diaphragm picks up the higher-pitched sounds. Quality is a vaguer descriptor of murmurs, comparing the murmur to other sounds that are generally recognizable. For example, a murmur may be described as blowing or harsh in quality.

Friction rubs are sounds made by inflamed pericardial tissue. The rubbing of the inflamed tissues as the heart rocks in the pericardial cavity causes harsh sounds that are somewhat "scratchy" in nature. The sound of a pericardial friction rub is similar to a pleural rub. To differentiate between a pericardial and a pleural rub, the nurse asks the patient to hold his breath for a couple of seconds. If the rub disappears during holding the breath, then it is a pleural friction rub. The most common cause of pericardial friction rub is pericarditis.

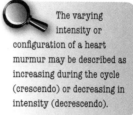

The varying intensity or configuration of a heart murmur may be described as increasing during the cycle (crescendo) or decreasing in intensity (decrescendo).

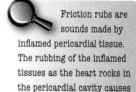

Friction rubs are sounds made by inflamed pericardial tissue. The rubbing of the inflamed tissues as the heart rocks in the pericardial cavity causes harsh sounds that are somewhat "scratchy" in nature.

Laboratory and Diagnostic Tests

A variety of tests are used to assess the functioning of the cardiovascular system. Some tests are more invasive and require more recovery time than others. The nurse's role is to understand the implications for the test and the patient's experience. Nurses teach patients about the tests, the required preparation, what to expect during the tests, and what is involved in recovering from the tests. Patients will also want to know what the tests will reveal and how soon they will have information about their health. The nurse addresses these issues prior to the testing to alleviate some anxiety.

Common tests of cardiovascular functioning include the following:

- Blood tests
- Chest radiology
- Electrocardiogram (EKG)
- Stress test
- Echocardiograms, ultrasound, and Doppler studies
- Arteriogram
- Cardiac catheterization
- Radionuclide scans
- Hemodynamic monitoring

Blood Tests

Laboratory blood work may be done by simple venipuncture in the outpatient or acute care setting. Preparation depends on the type of blood test. For example, serum cholesterol is best obtained in the morning after fasting during the previous night. Refer to the guidelines of the facility or contact the laboratory for test-specific preparation.

The following are blood tests that are commonly performed to evaluate the cardiovascular system:

- Electrolytes—Sodium, potassium, magnesium, calcium, and phosphorus are involved in the maintenance of fluid balance, blood vessel tone, and cardiac muscle contractility. Blood glucose may be drawn if there is a question about diabetes.
- Cholesterol and triglycerides—To assess changes that could signal hyperlipidemia and risk factors for arteriosclerosis
- Cardiac enzymes—Troponin T, creatine phosphokinase (CPK), and CPK-MB fraction to assess cardiac muscle damage, lactic acid dehydrogenase (LDH), serum glutamic oxoloacetic transaminase (SGOT), and aspartate amino transferase (AST)
- Hematologic tests—Complete blood count (CBC), C reactive protein, coagulation times (activated partial thromboplastin time—APTT, and prothrombin time—PT), and erythrocyte sedimentation rate (ESR)
- Arterial blood gases— Used to determine oxygenation of tissues, carbon dioxide levels, and acid–base balance (see Chapter 2 for more information on acid–base balance).

Chest Radiology

Chest X-rays are routinely used to assess the shape, size, and location of the heart. Anterior-posterior films can be taken in a radiology department or at the bedside. Left lateral views may also be taken to provide more information about the heart. The X-rays provide information about cardiac and left-ventricular enlargement, pulmonary edema, and the placement of catheters and endotracheal tubes.

Electrocardiograms

Electrocardiograms (EKG or ECG) are noninvasive tests that produce graphic representations of the electrical activity in the heart. The cardiac muscle contracts because of an electrical signal traveling along the conduction pathways of the heart. The electrical activity changes the polarity (negativity and positivity) of the cardiac muscle cells. The depolarization of the cells (i.e., a wave of positive charge) occurs just prior to and during contraction with a return to their negative charge after contraction. This change in polarity caused by the electrical stimulation can be captured and traced onto timed graph paper to provide a visual record of the heart's contractility, function, and structure. Electrodes are placed on the skin of the chest and extremities to capture these electrical changes. The electrodes are connected to an EKG machine or telemetry unit where a graphic record is recorded. EKG can also be monitored by ambulatory units (**Holter monitor**) to assess patients with suspected cardiac dysrhythmias over longer periods of time.

The cardiac rate, rhythm, and variations in the pattern can be read to reveal changes such as angina or myocardial infarction. A normal EKG (see Figure 6-6) means that the heart has intact conduction pathways. A standard 12-lead EKG evaluates anterior, inferior, and lateral walls of

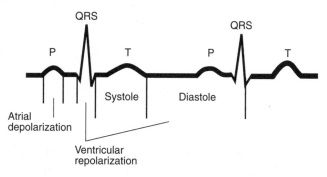

Figure 6-6 Normal EKG with labels (P, Q, R, S, T) for common features.

the heart. Additional leads (e.g., 15- or 18-lead EKG) may be necessary to evaluate the right ventricle and posterior wall. EKGs can also detect premature beats, blockages in the conduction system, myocardial ischemia, or electrolyte imbalances.

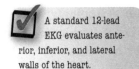

A standard 12-lead EKG evaluates anterior, inferior, and lateral walls of the heart.

Characteristic changes to the EKG occur during chest pain from angina and disappear when the pain subsides. Specific EKG changes in certain leads can identify an ischemic portion of the heart and follow evolution of a myocardial infarction.

An EKG can be displayed on a cardiac monitor so that the heart rate and rhythm can be continuously monitored and dysrhythmias can be quickly detected and treated. A printout of the EKG on special paper allows for more careful analysis of the heart's electrical activity. The paper is

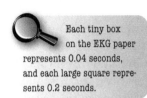

Each tiny box on the EKG paper represents 0.04 seconds, and each large square represents 0.2 seconds.

marked with squares allowing for rapid calculation of the heart rate and measurement of distances between landmarks on the waveform. Each tiny box on the EKG paper represents 0.04 seconds, and each large square represents 0.2 seconds. At the top of the EKG are vertical marks at every 3 seconds.

The tracings of an EKG indicate electrical changes within the myocardial cells. Electrical depolarization of the myocardial cells occurs immediately before contraction (systole). Repolarization of the myocardium occurs after contraction (diastole) as the intracellular environment regains its normal electrical charge. Myocardial cells must repolarize before they can effectively depolarize and contract again.

The following are the basic landmarks of an EKG:

- P wave—Indicates SA node function and atrial depolarization
- P-R interval—Indicates AV node conduction time (normal time 0.12 to 0.2 seconds)
- QRS complex—Indicates ventricular depolarization (normal time 0.06 to 0.10 seconds)
- ST segment—Indicates time between complete depolarization of the ventricles and complete repolarization
- T wave—Indicates ventricular repolarization

The bibliography at the end of the text lists additional readings about EKGs. Although it is beyond the scope of this book to describe all the different types of cardiac rhythms, all nurses should take a course on reading EKGs so they can provide more comprehensive care to their patients.

Stress Tests

Stress tests, or exercise EKGs, are noninvasive tests used to evaluate cardiac function and perfusion with increasing levels of activity. They are useful in diagnosing ischemic heart disease. Electrodes are placed on the chest to monitor the heart rate and rhythm, and the blood pressure is monitored while the patient exercises on a treadmill or stationary cycle. If the patient develops chest pain, hypotension, or EKG changes during a stress test, he or she may have coronary artery disease. A positive stress test indicates that more invasive tests may be needed. Stress tests also provide guidelines for safe activity levels to patients with known coronary artery disease.

 If the patient develops chest pain, hypotension, or EKG changes during a stress test, he or she may have coronary artery disease.

Echocardiograms, Ultrasound, and Doppler Studies

Echocardiograms are noninvasive tests used to assess left ventricular and valvular function. Using ultrasound waves, they can also visualize all four chambers of the heart, evaluate the motion of the left ventricular wall, and calculate the ejection fraction and **left ventricular end diastolic pressures (LVEDP)**. An ultrasound transducer is moved along the skin of the thorax over the thoracic structures. A water-soluble gel is used to enhance transmission of the ultrasound waves. **Transesophageal echocardiography** involves placing a transducer into the esophagus to evaluate the wall motion of the cardiac chambers. While this method requires local anesthesia and sometimes sedation, it provides clearer images of the motility of the heart.

As previously described in the section on assessment of pulses, Doppler ultrasound can aid in diagnosing problems with blood flow in the heart and the extremities. Color Doppler studies are useful in evaluating

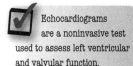
Echocardiograms are a noninvasive test used to assess left ventricular and valvular function.

blood flow in the heart, especially in cases of congenital anomalies or valvular regurgitation (backward flow). In the extremities, the test involves using a pressure cuff and ultrasound to detect the blood flow rates at different pressures.

Arteriograms

Arteriograms are commonly used to study the aorta, cardiac valves, femoral arteries, and carotid arteries. (Coronary artery studies, a type of arteriogram, will be described in the next section on cardiac catheteriza-

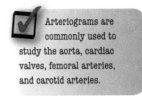

Arteriograms are commonly used to study the aorta, cardiac valves, femoral arteries, and carotid arteries.

tion.) During an arteriogram, an intravenous catheter is inserted into a large artery, a radiopaque dye is injected into the artery, and then X-ray pictures are taken to visualize the anatomy of the artery and the flow of blood through the artery. The blood vessel anatomy and valvular function are captured on film and help in diagnosing aortic aneurysm, valvular defects, and arterial blockages.

Nursing care of patients undergoing arteriography includes the following:

1. Obtain informed consent.

2. Assess the patient's vital signs before and during the procedure, and watch for reactions to the dye (dyspnea, numbness, or tingling).

3. Assess the puncture site after the procedure for signs of bleeding, and use sandbags for pressure as ordered.

4. Evaluate peripheral pulses distal to the perforation site to assess adequacy of circulation.

5. Ensure adequate hydration after the arteriogram to facilitate elimination of the dye and prevent kidney damage from the dye.

Cardiac Catheterization

Cardiac catheterization is performed to evaluate the coronary arteries and valves. It is an invasive procedure, requiring admission to an outpatient or short-stay unit in an acute care setting. Admission to an acute care facility is necessary because emergent surgery may be required if substantial blockages are detected.

Nursing care *prior* to cardiac catheterization includes the following:

1. Obtain informed consent.

2. No oral intake of food for 8 to 12 hours before the test.

3. Assess patient for allergies to dyes, iodine, or shellfish.

4. Evaluate peripheral pulses prior to catheterization.

5. Record vital signs, height, and weight before the test.

6. Inform the patient about sensations he or she may feel during the procedure, including a fluttering feeling as catheter is inserted. Encourage the patient to report dyspnea, itching, or numbness, which could signal an allergic reaction to the radiopaque dye.

> Encourage the patient to report dyspnea, itching, or numbness during cardiac catherterization, which could signal an allergic reaction to the radiopaque dye.

During cardiac catheterization, a catheter is inserted in a large blood vessel and threaded up to the heart. If a right heart catheterization is being performed, the catheter is inserted into the antecubital vein and threaded into the superior vena cava and into the right heart. Right heart catheterization allows monitoring of pressures in the right atria, ventricles, and pulmonary arteries, and the calculation of cardiac output. Continuous monitoring of circulatory pressures is useful in critically ill patients. Special hemodynamic catheters can be left in place after the catheterization to measure pressures and cardiac output in the intensive care setting.

> Right heart catheterization allows monitoring of pressures in the right atria, ventricles, and pulmonary arteries, and calculation of cardiac output.

If a left heart catheterization is being performed, a radiopaque catheter is inserted into the femoral or brachial artery and threaded into the aorta and left heart. The most common application of left heart catheterization is selective arteriography of the coronary arteries. This allows the evaluation

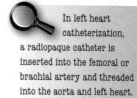

> In left heart catheterization, a radiopaque catheter is inserted into the femoral or brachial artery and threaded into the aorta and left heart.

of the patency of the coronary arteries and visualization of stenosis or blockage of the arteries. Other measurements may be taken during the procedure, including pressures in the chambers and great vessels, and an ejection fraction. Cardiac catheterization can be combined with interventions, such as balloon angioplasty or direct injection of thrombolytics (e.g., streptokinase, TPA) to reopen blocked coronary arteries.

Nursing care of patients *after* cardiac catheterization includes the following:

1. Maintain bed rest (including straight leg for 8 hours) and then increasing activity levels per cardiologist; patients are at risk for bleeding at the arterial puncture site, and bed rest allows time for adequate clot formation at the puncture site.

2. Assess puncture site for bleeding, including under the patient. Use sand bags for pressure on site as ordered (sandbags are used to apply steady pressure and prevent bleeding at the site).

3. Evaluate peripheral pulses (every 15 minutes for 1 hour, every 30 minutes for 1 hour, and every hour for 2 hours) distal to the puncture site to ensure adequate perfusion as patients are at risk for arterial occlusion at the puncture site, which could severely diminish blood flow to the periphery. Decreased blood flow would be demonstrated by decreased or absent peripheral pulses, cyanosis, or coolness of the extremity.

4. Continue intravenous fluids (to aid in elimination of dye), and increase diet per orders.

5. Evaluate adequacy of urinary output after the procedure.

Radionuclide Scans

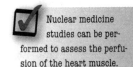

Nuclear medicine studies can be performed to assess the perfusion of the heart muscle.

Nuclear medicine studies can be performed to assess the perfusion of the heart muscle. Special dyes, such as Technetium 99m (T^{99m}) or Thallium-201 (Tl^{201}), are used to detect perfusion defects in the heart muscle and to localize areas of infarction. Thallium may also be injected into the bloodstream prior to exercise (treadmill) to evaluate the effect of exercise on coronary perfusion. Cameras in the nuclear medicine department are designed to measure the radioactivity given off by the dye in the tissues. Defects are seen as areas with little or no uptake of the dye indicating the area is poorly perfused.

Radionuclide scans can be combined with other diagnostic tests to evaluate the perfusion of the heart by the coronary arteries, ventricular wall motion, and ejection fraction. Scans may be combined with arteriography to measure right- or left-sided ejection fractions.

Multigated acquisition scanning (MUGA) combines the injection of technetium pertechnetate with scans to detect ventricular function, detect aneurysms, and evaluate coronary artery perfusion. An **ejection fraction (EF)** is the percentage of blood that fills the left ventricle ejected from the left ventricle during systole. A normal ejection fraction for the left ventricle is 65% to 75%, meaning that when the ventricle fills with blood, it ejects 65% to 75% of that blood with each contraction (systole).

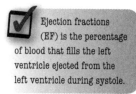

Ejection fractions (EF) is the percentage of blood that fills the left ventricle ejected from the left ventricle during systole.

Hemodynamic Monitoring

Hemodynamic monitoring provides information about pressures in the great vessels and the heart in seriously ill patients. Information about central pressures is useful in assessing cardiac function and volume status and directing and evaluating interventions (see Table 6-5).

A hemodynamic monitoring system requires a catheter, an infusion system, a transducer, and a monitor (see Figure 6-7). To directly monitor central pressures, invasive lines must be inserted into blood vessels such as external jugular vein and threaded toward the heart. A chest X-ray is needed to confirm the placement. The catheter is connected to a heparinized infusion system. The infusion system is delivered under pressure with a pressure bag to prevent back flow of blood into the catheter and possible occlusion of the catheter by thrombosis. The pressure in the catheter is relayed to a transducer that converts the mechanical pressure into electrical energy. The electrical energy is displayed as waveforms on a monitor. The transducer is calibrated according to the manufacturer's instructions and leveled to the patient's **phlebostatic axis**, the approximate location of the patient's right atrium (see Figure 6-8).

Hemodynamic monitoring provides information about the pressures of the heart and the systemic circulation. Different catheters, such as arterial lines, central venous lines, and pulmonary artery catheters are used to obtain specific information. Because of the risks involved, informed consent may be required from patients or their families prior to the insertion of these catheters.

Arterial lines Intra-arterial monitoring directly measures arterial blood pressure. A catheter is inserted into the radial artery (see Figure 6-7) and

Table 6-5 Hemodynamic Measurements

Measurement	Normal Values	Calculation/Significance
Blood pressure BP	Systolic (SBP): 90–130	>130SBP = hypertension
	Diastolic (DBP): 60–90	< 90 SBP = hypotension
Heart rate (HR)	60–100 beats/min or bpm	< 60 bpm = bradycardia
		> 100 bpm = tachycardia
Pulse pressure (PP)	40 mmHg	PP = SBP – DBP
		Measures force of pulse
Cardiac output (CO)	4–8 L/min	Heart rate × SV /1000
		Evaluates hemodynamic function
Pulmonary artery pressure (PAP)	Systolic: 18–30 mmHg	Useful in measuring pulmonary vascular resistance
	Diastolic: 6–15 mmHg	
Central venous pressure (CVP)	2–6 mmHg	Mean right atrial pressure— estimates right ventricle preload
Pulmonary capillary wedge pressure (PCWP)	4–12 mmHg	Estimates left ventricle filling and preload
Mean arterial pressure (MAP)	85–100 mmHg	SBP + (2 × DBP)/3 Used to calculate SV
Ejection fraction (EF)	65–75%	Cardiac function relative to contractility
Systemic vascular resistance (SVR or SV)	15–20 mmHg/L/min	(MAP – CVP)/CO

connected to a transducer that constantly reads the blood pressure onto a monitor. Directly measured blood pressures by intra-arterial monitoring are usually 10 to 15 mmHg higher than indirect measurements taken with a stethoscope and a sphygmomanometer. Intra-arterial catheters can also be used to obtain arterial blood gas samples and other blood tests. Assessment of the intravenous dressing over the puncture site in the radial artery must be done frequently because of the risk of bleeding.

Directly measured blood pressures by intra-arterial monitoring are usually 10 to 15 mmHg higher than indirect measurements taken with a stethoscope and a sphygmomanometer.

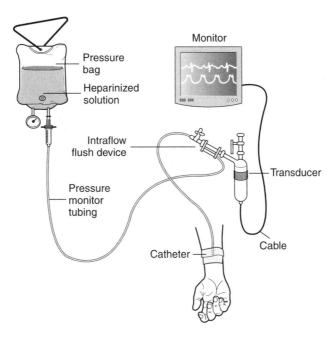

Figure 6-7 Components of hemodynamic monitoring system.

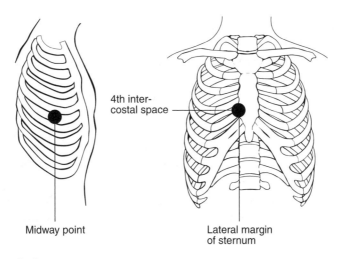

Figure 6-8 Phlebostatic axis.

Central venous pressure A pulmonary artery catheter or a central venous catheter monitors the **central venous pressure (CVP)**. A catheter is inserted into the venous system and threaded into the right atrium. A chest X-ray is needed to verify placement. The intravenous infusion system is connected to a transducer and a monitor (see Figures 6-9 and 6-10).

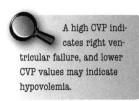
A high CVP indicates right ventricular failure, and lower CVP values may indicate hypovolemia.

A normal CVP reading is 1 to 6 mmHg (see Table 6-3). A high CVP indicates right ventricular failure, and lower CVP values may indicate hypovolemia. The insertion site must be carefully observed and the dressing changed according to the protocol of the facility. Because the CVP catheter is centrally placed, it can be a source of infection, thrombosis, and hemorrhage.

Because the CVP catheter is centrally placed, it can be a source of infection, thrombosis, and hemorrhage.

Pulmonary artery catheters Pulmonary artery catheters are triple or quadruple lumen catheters that are inserted into a large vein, such as the jugular vein, to measure pressures in the great vessels and the heart (see Figure 6-11). These catheters can measure right atrial pressures (CVP) directly and can indirectly measure pressures in the left side of the heart. The catheter has three ports—one at the tip to measure **pulmonary artery wedge pressure (PAWP)**, one in the right atrium to measure right atrial pressure, and one that can be used for cardiac output injectate. The right atrial pressure may be constantly observable on the monitor. Other calculations such as the PAWP, may be done intermittently to assess the effectiveness

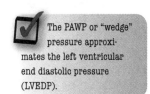
The PAWP or "wedge" pressure approximates the left ventricular end diastolic pressure (LVEDP).

of the interventions or to evaluate a change in status. The **PAWP** or "wedge" pressure approximates the **left ventricular end diastolic pressure (LVEDP)**. It is measured by inflating a balloon at the end of the catheter and allowing it to float through the heart and into the pulmonary circulation until it occludes a branch of the pulmonary artery. The sensor then reads pressures in the left side of the heart.

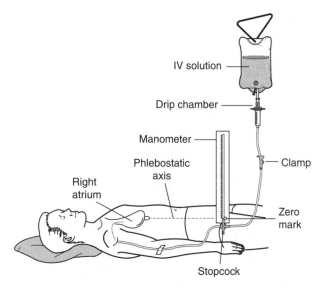

Figure 6-9 CVP monitoring.

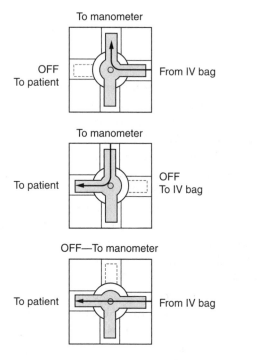

Figure 6-10 Stopcock to a water manometer for reading CVP.

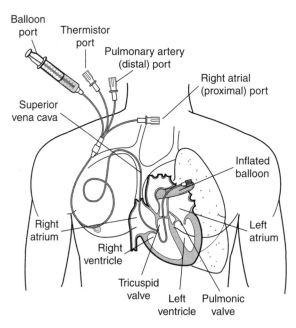

Balloon port
Thermistor port
Pulmonary artery (distal) port
Right atrial (proximal) port
Superior vena cava
Inflated balloon
Right atrium
Left atrium
Right ventricle
Tricuspid valve
Left ventricle
Pulmonic valve

Figure 6-11 Pulmonary artery catheter for hemodynamic monitoring. The inflated balloon in a pulmonary artery indirectly reads pressure on the left side of the heart.

Elevated PAWP may indicate left ventricular failure, cardiogenic shock, hypervolemia, shunting, or mitral valve regurgitation. A decreased PAWP may develop with hypovolemia and septicemia. Periodic measurements of the PAWP allow the healthcare team to follow trends in the patient's condition and assess the effectiveness of the treatments.

Measures of **cardiac output (CO)** can also be obtained with the **pulmonary artery catheter** using the thermodilution technique. A known amount of D_5W at either cooled or room temperature is injected into the port. The thermistor on the catheter measures the mixing of D_5W into the circulation. Cardiac output is calculated by machine and is useful in determining the functioning of the left ventricle. A normal CO is 4 to 8 L/min (see Table 6-3). The normal homeostatic mechanisms adjust the cardiac output to respond to increased tissue demands for oxygen. Low resting cardiac output may indicate inadequate filling of the

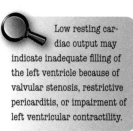

Low resting cardiac output may indicate inadequate filling of the left ventricle because of valvular stenosis, restrictive pericarditis, or impairment of left ventricular contractility.

left ventricle because of valvular stenosis, restrictive pericarditis, or impairment of left ventricular contractility. High resting CO occurs in fever, sepsis, anxiety, thyrotoxicosis, and arteriovenous fistula.

The delivery of oxygenated blood to the tissues is dependent on the functioning of the cardiovascular system. Assessment of the cardiovascular system involves evaluating the adequacy of the heart's pumping ability and the perfusion of tissues throughout the body. The cardiovascular system is responsive to changes in the tissue demands and usually can alter blood flow to meet the demands of the body. Many assessment strategies are available to examine the anatomy and functioning of the heart and blood vessels and to determine if the cardiovascular system meets the needs of the body. Hemodynamic monitoring provides current measurements of the patient's status allowing rapid adjustments to the interventions. Assessment strategies provide information about the patient's status and allow healthcare providers to measure the effectiveness of interventions to improve oxygenation.

ANSWERS TO THE CASE STUDY QUESTIONS

- How would you explain the purpose of the cardiac catheterization to Mr. H?

Cardiac catheterization is used to locate the area of the heart where the circulation is blocked and direct the appropriate treatment. The nurse should use drawings or diagrams as necessary to explain the procedure to the patient and his family.

- What allergies would you ask Mr. H about prior to the procedure?

The nurse should ask the patient about his allergies and check the medical record for evidence of sensitivity to intravenous dyes or shellfish prior to the cardiac catheterization.

- What feelings should Mr. H report to the nurses in the catheter lab during the procedure?

During the cardiac catheterization, Mr. H should report any pain to the nurse or physician. He should also tell them if he has any difficulty breathing or itchiness, which could indicate a sensitivity to the dye.

• Why is bed rest important after the catheterization?

Bed rest is important after cardiac catheterization because of the risk of bleeding from the catheter insertion site. Sandbags are used to apply pressure to the site. Vital signs as well as site assessment are performed every 15 minutes for 1 hour, every 30 minutes for 1 hour, and then every hour for 2 hours.

CHAPTER 6 MULTIPLE-CHOICE QUESTIONS

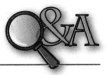

1. During the first heart sound, S1 or "Lub," what valves are closing?
   a. Aortic and pulmonic
   b. Tricuspid and mitral
   c. Aortic and mitral
   d. Mitral and pulmonic

2. All of the following are true about S3 except:
   a. It sounds like "Kentucky" with the other heart sounds.
   b. It falls after S2.
   c. It is called a ventricular gallop.
   d. S3 may indicate congestive heart failure.

3. Nursing care prior to cardiac catheterization includes all of the following except:
   a. Assessment for allergies to dyes or iodine
   b. Evaluation of peripheral pulses
   c. Obtaining informed consent
   d. Clear liquids prior to the test

4. A normal central venous pressure (CVP) is:
   a. 15 to 26 mmHg
   b. 6 to 10 cmHg
   c. 2 to 6 mmHg
   d. 25 to 35 mmHg

5. Pulmonary artery wedge pressures (PAWP) are used as a way to approximate:
   a. Right ventricular pressures
   b. Central venous pressure
   c. Left ventricular end diastolic pressure
   d. Systemic blood pressure

CHAPTER 6 ANSWERS AND RATIONALES

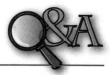

1. **b.**

   Rationale: The tricuspid and mitral valves are closing in preparation for systole.

2. **a.**

   Rationale: It sounds like "Tennessee" with the other heart sounds.

3. **d.**

   Rationale: The patient having a cardiac catheterization should have nothing by mouth for at least 8 hours prior to the test.

4. **c.**

   Rationale: A normal CVP is 2–6 mmHg.

5. **c.**

   Rationale: PAWP are used to approximate the left ventricular end diastolic pressure by filling a balloon that is wedged in a pulmonary artery and sensing the pressure ahead of the catheter.

This chapter will discuss the following disorders of the cardiovascular system as they pertain to the process of oxygenation:

- Atherosclerosis

- Coronary artery disease

- Heart failure

- Pulmonary edema

- Peripheral arterial disease

7

Disorders of the Cardiovascular System: Impact on Oxygenation

TERMS
- [ ] artherosclerosis
- [ ] plaque
- [ ] hypertension
- [ ] angina pectoris
- [ ] myocardial infarction
- [ ] coronary artery bypass graft
- [ ] heart failure
- [ ] percutaneous transluminal angioplasty
- [ ] pulmonary edema
- [ ] thrombolytic agents

CASE STUDY

Mr. K arrives in the emergency department with chest pain. He is 64 years old, has a history of hypertension, a significant smoking history (50 pack-years), and is moderately obese. Today, his blood pressure is 160/93, heart rate 100, respiratory rate 24, and oxygen saturation 94%. Per protocol, he receives aspirin, oxygen at 2 L/min via nasal prongs and intravenous morphine. His pain is somewhat relieved by nitroglycerine and morphine, but his EKG shows ST elevations. An emergent cardiac catheterization shows an 80% stenosis of the left anterior descending artery, and angioplasty is performed with stent placement. Mr. K's pain subsides quickly after reperfusion, and he is discharged 2 days later. His discharge medications include propanolol and sublingual nitroglycerine. Mr. K returns to the office for a follow-up 1 week later.

Important Questions to Ask

♦ What are the risk factors for coronary artery disease?
♦ Why does Mr. K's pain subside after stent placement?
♦ How does propanolol help patients with coronary artery disease?
♦ What teaching will you do regarding the use of sublingual nitro-glycerine?
♦ Which cardiovascular risk factors are modifiable, and how will you incorporate these into your teaching with Mr. K?

The functioning of the cardiovascular system is integral to the process of oxygenation. The cardiovascular system perfuses tissues with oxygenated blood and removes the waste products of cellular metabolism. Without a delivery system of blood vessels and a pumping heart, the process of breathing would be useless to the body. The respiratory and cardiovascular systems work together in the process of oxygenation.

There are many disorders of the cardiovascular system, but not all of them are appropriately covered in a book that focuses on oxygenation. This chapter will focus on selected cardiovascular disorders that affect the delivery of oxygen to the cells. Atherosclerosis, coronary artery disease, heart failure, peripheral arterial disease, and cardiogenic shock will be covered in this chapter. Cardiovascular disorders require collaborative interventions by members of the healthcare team to facilitate patient recovery from acute conditions, to minimize complications for patients with chronic conditions, and to maximize the patient's functional abilities.

 # ATHEROSCLEROSIS

Atherosclerosis is the most common cause of arterial obstruction and can lead to peripheral arterial disease, coronary artery disease, and cerebrovascular accidents (CVA). **Arteriosclerosis** is a general term to describe a number of disorders in which the arterial walls thicken and lose elasticity. Where arteriosclerosis is a generalized disorder, **atherosclerosis** refers to the thickening of large and medium-size arteries with the deposition of fatty streaks or plaques that decrease the lumen of the artery (see Figure 7-1).

Causes of atherosclerosis include the following:

- Accumulation of lipids in the connective tissue
- Overgrowth of smooth muscle and accumulation of macrophages and T cells
- Formation of a matrix of connective tissue within the intima of the vessel

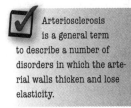
Arteriosclerosis is a general term to describe a number of disorders in which the arterial walls thicken and lose elasticity.

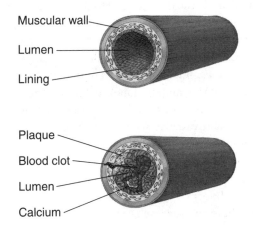

Muscular wall
Lumen
Lining

Plaque
Blood clot
Lumen
Calcium

Figure 7-1 Atherosclerotic plaque narrowing the artery.

Atherosclerosis is usually a silent disorder until the blood flow is severely diminished. When the lumen of an artery is obstructed to the point where blood flow is inadequate to meet the tissue demands, hypoxia and ischemia develop distal to the blockage because of an insufficient supply of oxygen. Without sufficient oxygen, the tissue converts from aerobic to anaerobic metabolism. Lactic acid and other caustic waste products result from anaerobic metabolism, causing irritation and pain in the local tissues. When an artery becomes blocked by plaques, thrombosis, or embolism, tissue necrosis or death may occur.

The process of fatty deposition and plaque formation seems to be enhanced by other factors, such as genetic predetermination, diseases such as diabetes and hypertension, and lifestyle habits such as high fat intake and smoking.

The etiology of atherosclerotic changes is unknown but many theories exist. One theory is that the intimal (inner) wall of an artery is damaged and platelets cluster or aggregate over the injury (the so-called **platelet aggregation theory**). The platelets stimulate proliferation of smooth muscle in the vessel wall, blocking the lumen of the artery. Another theory hypothesizes that lipids deposit over the injury on the intimal wall of the arteries and a fibrous plaque forms over this fatty core (the **chronic endothelial injury theory**.) The process of fatty deposition and plaque formation seems to be enhanced by other factors, such as genetic predetermination, diseases such as diabetes and hypertension, and lifestyle habits such as high fat intake and smoking.

Over years, the atherosclerotic process progresses and the arteries may become narrowed. The tissues distal to the blockage are increasingly deprived of oxygenated blood. Arteries around the heart may become blocked, causing angina and myocardial infarction. Arteries in the legs may become narrowed, and nonhealing ulcers or gangrene may develop on the feet and toes. Infection in the gangrenous tissue may become life-threatening, requiring amputation of the limb. Plaque in the carotid arteries can break off and block cerebral arteries, causing transient ischemic attacks or cerebrovascular accidents (CVAs or strokes.) The ramifications of atherosclerosis are astounding in terms of loss of function, quality of life, and even death.

Atherosclerosis is a silent disease until years of damage to the vessels have been done. Abnormal levels of fats in the blood or **dyslipidemia** appear to contribute to atherosclerosis. Dyslipidemia refers to disorders of fat or lipoprotein metabolism including lipoprotein overproduction or deficiency. Dyslipidemias may be manifested by elevation of the total cholesterol, the "bad" **low-density lipoprotein (LDL)** cholesterol and the triglyceride concentrations, and a decrease in the "good" **high-density lipoprotein (HDL)** cholesterol concentration in the blood. Two genetic predispositions to dyslipidemia are e-4 allele and the pattern B form of high low-density lipoprotein (LDL) levels.

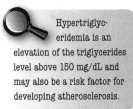

Hypertriglyceridemia is an elevation of the triglycerides level above 150 mg/dL and may also be a risk factor for developing atherosclerosis.

Triglycerides, another fatty substance in the blood, are measured separately from cholesterol levels. **Hypertriglyceridemia** is an elevation of the triglycerides level above 150 mg/dL and may also be a risk factor for developing atherosclerosis. Hypertriglyceridemia is thought to be a congenital disorder, and its affect on the development of atherosclerosis is being studied. Triglycerides may also be elevated with excessive alcohol consumption and disorders of carbohydrate metabolism.

To screen for congenital dyslipidemia, total serum cholesterol should be performed on all people over the age of 20. The National Cholesterol Education Program (2004) set aggressive guidelines for lowering LDL levels based on a patient's risk profile, LDL, HDL, and triglyceride levels. Detection of dyslipidemia in early adulthood allows time for lifestyle changes, dietary modifications, and possibly medications to correct elevations or disproportions in lipoprotein levels (see Table 7-1).

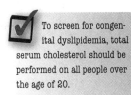

To screen for congenital dyslipidemia, total serum cholesterol should be performed on all people over the age of 20.

Atherosclerosis can lead to high blood pressure or **hypertension**. The diminished elasticity of the arteries and the thickening caused by plaque formation and smooth muscle proliferation can make the vessels less responsive to changes in blood pressure. Conversely, hypertension may cause atherosclerotic changes in the vessel walls because of consistently high pressure and tension exerted on the intimal membranes of the vessels.

Hypertension does not directly decrease oxygen supply to the tissues, but it is a risk factor for the development of atherosclerosis. Controlling hypertension is an essential component of preventing atherosclerosic changes to the blood vessels. However, because hypertension does not directly affect oxygenation, it will not be reviewed in this book.

Table 7-1 Therapeutic Lifestyle Changes to Improve Dyslipidemia

- Reduce weight—Maintaining the appropriate weight is important for reducing lipids. Being overweight is a risk factor for high blood pressure and cardiovascular disorders.

- Modify diet—Decreasing total fat intake, and especially saturated fats and cholesterol, can lower LDLs, particularly in patients with congenital hyperlipidemia. If LDLs are between 130 to 159, a fat-modified diet is usually prescribed. If LDLs are greater than 160, both saturated fat and cholesterol intake need to be reduced. The American Heart Association recommends the following dietary proportions to decrease fat intake and serum cholesterol:

    Step 1: Diet—Reduce total daily fat intake to less than 30% of total daily caloric intake, saturated fat intake to less than 10%, and total cholesterol to less than 300 mg/day.

    Step 2: Diet (if LDLs remain elevated after Step 1 diet)—Reduce saturated fat intake to less than 7% and total cholesterol to less than 200 mg/day.

- Exercise—Moderate exercise (30 minutes a day, three to five times a week) appears to promote optimal lipid levels and decrease the risk of cardiovascular disease. Exercise may also promote collateral circulation and plaque regression. A stress test may be prescribed before starting an exercise program.

- Stop smoking—Smoking increases the risks for peripheral arterial disease, hypertension, low HDL levels (the "good cholesterol"), and cardiovascular disease. Even half a pack of cigarettes a day can significantly increase the chances of a person dying from heart disease. Encourage all patients to quit smoking and especially those with hyperlipidemia.

- Control hypertension—Take blood pressure medication regularly, and get follow-up blood pressure measurements as prescribed.

- Take cholesterol-lowering medications regularly (if prescribed after dietary interventions alone are not working) to decrease total lipids—Types of medications include the following:
  - Bile-acid sequestrants (cholestyramine)
  - Nicotinic acid (niacin)
  - Fibric acid (gemfibrozil)
  - HMG-CoA reductase inhibitors (Lovastatin)

- Control diabetes—Follow prescribed dietary and medical treatment for diabetes if this is also a problem. Consultation with a dietician or diabetic teaching nurse may help the patient understand the disease and facilitate better control of blood sugar.

CORONARY ARTERY DISEASE

Changes to the coronary arteries brought on by atherosclerosis can result in diminished blood flow to the myocardium. If the heart muscle does not receive an adequate blood supply with the necessary oxygen and nutrients, ischemia can result. Patients with myocardial ischemia often have chest pain or **angina**. If the ischemia is prolonged, tissue death occurs and the patient has a **myocardial infarction** (MI or heart attack).

Atherosclerotic changes in the coronary arteries develop silently until the lumen of the artery is blocked more than 70%. At this point, the decrease in blood flow to the myocardial tissue becomes more evident when the patients exercise or increase activity levels, thus increasing the myocardial oxygen demands. The narrowed or obstructed

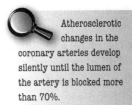

Atherosclerotic changes in the coronary arteries develop silently until the lumen of the artery is blocked more than 70%.

coronary artery can not supply enough blood to meet the myocardial demands, and the result is tissue hypoxia and ischemia. Patients experience chest pain or tightness that usually subsides once the activity level is decreased and the demand for oxygen subsides.

Angina

When the myocardium is ischemic, the patient feels chest pain or angina. The Latin phrase **angina pectoris** means "strangling of the chest." Patients may describe their pain differently. Some common descriptions are tightness, burning, boring, or aching. Careful assessment of symptoms is necessary because women are more apt to describe angina as indigestion and nausea or vague sensations of not feeling well. Angina is classified into two groups:

- Stable angina—Chest pain that occurs with exercise and disappears with rest
- Unstable angina—Chest pain at rest or with minimal exertion

Careful assessment of symptoms is necessary because women are more apt to describe angina as indigestion and nausea or vague sensations of not feeling well.

Angina is a clinical diagnosis based on a history of chest pain brought on by exertion and relieved by rest. Chest pain relieved by nitroglycerine is also characteristic of angina. Exercise stress tests and radionuclide scans may be performed to establish the diagnosis. EKG findings may occur during an episode of angina and disappear after the attack. Coronary arteriography may be used to examine the extent of the coronary artery disease and determine whether other interventions are necessary.

Treatment of Angina

Patients with angina are at risk for unstable angina, myocardial infarction, and sudden death. Treatment involves relieving the symptoms, modifying risk factors, treating underlying coronary artery disease and starting the appropriate medications. Nonpharmacologic treatment is directed at modifying risk factors through weight loss, exercise, and stress reduction. Some ways to reduce stress include lifestyle modification, massage, yoga, and meditation.

> Patients with angina are at risk for unstable angina, myocardial infarction, and sudden death.

Pharmacologic treatment for angina includes short- and long-acting nitroglycerine, beta-blockers (metoprolol, atenolol, and propanolol), and calcium channel blockers (nifedipine, verapramil, and dilitiazem). Patients are instructed to carry sublingual nitroglycerine with them at all times. Antiplatelet drugs such as aspirin and clopidogrel are used to decrease platelet aggregation. If symptoms persevere despite lifestyle changes, risk reduction and pharmacologic therapies, then surgical intervention (balloon angioplasty or coronary artery bypass surgery) may be required to reperfuse the myocardium and prevent life-threatening damage to the heart muscle.

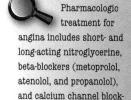

Pharmacologic treatment for angina includes short- and long-acting nitroglycerine, beta-blockers (metoprolol, atenolol, and propanolol), and calcium channel blockers (nifedipine, verapramil, and dilitiazem).

Heart Disease

The New York Heart Association (NYHA) has classified heart disease depending on the amount of dysfunction (see Table 7-2).

Unstable angina is treated more aggressively because of the increased risk of myocardial infarction and sudden death. Aspirin and heparin may

Table 7-2 New York Heart Association Classification of Heart Disease

Class	Patient Symptoms
Class I (Mild)	No limitation of physical activity. Ordinary physical activity does not cause undue fatigue, palpitation, or dyspnea (shortness of breath).
Class II (Mild)	Slight limitation of physical activity. Comfortable at rest, but ordinary physical activity results in fatigue, palpitation, or dyspnea.
Class III (Moderate)	Marked limitation of physical activity. Comfortable at rest, but more than ordinary activity causes fatigue, palpitation, or dyspnea.
Class IV (Severe)	Unable to carry out any physical activity without discomfort. Symptoms of cardiac insufficiency at rest. If any physical activity is undertaken, discomfort is increased.

be used to prevent MI. Balloon angioplasty and coronary artery bypass surgery (CABG) may provide excellent relief if the patient has localized disease and is a good candidate for surgery. (See section on CABG surgery later in this chapter.)

Myocardial Infarction

Myocardial infarction is the leading cause of death in the United States with approximately 800,000 people affected annually. Myocardial ischemia can progress to a myocardial infarction (MI) if a coronary artery is narrowed or occluded for too long. This may happen if a plaque ruptures, blocking a coronary artery, if platelets clump or aggregate on irregular surface (like an atherosclerotic plaque) inside the artery, or if a thrombus develops and occludes the artery. If a coronary artery is 80% to 90% occluded, then ischemia develops in the myocardium distal to the blockage. If the ischemia continues and the blood flow is not returned, then tissue necrosis or death occurs. This is called a myocardial infarction.

A myocardial infarction develops over several hours, and quick treatment may limit the extent of tissue death. Survival rates increase to 90–95% if patients are hospitalized with an MI. The most common cause of death from myocardial infarctions prior to hospitalization is cardiac

> Myocardial infarction is the leading cause of death in the United States with approximately 800,000 people affected annually.

arrest, usually due to ventricular dysrhythmias. Patients with chest pain should be brought into the healthcare system as soon as possible so that life-threatening dysrhythmias can be detected and treated quickly and myocardial oxygenation can be improved.

> The most common cause of death from myocardial infarctions prior to hospitalization is cardiac arrest, usually due to ventricular dysrhythmias.

Myocardial infarctions often begin with necrosis of the subendocardial layer of the heart but may progress through other layers of the myocardium. If the infarction spreads to all three layers of the heart, this is called a **transmural** ("through the wall") MI. Transmural MIs can affect ventricular wall motion and cardiac output. Left ventricular wall damage from transmural MIs can result in heart failure and cardiogenic shock.

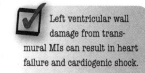
Left ventricular wall damage from transmural MIs can result in heart failure and cardiogenic shock.

Myocardial infarctions are often described in terms of the damage to the heart tissue. The myocardium that dies due to the infarction is divided into three sections: the **zone of necrosis**, surrounded by a **zone of injury** and, further out, a **zone of ischemia** (see Figure 7-2). Prompt treatment may provide oxygen to the outer two zones of an infarction and reduce the extent of myocardial necrosis.

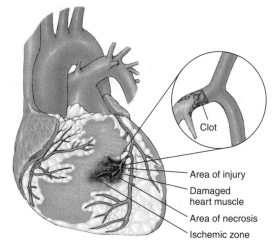

Clot
Area of injury
Damaged heart muscle
Area of necrosis
Ischemic zone

Figure 7-2 Zones of myocardial infarction.

Depending on the location and extent of the tissue death, the conduction system of the heart may be damaged, the cardiac output diminished, or the heart may stop beating. The type of response to an MI depends on which arteries are occluded (see Figure 7-3).

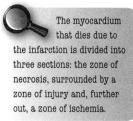

The myocardium that dies due to the infarction is divided into three sections: the zone of necrosis, surrounded by a zone of injury and, further out, a zone of ischemia.

The three most common coronary arteries to become obstructed during a myocardial infarction are the left anterior descending, circumflex, and right coronary arteries:

- Left anterior descending (LAD) artery—Supplies anterior wall and septum and usually produces anterior and septal MIs. Anterior wall MIs account for 25% of all infarctions and have the highest mortality rate. The left ventricular wall is frequently damaged in anterior MIs, resulting in ventricular failure and dysrhythmias.
- Circumflex artery—Supplies part of the left ventricular wall and portions of the conduction system
- Right coronary artery (RCA)—Perfuses the SA and AV nodes, and obstructions of this artery produce bradycardias and heart blocks. Blockage of the RCA usually causes an inferior MI.

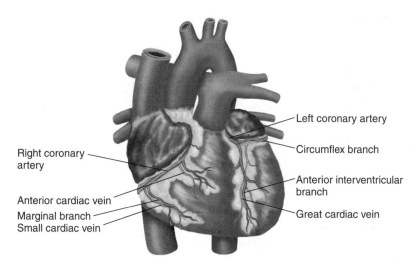

Figure 7-3 Coronary arteries.

Assessment of the Patient with Chest Pain

Assessment of a patient with chest pain who may be having an MI is divided into two parts. One is a quick assessment of the presenting pain. The second part of the assessment includes the family history and risk factors and is done when the patient is stable and comfortable.

The quick assessment is followed by physical assessment and treatment.

Quick Assessment

Rapid assessment of patients with chest pain is important as it provides information to direct interventions to minimize damage to the myocardium. Quick assessment includes the following:

- Type of pain (e.g., burning, aching, stabbing, pressure, or tightness)—Women may describe indigestion or vague sensations of not feeling well.
- Location of the pain (e.g., chest, left shoulder, left arm, or jaw should be noted)—Radiation of the pain to the jaw, shoulder, and back is more common during an MI than with angina.
- Intensity of pain—Graded on a scale of 1 to 10
- Pain duration—Pain from a myocardial infarction usually lasts more than 30 minutes and is relieved only by opioids. Chest pain from angina is usually relieved by nitroglycerine and rest.
- Relieving factors—What has the patient tried to relieve the pain and what has worked (e.g., nitroglycerine under the tongue will relieve anginal pain but not MI pain)? Rest may relieve anginal pain but not MI pain.
- Precipitating factors—What makes the chest pain come on or become more intense? Anginal pain may be brought on by exertion or stress. MI pain may occur without cause and commonly starts early in the morning.

What has the patient tried to relieve the chest pain and what has worked (e.g., nitroglycerine under the tongue will relieve anginal pain but not MI pain)?

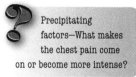

Precipitating factors—What makes the chest pain come on or become more intense?

Patients with chest pain may have additional symptoms such as nausea, vomiting, diaphoresis, dizziness, palpitations, shortness of breath, and headache. Note any additional symptoms that are not necessarily classic chest pain. It is important to remember that women may experience chest pain and describe it differently from men. Women more often report other symptoms that are more general such as indigestion and dizziness, resulting in overlooked cardiac problems. Careful screening questions and an open mind are important in accurately assessing all patients with chest pain.

 Women more often report other symptoms that are more general such as indigestion and dizziness, resulting in overlooked cardiac problems.

Physical Assessment

Physical assessment should proceed quickly and perhaps occur during questioning:

1. Vital signs—Blood pressure, heart rate, respiratory rate, temperature, and oxygen saturation. In patients with an MI, decreased cardiac output may be manifested by hypotension, tachycardia, diaphoresis, diminished peripheral pulses bilaterally, and cool skin. Temperature may be elevated to as high as 102°F (38.9°C) for several days after an MI.

2. Cardiac monitor and 12-lead EKG—The patient should be connected to a cardiac monitor to assess for dysrhythmias. Sinus tachycardia with frequent premature beats occurs early in the course of an MI because of ischemia. A 12-lead EKG provides further information about the location of ischemia and necrosis. Changes in the S-T segment, T waves, and Q waves may be seen on the EKG during an MI. (In-depth analysis of EKGs is beyond the scope of this book. See the bibliography.)

3. Vascular access—The patient should have an IV placed as soon as possible for intravenous medications and fluids.

The diagnosis of myocardial infarction is based on symptoms, history, EKG changes, and elevation of troponin T and cardiac isoenzymes. MIs are usually caused by blockage of a coronary artery by a plaque or thrombus, but they can also be caused by vasospasm of a coronary artery, prolonged hypotension,

> A 12-lead EKG provides further information about the location of ischemia and necrosis. Changes in the S-T segment, T waves, and Q waves may be seen on the EKG during an MI.

and excessive metabolic demands. MIs are often divided into Q wave and non-Q wave infarctions. The Q wave is seen on the EKG, and its presence is associated with prolonged myocardial ischemia and necrosis. Non-Q wave MIs are associated with early reperfusion of the ischemic myocardium and better outcomes. Diagnostic tests for MI include laboratory blood work, exercise stress test, thallium scan, and cardiac catheterization.

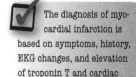
The diagnosis of myocardial infarction is based on symptoms, history, EKG changes, and elevation of troponin T and cardiac isoenzymes.

Cardiac enzymes are useful laboratory blood tests that can confirm that an MI has occurred. **Creatine phosophokinase (CPK)** is a cardiac enzyme that rises within 3 hours of an MI, peaks in 24 hours, and returns to normal in 48 to 72 hours. CPK is released when muscle tissue has been damaged. A specific component of CPK, the **CPK-MB isoenzyme**, is released into the bloodstream when the cardiac muscle is damaged. CPK-MB levels are elevated for 24 hours after an MI. **Lactic dehydrogenase (LDH)** also rises after an MI and remains elevated for a week after the MI. A complete blood count is also done to rule out other disorders such as anemia. White blood cells may be elevated (up to 1500/mL) on days two to seven after an MI. **Troponin** is a newer serum indicator of myocardial damage. Troponin I and T may rise earlier than the CPK and remain elevated longer than CPK-MB, allowing for diagnosis of MI after the initial 24-hour peak of CPK-MB. Exercise stress tests may be done after the acute stage of an MI to assess the extent of ischemia and necrosis and to determine the need for more invasive therapies such as cardiac catheterization, angioplasty, or bypass surgery (see Table 7-3).

Thallium scans are also useful in imaging the areas of ischemia and necrosis. Thallium is injected intravenously and is "picked up" by the per-

Table 7-3 Normal Values of Blood Tests to Detect Myocardial Infarction

Laboratory Test	Normal Values
Total creatinine phosphokinase (CPK)	30–200 U/L
CPK, MB fraction	0.0–8.8 ng/mL
CPK, MB fraction percent of total CPK	0–4%
CPK, MB2 fraction	< 1 U/L
Troponin I	0.0–0.4 ng/mL
Troponin T	0.0–0.1 ng/mL

fused myocardium. Areas of decreased perfusion in the heart pick up less thallium and
are imaged as "cold spots" on the scan.

Cardiac catheterization (as described in
Chapter 6) is used to visualize the coronary
arteries and locate occlusions. Not only does
cardiac catheterization provide visualization
of the coronary arteries, it may also provide
a route for invasive interventions such as angioplasty, stent placement, and laser removal of obstructions.

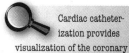

Cardiac catheter-
ization provides
visualization of the coronary
arteries. It may also provide
a route for invasive interventions such as angioplasty,
stent placement, and laser
removal of obstructions.

Treatment

Treatment of angina and MI begins in a similar manner while further
diagnostic testing for an MI is being conducted.

The goals of treatment are the following:

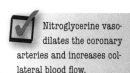

Nitroglycerine vaso-
dilates the coronary
arteries and increases collateral blood flow.

♦ Relieve pain.
♦ Increase myocardial oxygen supply.
♦ Decrease myocardial oxygen demand.
♦ Minimize damage to myocardium.

Pain relief is an essential part of early treatment. The experience of pain
results in a catecholamine release that increases the heart rate, blood pressure, and myocardial oxygen demand. The first treatment for chest pain
whether from angina or infarction is nitroglycerine 0.3 to 0.4 mg sublin-
gually. Intravenous nitroglycerine is a potent vasodilator and can rapidly
decrease the blood pressure (see Table 7-4). It may also be given topically
in an ointment for longer-acting relief than sublingual administration.
Nitroglycerine vasodilates the coronary arteries and increases collateral
blood flow. If the pain is from ischemia (anginal pain), sublingual nitroglycerine will bring prompt relief. If the pain is not relieved and the systolic
blood pressure remains above 100 mmHg, then sublingual nitroglycerine
may be repeated every 5 minutes for a total of three doses. Side effects of
nitroglycerine include rapid onset of hypotension and headache. Patients
should be instructed to lie down before taking nitroglycerine. For many patients with angina, sublingual nitroglycerine and cessation of activity bring
rapid relief of their chest pain.

If three doses of nitroglycerine do not relieve the pain or if the pain
is very severe, then intravenous morphine is given to decrease the pain

Table 7-4 Nursing Care of the Patient with Chest Pain

1. Assess signs and symptoms of chest pain. Include location, severity, radiation, onset, precipitating factors, relieving factors, and associated symptoms.
2. Relieve pain with collaborative interventions (nitroglycerine, morphine) and nonpharmacologic methods such as massage, deep breathing, and a calming atmosphere.
3. Provide supplemental oxygen at 2 to 4 L/min (if not contraindicated) to improve myocardial oxygenation.
4. Place the patient in the semi-Fowler's or high Fowler's position to promote comfort and breathing.
5. Decrease myocardial oxygen demands by promoting rest, controlling pain, and talking with the patient and his or her family in a calm and reassuring manner.

and diminish the myocardial oxygen demand. Side effects of morphine include respiratory depression, hypotension, and vomiting. Morphine is given intravenously because it provides prompt relief, can be titrated to achieve adequate pain control, and it does not damage muscle tissue as an intramuscular injection. Remember that damaged muscle tissue releases creatine phosphokinase (CPK), one of the diagnostic measures for determining the occurrence of an MI. Nursing interventions for the patient experiencing chest pain are found in Table 7-4.

 Side effects of morphine include respiratory depression, hypotension, and vomiting.

Increasing available oxygen improves the chances for the recovery of ischemic and injured myocardium. Oxygen via nasal cannula is often administered at 2 to 4 L/min. If the patient is also in respiratory distress from heart failure as evidenced by a rapid respiratory rate, low Pao_2 or Sao_2, then he may require intubation and mechanical ventilation to maintain adequate oxygen levels.

Decreasing myocardial oxygen demands is accomplished through pain relief, rest, and reassurance. Pain and anxiety, as previously discussed, increase catecholamine release. The nurse should provide a calm atmosphere and speak in a reassuring manner when explaining all interventions to the patient. Try to stay with the patient and incorporate a family member in discussions about the patient's care.

Patients with myocardial infarctions are usually admitted to intensive care or the coronary care unit. Their care includes close cardiac monitoring, rest, analgesia, oxygen therapy, and treatment of dysrhythmias and heart failure. Medications for myocardial infarction are used to decrease the myocardial oxygen demands, increase the cardiac output, and improve oxygenation of the myocardial tissue.

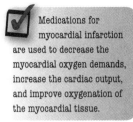

Medications for myocardial infarction are used to decrease the myocardial oxygen demands, increase the cardiac output, and improve oxygenation of the myocardial tissue.

Commonly used medications during myocardial infarction include the following:

- Nitrates—Vasodilate coronary and other arteries (sublingual and intravenous nitroglycerine). Side effects include hypotension and headache.
- Isosorbide dinitrate—Promotes vasodilation. Side effects include hypotension and dizziness.
- Beta-blockers (propanolol, atenolol)—Decrease heart rate, blood pressure, and cardiac output. A decreased heart rate allows for a longer period of diastole, which is when the heart perfuses itself. Side effects include bradycardia and bronchoconstriction. (*Note:* Beta-blockers may contribute to the development of heart failure in patients with myocardial infarction.)
- Aspirin and other antiplatelet agents—Decrease inflammatory response and prevent platelet aggregation. Side effects include gastric irritation and tinnitus (at high doses). Newer agents include platelet IIb and IIIa receptor blockers.
- Angiotensin-converting enzyme (ACE) inhibitors (enalapril)— Decrease the work of the heart by decreasing systemic blood pressure and afterload. ACE inhibitors also affect ventricular remodeling after MI. Side effects include hypotension, cough, and edema.
- Sympathomimetics (dobutamine and dopamine)—Increase blood pressure in patients who are hypotensive but not in shock. Side effects include dysrhythmias, increased heart rate, and blood pressure. Sympathomimetics are titrated in an intensive care setting with hemodynamic monitoring.

Beta-blockers may contribute to the development of heart failure in patients with myocardial infarction.

More invasive strategies may be used to treat myocardial infarction depending on the symptoms, EKG findings, catheterization results, or other diagnostic test findings. Interventions include the administration of thrombolytic agents, percutaneous transluminal angioplasty (PTCA), stent placement, laser treatment of lesions in the coronary arteries, and coronary artery bypass surgery.

Thrombolytic Agents

Thrombolytic agents are used to dissolve thrombi that are occluding coronary arteries. Because myocardial infarctions evolve over a period of hours, there is often a window of opportunity to open the artery and reperfuse ischemic myocardium. Thrombolytic agents are most effective if given within 6 hours of the coronary event. These agents are administered intravenously or via a coronary route during cardiac catheterization. Some examples are streptokinase, tissue plasminogen activator (tPA), and anisoylated plasminogen-streptokinase activator complex (APSAC).

Nursing Care for Patients Receiving Thrombolytic Therapy

Nursing care for the patient receiving thrombolytic therapy entails understanding the nature of these medications. Thrombolytics affect the clotting mechanism of the blood all over the body. Clots form when platelets and fibrin threads create a mesh that captures red blood cells. Thrombolytics facilitate the breakdown of clots by accelerating the conversion of plasminogen to plasmin, a clot dissolver (see Figure 7-4). Streptokinase in particular is not fibrin-specific and may cause systemic bleeding problems. Because of this risk, patients with known bleeding in the gastrointestinal or cerebrovascular system are not candidates for this treatment.

 Streptokinase is not fibrin-specific and may cause systemic bleeding problems.

Nursing interventions for patients receiving thrombolytic therapy include the following:

1. Assess indications of reperfusion after injection of thrombolytic agent (i.e., relief of chest pain, reversal of EKG changes, and sudden onset of ventricular ectopy, sometimes referred to as reperfusion dysrhythmias).

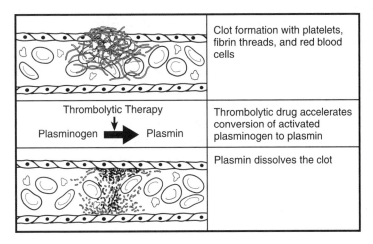

	Clot formation with platelets, fibrin threads, and red blood cells
Thrombolytic Therapy Plasminogen ➡ Plasmin	Thrombolytic drug accelerates conversion of activated plasminogen to plasmin
	Plasmin dissolves the clot

Figure 7-4 Thrombolytic therapy.

2. Observe for signs of hypersensitivity to the thrombolytic agent (e.g., itching, hives). Premedication with steroids and antihistamines is often done, particularly before treatment with streptokinase.

3. Assess for signs of bleeding, including neurological changes, abdominal pain, changes in color of urine and stool, changes in hemoglobin, and hematocrit values from pretreatment values.

4. Assess blood pressure and heart rate during and after injection of the thrombolytic agent and compare to pretreatment values.

After reperfusion, the physician usually prescribes heparin and intravenous nitroglycerine for several days to maintain the patency of the reopened coronary artery. Long-term therapy includes daily aspirin to decrease the incidence of platelet aggregation or clopidogrel, a platelet aggregation inhibitor.

Cardiac Catheterization

Cardiac catheterization is frequently performed after the acute phase of angina or myocardial infarction has resolved. Using injected dye, the coronary arteries and their blockages or lesions can be visualized. If the patient is shown to have a treatable lesion in a coronary artery, **percutaneous transluminal angioplasty (PTCA)** can be performed. The best candidates for PTCA have one or two vessel disease with proximal, noncalcified lesions. PTCA involves catheterization of the left side of the heart from the femoral artery and fluoroscopic insertion of a balloon-tipped catheter to the area of the lesion (see Figure 7-5). The balloon is then inflated to compress the plaque against the vessel wall. Balloon inflation may be repeated to maintain the patency of the artery. A stent may be placed to maintain the opening by providing stiffer scaffolding in the newly opened artery. Laser angioplasty and arthrectomy may also be used to remove atherosclerotic plaque in the artery during cardiac catheterization.

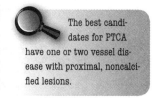

The best candidates for PTCA have one or two vessel disease with proximal, noncalcified lesions.

Coronary Artery Bypass Grafting

Invasive surgery may be needed to perfuse the myocardium. **Coronary artery bypass graft surgery (CABG)** can bypass occluded vessels and provide blood flow to the myocardium. CABG may be needed when patients do not respond to medical management or when the symptoms or diagnostic tests show disease progression. Indications for coronary artery bypassing include the following:

- Unstable angina with severe two or three vessel disease
- Left main coronary artery disease with angina
- Acute myocardial infarction
- Signs of impending MI after PTCA
- Ischemia with heart failure

Bypass surgery involves grafting a piece of blood vessel (the saphenous vein or internal mammary artery are common donor vessels) from the aorta to an area distal to the occlusion in the coronary artery (see Figure 7-6). CABG surgery may be done on an immediate basis if the patient's condition warrants it, or it may be scheduled after the acute phase of a myocardial infarction. Several vessels may be bypassed during the surgery.

CABG is accomplished by splitting the sternum (medial sternotomy) and opening the thoracic cage to reveal the heart. CABG may be performed with the patient on **cardiopulmonary bypass** (extracorporeal circulation) or with the heart beating (so-called "beating-heart" surgery). If cardiopulmonary bypass is used, then the heart is stopped with a cold cardioplegia solution to decrease the metabolic (and oxygen) re-

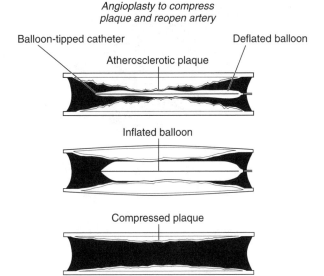

*Angioplasty to compress
plaque and reopen artery*

Balloon-tipped catheter

Atherosclerotic plaque

Deflated balloon

Inflated balloon

Compressed plaque

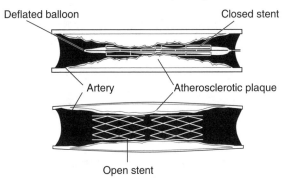

*Stent placement after angioplasty
to maintain arterial patency*

Deflated balloon

Closed stent

Artery

Atherosclerotic plaque

Open stent

Figure 7-5 Angioplasty and stent placement.

quirements of the heart. The body is also cooled to reduce its metabolic requirements. Electrodes are left on the atria and ventricles in case temporary pacing is needed after the surgery. Chest tubes are placed in the mediastinum and thorax to drain fluid and promote lung reexpansion. Postoperative complications of CABG include myocardial infarction,

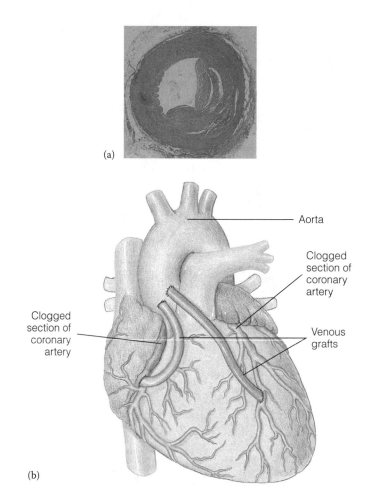

Figure 7-6 Coronary artery bypass grafting. (a) Atherosclerotic plaque in coronary arteries can block the flow of blood to heart muscle. (b) Venous grafts bypass coronary arteries blocked by atherosclerotic plaque. *Source:* Part A © William Ober/Visuals Unlimited.

dysrhythmias, heart failure, cardiac tamponade (bleeding), pneumothorax, impaired renal function, thromboembolism, and cerebral vascular accidents.

Postoperative complications of CABG include myocardial infarction, dysrhythmias, heart failure, cardiac tamponade (bleeding), pneumothorax, impaired renal function, thromboembolism, and cerebral vascular accidents.

Nursing Care of the Patient Undergoing Bypass Surgery

Nursing care preoperatively involves allaying the patient's anxiety. Because surgery involves the heart, many patients fear dying during the surgery. Focusing on postoperative care may help the patient feel he or she is going to get through the surgery. Explain the intensive care unit, ventilator, chest tubes, intravenous lines, cardiac monitoring, and pain relief. Take time to explain the surgery to the patient and his or her family and show the family where to wait and how to contact their surgeon after the surgery. Families benefit from seeing their loved one as soon as possible after surgery.

The care of the patient undergoing coronary artery bypass grafting fills entire books and is beyond the scope of this text. Refer to the bibliography at the end of the text for further information.

HEART FAILURE

Heart failure is the result of the heart's inability to pump sufficient amounts of blood to meet the metabolic needs of the body. There are many causes of heart failure, including myocardial ischemia and infarction, valvular dysfunction, hypertension, dysrhythmias, and constrictive pericarditis. If the body has compensated for the heart failure, sympathetic stimulation will increase the heart rate and blood pressure. Increased antidiuretic hormone (ADH) secretion will activate the renin-angiotensin-aldosterone

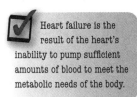

Heart failure is the result of the heart's inability to pump sufficient amounts of blood to meet the metabolic needs of the body.

system, resulting in salt and water retention. If the body can no longer compensate for the failing heart, the pulmonary artery pressures will increase and the ejection fraction will fall.

Heart failure can be divided in many ways, including right- and left-sided failure, backward and forward failure, and systolic and diastolic failure:

- Right-sided failure (cor pulmonale)—Reduced emptying of the right ventricle with systemic venous congestion and major organ engorgement
- Left-sided failure—Decreased emptying of the left ventricle with decreased tissue perfusion and backup of blood in the pulmonary vasculature

- Backward failure—Inadequate emptying of the ventricle
- Forward failure—Caused by low cardiac output
- Systolic failure—Decreased ventricular emptying and ventricular dilation
- Diastolic failure—Impaired relaxation of the ventricle and decreased filling

Symptoms of heart failure are dependent on which side of the heart is failing and whether the failure is backward or forward. This chapter will focus on left-sided heart failure and right-sided heart failure, particularly cor pulmonale. Some general signs and symptoms of heart failure include the following:

- Blood pressure—High or low depending on sympathetic stimulation, fluid volumes, and degree of failure
- Respiratory pattern—Dyspnea, rapid and shallow respirations, cough
- Heart rate—Tachycardia
- Lung sounds—Crackles, perhaps wheezes, decreased breath sounds
- Heart sounds—S3 may be present.
- General symptoms—Cool and clammy skin, fatigue, restlessness, dizziness
- Circulation—Cyanosis, decreased peripheral pulses, perhaps peripheral edema, jugular vein distention, abdominal tenderness over the upper right quadrant

Left-Sided Heart Failure

The left side of the heart is the pump for circulating oxygenated blood throughout the systemic vasculature. Effective pumping may be impeded if the walls of the left ventricle have areas of necrotic and inactive tissue from myocardial ischemia and infarction or degeneration. The first signs of **left-sided heart failure** are dyspnea, diffuse pulmonary crackles, and arterial hypoxemia (see Figure 7-7). The crackles are more pronounced in the dependent regions of the lungs. These signs develop as a result of blood backing up behind the left side of the heart and into the pulmonary vasculature. The pressure in the pulmonary vessels is so high that fluid leaks out of the capillaries into the alveoli causing pulmonary edema. Systemic blood pressure may initially be elevated as a response to chest pain if an MI has occurred but may decrease as the left ventricle fails. Compensatory mechanisms respond to the falling blood pressure and stimulate the sympathetic system to increase the heart rate. Gallop rhythms (S3) may develop as the heart fails. The patient

The first signs of left-sided heart failure are dyspnea, diffuse pulmonary crackles, and arterial hypoxemia.

may complain of fatigue at rest, weakness, cold intolerance, and difficulty breathing with mild exercise. He may be anxious and restless. His skin may be pale and clammy or overtly diaphoretic.

Left-ventricular failure may lead to gradual or abrupt onset of pulmonary edema. Pulmonary hypertension results in movement of fluid from the pulmonary capillaries into the alveoli. With less alveolar surface area for gas exchange, the patient becomes hypoxemic and may have signs of cyanosis. The pulse may be thready (weak and low pressure), and the blood pressure may be difficult to obtain.

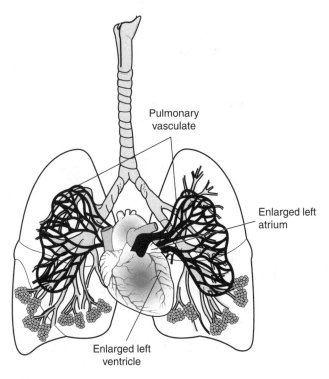

Figure 7-7 Left-sided heart failure.

Left-ventricular failure may lead to gradual or abrupt onset of pulmonary edema.

Right-Sided Heart Failure (Cor Pulmonale)

Cor pulmonale and **right-sided heart failure** may develop because of left-sided heart failure, chronic respiratory disorders such as COPD, obesity, or primary vascular disorders (such as pulmonary emboli). Left-sided heart failure is the most common cause of right-sided heart failure. The right ventricle wearies from pushing against the increased pressures in the pulmonary circulation. With pressures increasing behind a failing right side of the heart, the venous system becomes engorged, with the patient experiencing related symptoms such as increasing dyspnea on exertion. He may complain of fullness in the neck (related to jugular venous distention), tenderness over the right upper quadrant (liver fullness), and ankle swelling (peripheral edema).

In patients with chronic obstructive respiratory disorders, 25% will develop cor pulmonale as a long-term effect of chronic pulmonary hypertension. When the heart can no longer compensate for the increased pulmonary vascular resistance caused by the underlying respiratory disorder, the right ventricle becomes hypertrophied. Peripheral edema and liver enlargement may develop as the failure progresses.

Symptoms of cor pulmonale include fatigue and weakness, chronic cough, exertional dyspnea, dependent edema, distended neck veins, and liver enlargement.

Treatment of Heart Failure

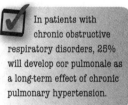
In patients with chronic obstructive respiratory disorders, 25% will develop cor pulmonale as a long-term effect of chronic pulmonary hypertension.

The nursing care of patients with heart failure requires a collaborative approach and should be customized to the patient's diagnosis and functional abilities (see Table 7-5). Treatment of heart failure involves identifying and treating the cause, reducing cardiac workload, supporting cardiac function, and improving oxygenation.

Collaborative interventions for heart failure may include the following:

• Diuretics —Decrease preload and sodium and water retention.

Table 7-5 Nursing Care of Patients with Heart Failure

1. Decrease the cardiac workload:
   - Place the patient in the semi-Fowler's position, avoid Valsalva's maneuver, avoid breath holding (increases venous return and the workload of the heart during exhalation). Administer nasal oxygen to increase inspired O_2 content.
   - Promote rest, both physical and emotional, and increase activity as ordered.
   - Provide small frequent meals to prevent excessive blood flow to the gastrointestinal tract. Avoid caffeine (a cardiac stimulant). Follow fluid and salt restrictions as ordered to reduce fluid volume excess. Monitor intake and output.
   - Do not allow smoking—nicotine is a cardiac stimulant and a vasoconstrictor.
2. Medicate to increase cardiac output and decrease fluid volume excess:
   - Administer positive inotropic agents (digitalis, dobutamine, amrinone) to increase myocardial contractility.
   - Use vasodilators (sodium nitroprusside, nitroglycerine, isosorbide, ACE inhibitors) to decrease vascular resistance and cardiac workload.
   - Administer diuretics (furosemide) to decrease preload by decreasing sodium and fluid excess.
3. Use balloon pump (counterpulsation) to increase left ventricular emptying.
4. Assessment of fluid balance:
   - Daily weights—If greater than 2% increase, then a follow-up is required.
   - Vital signs—Check blood pressure, heart rate and rhythm (check for S3, tachycardia as signs of failure), respiratory rate (increase may indicate increasing failure).
   - Intake and output—Imbalance may indicate fluid retention or kidney failure.
   - Pulmonary status—Crackles (including a gravitational component), dyspnea, orthopnea (indicates failure or fluid volume excess)
   - Jugular venous distension (JVD) and central venous pressure to follow intravascular volume, preload, and right-sided pressures
   - Third spacing—Check edema and ascites.
   - Chest X-ray—Shows pulmonary edema and cardiac dilation
   - Laboratory results—Hematocrit (low if blood diluted by fluid excess), potassium and sodium values (diuretics may result in depletion of these electrolytes)
5. Restore fluid balance:
   - Restrict fluid and sodium as ordered; carefully monitor intake and output measurement.
   - Medicate with diuretics as ordered to increase water excretion; watch serum potassium levels if using furosemide. Assess for signs of hyponatremia.
   - Medicate with vasodilators to increase cardiac output and improve renal blood flow.
   - Prevent third spacing; supplement dietary protein to increase serum albumin and increase colloidal osmotic pressure.
   - Thoracentesis to remove excessive pleural fluid

- Positive inotropic agents (digitalis, dobutamine, amiodarone)—Increase myocardial contractility.
- Vasodilators (sodium nitroprusside, nitroglycerine, isosorbide, ACE inhibitors such as captopril)—Decrease vascular resistance and cardiac workload.
- Oxygen—Improve arterial oxygenation with careful titration of oxygen to avoid respiratory depression in the patient with COPD.
- Balloon pump (counterpulsation)—Improve cardiac output by assisting in left ventricular emptying.
- Salt-restricted diet (less than 2 g per day)—Reduce fluid retention and intravascular volume.
- Rest—Reduce the workload of the heart, including sedation with morphine or sedatives as needed.
- Complementary therapies—Enhance relaxation using such therapies as music therapy, massage, and guided imagery.

Oxygen should be delivered carefully to patients with COPD and heart failure as high doses of oxygen may suppress the hypoxic drive and cause respiratory depression.

PULMONARY EDEMA

Pulmonary edema, the accumulation of fluid in the extravascular spaces of the lung, is a common complication of heart failure, pneumonia, inhalation injury, and pulmonary embolism. Increased pressure in the pulmonary vasculature due to left-sided heart failure increases the capillary hydrostatic pressure, pushing fluid into the alveoli. Membranes damaged by inflammation or trauma may increase capillary permeability and allow fluid to seep from the intravascular spaces into the alveoli. The flooded alveoli have less surface area to participate in gas exchange across the alveolar membrane.

 Pulmonary edema, the accumulation of fluid in the extravascular spaces of the lung, is a common complication of heart failure, pneumonia, inhalation injury, and pulmonary embolism.

Patients with pulmonary edema present with symptoms related to the underlying condition. Usually, they are short of breath and complain of chronic cough and exertional dyspnea. They may be tachy-cardic and have decreasing blood pressure. Their sputum may be frothy or blood tinged. On examination, their skin may be cool and clammy. Auscultation of the lungs reveals crackles and perhaps wheezes. There may be an S3 on the cardiac exam. The patient may be restless and anxious.

Diagnostic tests include chest X-ray, arterial blood gases, pulse oximetry, pulmonary artery catheterization and EKG. After diagnosis, treatment for pulmonary edema needs to be instituted quickly to prevent progression to respiratory and/or cardiac arrest. Interventions are focused on reducing fluid volume, supporting cardiac functioning and improving gas exchange while treating the underlying disorder.

Collaborative Interventions for Patients with Pulmonary Edema

1. Place patient in semi-Fowler's position (or high Fowler's if the patient can tolerate it) to improve chest expansion and help breathing.

2. Provide supplemental oxygen to improve hypoxia or proceed with intubation and mechanical ventilation if necessary.

3. Monitor condition. Assessment of vital signs, intake and urine output, EKG monitoring, oxygen saturation, electrolytes, and arterial blood gases helps direct treatment. If hemodynamic monitoring is being used, watch pulmonary artery and wedge pressures as increases may indicate worsening heart failure.

4. Administer morphine to promote comfort and relieve distress or breathlessness. *Note:* Watch for respiratory depression from morphine and have resuscitation equipment available.

5. Administer medications to improve cardiac function (nitroprusside), improve contractility (digoxin), improve bronchodilation (aminophyilline), and decrease preload (diuretics such as furosemide).

6. Use rotating tourniquets as ordered.

7. Support patient and family. Extreme dyspnea is frightening for both the patient and family.

PERIPHERAL ARTERIAL DISEASE

Narrowing and blockage of an artery can result in tissue hypoxia distal to the occlusion. The blockage may be due to a clot or, more commonly, an atherosclerotic plaque. **Peripheral arterial insufficiency**, a decrease in blood flow to the extremities, is most commonly caused by atherosclerotic changes. The femoral artery is the most common site for arterial narrowing and occlusion. As with coronary arteries with atherosclerotic changes, the tissues in the legs and feet receive less blood flow, and therefore less oxygen. Progressively, increased tissue demands for oxygen during activity cannot be met. The cells begin anaerobic metabolism with subsequent lactic acid build-up in the tissues.

 One of the first symptoms of arterial insufficiency is intermittent claudication—pain or cramping that occurs in an extremity during activity that is relieved by rest.

The signs and symptoms of peripheral arterial disease are related to the tissue hypoxia. One of the first symptoms of arterial insufficiency is **intermittent claudication**—pain or cramping that occurs in an extremity during activity and is relieved by rest. It occurs most commonly in the calf but can be felt in the foot, thigh, or hip. A common description of intermittent claudication is that a patient feels fine when he begins to walk and develops pain and cramping in his calves after 10 minutes. When he stops, the pain subsides. He begins walking again and the same pain occurs. Ask the patient to describe the pain pattern—the onset, precipitating factors, quality, location, and alleviating factors. Note any rubbing of the affected extremity and facial expressions during activity. It is often useful to have the patient use a pain scale (0 = no pain to 10 = worst pain ever) when describing his symptoms.

As the arterial occlusion progresses, the pain may occur earlier during exercise or even at rest (so-called **rest pain**). Rest pain may be unrelenting, especially when the affected limb is elevated, such as at bedtime. The patient may get relief by hanging his leg over the bed (gravity increases the blood flow to the extremity). Nonhealing openings or ulcers may develop on the affected extremity as the result of long-term tissue hypoxia. Severe disease may progress to **gangrene** of the extremity. Amputation

 As the arterial occlusion progresses, the pain may occur earlier during exercise or even at rest (so-called rest pain).

may be the only solution to prevent life-threatening infection or gangrene of the extremity.

Assessment

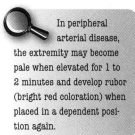

In peripheral arterial disease, the extremity may become pale when elevated for 1 to 2 minutes and develop rubor (bright red coloration) when placed in a dependent position again.

Assessment of the patient with suspected **peripheral arterial disease** reveals physical evidence of arterial insufficiency. Pulses in the extremity may be weak or absent. In peripheral arterial disease, the extremity may become pale when elevated for 1 to 2 minutes and develop **rubor** (bright red coloration) when placed in a dependent position again. If severe ischemia exists, then the foot may be pale and cool. The skin of the lower leg and foot may be hairless and scaly with poor toenail growth.

A diagnosis of peripheral arterial disease is made by combining the patient's history of symptoms with the results of the diagnostic tests. Tests may include Doppler ultrasound of the artery, plethysmography, MRI, arteriography of the extremity, and segmental limb pressure measurements.

Treatment

Conservative treatment of patients with peripheral arterial disease with intermittent claudication involves joint decision making with the patient to formulate a plan of care. Nursing care of patients with peripheral arterial disease is summarized in Table 7-6.

When conservative therapy fails to relieve the symptoms or the disease progresses, surgical intervention may be necessary to improve tissue perfusion. Worsening symptoms, pain at rest, and ischemic ulcers are all indications of significant arterial occlusion.

Worsening symptoms, pain at rest, and ischemic ulcers are all indications of significant arterial occlusion.

In contrast to the gradual progression of atherosclerotic peripheral arterial disease, acute ischemia of an extremity occurs when an artery is suddenly blocked by a clot or ruptured plaque and requires immedi-

Table 7-6 Nursing Care of Patients with Peripheral Arterial Disease

1. Follow a foot care regimen—The patient should be taught the following steps:
   - Inspect feet daily, including between the toes and the bottoms of the feet for cracks, calluses, ulcers, or fissures.
   - Wash feet with lukewarm water and mild soap and gently pat dry.
   - Moisturize with a lubricant such as lanolin.
   - Use a podiatrist to treat calluses, cut nails, and prescribe correctly fitting shoes if necessary.
   - Use white cotton socks and change them daily. Loose wool socks may be used in the winter to keep feet warm.
   - Avoid hot water bottles and electric pads.
   - Always wear shoes (never go barefoot), and make sure they fit correctly.
2. Walk for 60 minutes a day—Stop if the pain develops and then begin again. (This can help develop better circulation and lessen the pain.)
3. Eliminate all tobacco products.
4. Take medications as directed—Medications such as pentoxifylline, calcium channel blockers, and thromboxane inhibitors may improve circulation.
5. Control diabetes. Use care if this condition coexists with peripheral arterial disease, which it frequently does.
6. Use analgesics as necessary to control pain.
7. Elevate the head of the bed 4 to 6 inches (this allows gravity to increase blood flow to the extremity), or sleep in a recliner.

ate treatment. The pain is sudden in onset and severe, with coldness and numbness of the extremity. Pulses are absent distal to the blockage. Immediate treatment includes thrombolytics such as PTA (percutaneous transluminal angioplasty) stents placement or surgical intervention such as femoral artery bypass surgery.

 In contrast to the gradual progression of atherosclerotic peripheral arterial disease, acute ischemia of an extremity occurs when an artery is suddenly blocked by a clot or ruptured plaque and requires immediate treatment.

Invasive treatment involves surgically cleaning the plaque from the artery (**endarterectomy**) or bypassing the occluded artery with a synthetic or autologous vein graft, such as the saphenous vein. Plaque removal or endarterectomy may be performed with lasers or surgical excision. Grafts are used to bypass the area of the occlusion beginning above the occlusion and then distal to the occlusion (see Figure 7-8). The most common graft for peripheral arterial disease is the **femoral-popliteal bypass graft**. Other types include the axillo-femoral, femoral-femoral, and axillo-bifemoral bypass grafts.

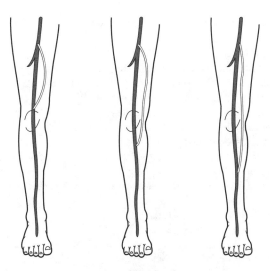

Figure 7-8 Bypass grafts for peripheral vascular insufficiency.

Care of the patient undergoing bypass grafts for peripheral vascular insufficiency is focused on maintaining tissue perfusion of the extremity. Of course, maintaining comfort, allaying anxiety, and teaching about self-care after surgery are all important nursing care goals for the patient undergoing surgery. Interventions for the patient with bypass surgery integrate the physiologic changes of peripheral arterial disease with improved perfusion and oxygenation of the extremity after surgery (see Table 7-7).

Potential complications of bypass grafting include graft occlusion (by a clot or kink in the graft) and **compartment syndrome** (compression of tissues and blood vessels from swelling around the incision and in the reperfused muscles).

ANSWERS TO THE CASE STUDY QUESTIONS

♦ What are the risk factors for coronary artery disease?

The risk factors for coronary artery disease (CAD) include familial history of CAD, hypertension, diabetes, obesity, hypercholesterolemia, cigarette smoking, male gender, increased stress, and sedentary lifestyle.

Table 7-7 Nursing Care of the Patient Undergoing Femoral-Popliteal Bypass Graft

1. Assess for alteration in blood flow in the bypassed extremity:
   - Increased pain or intermittent claudication with less activity
   - Diminished or absent pulses in the extremity
   - Increasing pallor, coolness, or numbness
   - Longer capillary refill time (greater than 3 seconds)
2. Prevent decreases in tissue perfusion:
   - Avoid crossing legs, pillows under the knees, sitting for long periods, 90° flexion at the hip.
   - Control pain and minimize stress (decrease sympathetic stimulation and vasoconstriction).
   - Eliminate all tobacco products.
   - Keep patient warm.
   - Progress activity as ordered, starting with foot exercises every 1 to 2 hours and progressing to short walks as ordered.
3. Implement measures to maintain graft perfusion:
   - Heparin intravenously for 24 to 48 hours—monitor PTT (partial thromboplastin levels).
   - Maintain a regular exercise program, such as short walks as ordered. Have patient time activities to establish predictable times to stop and rest. Medicate with analgesics as necessary to maintain comfort during activity.
   - Medicate with pentoxifylline if ordered.
   - Avoid constrictive stockings, such as knee-highs and garters.
   - Teach patient the signs of changing perfusion in the grafted extremity: increasing pain, numbness, tingling, coolness, paleness, or difficulty moving the extremity.
   - Reduce cholesterol levels with a low-fat diet and medication as ordered to prevent further atherosclerotic damage to the arteries.

- Why does Mr. K's pain subside after stent placement?

Mr. K's pain subsides after stent placement because the perfusion through the stenosed coronary artery has been re-established, allowing more oxygenated blood to reach the hypoxic cardiac muscle.

- How does propanolol help patients with coronary artery disease?

Beta-blockers such as propanolol decrease the work of the heart by decreasing the heart rate, blood pressure, and myocardial contractility. With a diminished workload, the heart muscle also has decreased oxygen requirements.

- What teaching will you do regarding the use of sublingual nitro-glycerine?

Mr. K has been given a prescription for sublingual nitroglycerine (NTG) to use if his chest pain returns at home. He should carry the NTG with him at all times. If rest does not relieve the chest pain, Mr. K should take one NTG and wait 5 minutes. If pain is not relieved, he should take another NTG and wait 5 minutes. If the pain is still not relieved, he should take a third NTG and wait another 5 minutes. If the pain continues despite three NTGs in 15 minutes, he should dial 911 and/or his physician. Nitroglycerine can cause dizziness (orthostatic hypertension) and headache. Mr. K should lie down if he feels dizzy. NTG should be kept in a dark bottle because it is light sensitive. The prescription should be replaced every 3 to 5 months.

- Which risk factors are modifiable, and how will you incorporate teaching about these to Mr. K now that he has been diagnosed with coronary artery disease?

Modifiable risk factors are those that Mr. K can change to reduce his chances of having another MI. Mr. K's teaching should include weight reduction, quitting cigarette smoking, reducing dietary fat intake, increasing his exercise level as prescribed by his cardiologist, and reducing stress.

CHAPTER 7 MULTIPLE-CHOICE QUESTIONS

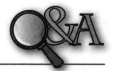

1. Atherosclerosis occurs because of all of the following except:
   a. Accumulation of lipids in connective tissue
   b. Overgrowth of smooth muscle
   c. Formation of connective tissue in the intima of the vessel
   d. Hormonal response with peripheral vasoconstriction

2. Three risk factors for developing peripheral arterial disease are:
   a. Smoking, hypercholesterolemia, obesity
   b. Age, gout, smoking
   c. Hypertension, diabetes, smoking
   d. Prior surgery, age, gout

3. All of the following may be sign(s) of myocardial infarction except:
   a. Pain between the shoulder blades
   b. Nausea and vomiting with jaw pain
   c. Chest pain lasting more than 30 minutes
   d. Chest pain relieved by one nitroglycerin tablet

4. Treatment of suspected myocardial infarction includes:
   a. Oxygen, aspirin, morphine, nitroglycerin
   b. Acetaminophen, bed rest, EEG
   c. Oxygen, cardiac catheterization
   d. Mechanical ventilation, CEA levels, acetaminophen

5. Thrombolytic agents are used to dissolve thrombi but have all of the following potential side effects except:
   a. Reperfusion dysrhythmia
   b. Bleeding
   c. Itching, hives, and hypersensitivity
   d. Renal failure

CHAPTER 7 ANSWERS AND RATIONALES

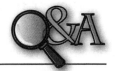

1. **d.**

   Rationale: Peripheral vasoconstriction does not cause atherosclerosis, but accumulation of lipids in connective tissue, overgrowth of smooth muscle, and formation of connective tissue in the intima of the vessel all contribute to the process.

2. **c.**

   Rationale: Hypertension, smoking, and diabetes are all associated with increased incidence of peripheral arterial disease.

3. **d.**

   Rationale: Chest pain relieved by sublingual nitroglycerine is characteristic of angina and not myocardial infarction.

4. **a.**

   Rationale: The treatment of chest pain and suspected myocardial infarction includes oxygen, aspirin, morphine, and sublingual nitroglycerine.

5. **d.**

   Rationale: Thrombolytic agents have multiple potential side effects but not renal failure.

This chapter will review the roles of the hematologic system in oxygen transport:

- Red blood cells and hemoglobin

- Laboratory tests of the hematologic system

8

The Role of the Hematologic System in Oxygen Transport

TERMS
- ☐ erythrocytes
- ☐ leukocytes
- ☐ thrombocytes
- ☐ hemoglobin
- ☐ oxyhemoglobin
- ☐ hematocrit
- ☐ anemia
- ☐ iron overload
- ☐ sickle cell anemia
- ☐ thalassemia

CASE STUDY

When Miss D comes into the campus health office, she is moving slowly. She states that she has no energy and just wants to sleep all the time. Miss D is a 20-year-old college student and has been into the office before because of heavy menstrual periods. She is thin, 5 feet 6 inches tall, and weighs 110 pounds. She has been skipping meals because of midterms, drinking diet soda, and eating popcorn in her room. Her blood work comes back with a hematocrit of 31 and a hemoglobin of 8.7.

Important Questions to Ask

- What lifestyle patterns would put Miss D at risk for anemia?
- What is the most common cause of anemia in young women?
- What interventions will improve Miss D's energy levels?

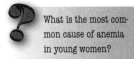

What is the most common cause of anemia in young women?

INTRODUCTION

Oxygen is transported throughout the body by the hematologic or hematopoietic system. This system is composed of blood, plasma, and lymph. Blood is composed of **plasma**, **red blood cells** (**erythrocytes**), **white blood cells (leukocytes)**, and **platelets (thrombocytes)**. The hematologic system has the following three important functions:

- Gas exchange (oxygen and carbon dioxide)
- Nutrient delivery to the cells
- Waste removal from the cells

Additionally, the hematologic system is involved in the acid–base balance, fluid and electrolyte balance, delivery of hormones, protection from foreign organisms, and temperature regulation.

The red blood cell (especially the **hemoglobin** molecule within the red blood cell) plays a crucial role in oxygen transport. The hemoglobin binds to oxygen in the pulmonary capillaries in the alveolar walls. Hemoglobin transports the oxygen through the arterial system, releasing it at the cellular level. Readily available oxygen allows the cells to create energy aerobically. Without sufficient oxygen, the cells produce energy anaerobically, creating lactic acid as an end product. Sufficient oxygen for aerobic metabolism is referred to as **critical oxygen (O₂ crit)**.

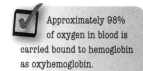

Approximately 98% of oxygen in blood is carried bound to hemoglobin as oxyhemoglobin.

The red blood cell, or erythrocyte, is the most numerous of the formed elements in blood. Red blood cells (RBC) are of particular interest in a text on oxygenation because they carry hemoglobin, the molecule that binds to oxygen during transport. Approximately 98% of oxygen in blood is carried bound to hemoglobin as **oxyhemoglobin**. RBCs make up about 40% to 50% of the total blood volume. This percentage is referred to as the **hematocrit**. RBCs are produced in the bone marrow and have a life span of about 120 days. Balanced production and destruction of red blood cells maintains a stable blood count. Every day, 1% of RBCs are produced by the bone marrow, and another 1% are destroyed by phagocytic cells in the liver, spleen, and bone marrow.

RBCs are released by the bone marrow as **reticulocytes** (immature RBC) and develop into erythrocytes in the circulating blood within 24 to 48 hours of their release from the bone marrow. The normal percentage of reticulocytes in the circulating blood is 1% to 1.5% of the total RBCs. Abnormally high percentages of reticulocytes may occur during times of rapid RBC production.

The bone marrow is stimulated to produce red blood cells by the hormone **erythropoietin** (see Figure 8-1). The kidneys produce this hormone when the capillary endothelial cells in the kidney sense hypoxia. Human erythropoietin is now produced using recombinant DNA technology (epoetin alpha). It is used to stimulate bone marrow production in severe anemia that occurs in conditions such as chronic renal failure.

RBCs make up about 40% to 50% of the total blood volume.

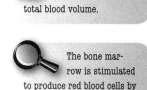

The bone marrow is stimulated to produce red blood cells by the hormone erythropoietin.

Hemoglobin is the master transporter of oxygen. It is composed of two pairs of polypeptide chains, each attached to a heme unit. The heme unit is made of iron. If iron stores are low due to nutritional deficiencies, then the red blood cells contain low levels of hemoglobin (iron deficiency anemia). Hemoglobin also contains the red pigment, **porphyrin**. This pigment combines with oxygen in hemoglobin and gives oxygenated blood the distinctive red color.

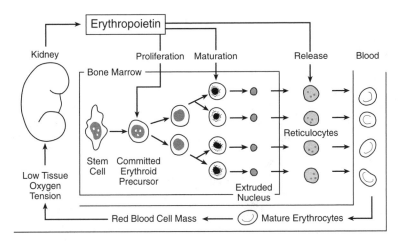

Figure 8-1 Red blood cell development.

Hemoglobin carries the majority of the oxygen to the capillaries, where it moves out of the red blood cell, into the plasma, across the capillary wall, and into the interstitial fluid, becoming available to the cells. Only a small portion (1–2%) of the blood's oxygen is dissolved in plasma; the rest is bound to hemoglobin. The portion of oxygen that is dissolved in plasma can be measured as the P_{O_2}. The oxygen that is combined with hemoglobin is measured as the percent of saturated hemoglobin (S_{O_2}).

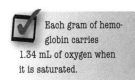

Only a small portion (1–2%) of the blood's oxygen is dissolved in plasma, the rest is bound to hemoglobin.

The hemoglobin-oxygen bond (oxyhemoglobin) is a loose bond that is quickly reversed in the capillaries at the cellular level. Each gram of hemoglobin carries 1.34 mL of oxygen when it is saturated. For oxygen to become available to the cells, the oxyhemoglobin bond must be broken (dissociated). Hemoglobin's affinity for oxygen or its capacity to bind to oxygen depends on the pH of the blood and the presence of specific enzymes. Hemoglobin binds more strongly to oxygen when the blood is alkaline and releases it more easily when the pH is more

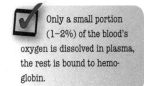

Each gram of hemoglobin carries 1.34 mL of oxygen when it is saturated.

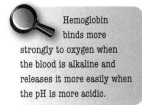

Hemoglobin binds more strongly to oxygen when the blood is alkaline and releases it more easily when the pH is more acidic.

acidic. This relationship or affinity between hemoglobin and oxygen is described in the oxygen-hemoglobin dissociation curve. (Refer to Chapter 2 for more on this topic.) The enzymes 2-3-DPG and G6PD also affect hemoglobin's affinity for oxygen.

Red blood cells and hemoglobin also function to remove carbon dioxide and other waste from the cellular level. Carbon dioxide is a waste product of aerobic metabolism and is transported away from the cells in three ways: dissolved in the plasma as carbon dioxide, attached to hemoglobin (**carbaminohemoglobin**), and as bicarbonate (HCO_3^-). Seventy to 80% of the carbon dioxide in the blood is carried as bicarbonate or dissolved in plasma.

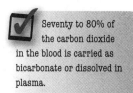

Seventy to 80% of the carbon dioxide in the blood is carried as bicarbonate or dissolved in plasma.

LABORATORY TESTS

The components of the hematologic system can be studied and measured in the laboratory. The hematocrit is the percentage of red blood cells in 100 mL of whole blood. A sample of blood is placed in a centrifuge and spun. The RBC, being he heaviest component of blood, falls to the bottom of the tube. The normal range for the hematocrit varies by age and sex. The hematocrit can be a deceiving measure of the actual RBC count because the amount of plasma and the intravascular volume can vary. If the intravascular volume falls because of dehydration or increases because of fluid shifts into the intravascular space, then the percentage of RBCs will increase or decrease while the actual count is unchanged.

The hematocrit can be a deceiving measure of the actual RBC count because the amount of plasma and the intravascular volume can vary.

Hemoglobin levels can also be measured in the laboratory and are often considered a more reliable measure of the oxygen-carrying capacity of the blood. It is measured in grams per 100 mL of blood. Hemoglobin is measured to screen for anemia and evaluate **polycythemia** (too many RBCs). The RBC count measures the total number of RBCs in a cubic millimeter of blood. RBC indices are tests to distinguish the color and size of the RBCs. The **mean corpuscular hemoglobin concentration (MCHC)** is the average concentration of hemoglobin in the RBCs.

It is often used to describe the color of the cells, but it is expressed as the ratio of the weight of hemoglobin to the volume of the RBC. For example, hypochromic anemia refers to RBCs of decreased color and is often a finding in iron deficiency anemia.

Another RBC index is the **mean corpuscular volume (MCV)**. It refers to the relative size of the RBCs, such as normocytic (normal), microcytic (small), or macrocytic (large). It is used to classify different anemias.

Finally, the **mean corpuscular hemoglobin (MCH)** is an RBC index used to measure the weight of hemoglobin in the RBC. It is a calculated value with an increase associated with macrocytic (large RBC) anemias and a decrease associated with microcytic (small RBC) anemias.

DISORDERS OF THE HEMATOLOGIC SYSTEM

Disorders of the hematologic system can affect the oxygen-carrying capacity of the blood. Although disorders can affect any component of the blood, this section will focus on problems with the RBC and hemoglobin: anemias and hemoglobinopathies.

Anemia reflects a reduction in the total hemoglobin concentration in the body. A decreased amount of hemoglobin diminishes the oxygen-carrying capacity of the blood. Anemia results from the following three main problems:

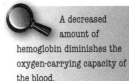

A decreased amount of hemoglobin diminishes the oxygen-carrying capacity of the blood.

- Decreased production of erythrocytes (e.g., iron deficiency, pernicious anemia, lead poisoning, and renal failure)
- Acute or chronic blood loss (e.g., trauma, chronic gastrointestinal bleeding)
- Increased destruction of erythrocytes (e.g., hemolytic anemias, physical trauma to blood such as extracorporeal "bypass" circulation)

The signs of anemia do not usually present until there is a substantial drop in the amount of hemoglobin or circulating RBCs. The signs and symptoms reflect the decrease in oxygen-carrying capacity of the blood and tissue hypoxia. They include the following:

- Fatigue, weakness, and muscle cramps
- Dyspnea and tachypnea

- Pallor of skin, conjunctiva, and mucus membranes
- Dizziness and syncope
- Tachycardia and palpitations
- Beefy red tongue, sore mouth, and anorexia
- Jaundice in hemolytic anemias
- **Petechiae** (small, red spots from bleeding) in aplastic anemia

 The signs of anemia do not usually present until there is a substantial drop in the amount of hemoglobin or circulating RBCs.

The most common cause of anemia is iron deficiency. Iron deficiency produces a microcytic, hypochromic RBC because insufficient iron is available to synthesize hemoglobin. Although body iron is retained from destroyed RBCs and reused, over time the iron stores can be depleted due to chronic loss. In men and in postmenopausal women, the most common cause of chronic loss and

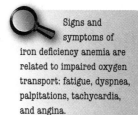
Signs and symptoms of iron deficiency anemia are related to impaired oxygen transport: fatigue, dyspnea, palpitations, tachycardia, and angina.

iron-deficiency anemia is gastrointestinal bleeding from ulcers, tumors, or hemorrhoids. In menstruating women, monthly periods, especially heavy or prolonged periods, can lead to anemia. Pregnant women also have increased iron needs. People at risk for hookworm may also have chronic blood loss as the parasite removes blood from the intestinal tract.

Signs and symptoms of iron deficiency anemia are related to impaired oxygen transport: fatigue, dyspnea, palpitations, tachycardia, and angina. Treatment is aimed at controlling blood loss, increasing dietary intake of iron, and administering supplemental iron either orally or intramuscularly as needed. Although an adequate diet includes 12 to 15 mg of indirect iron, only 1 mg is absorbed daily and another 1 mg is lost. Supplemental iron may be necessary to rebuild the iron stores. Interventions are aimed at teaching the patient to increase intake of iron-rich foods and pacing activities until the fatigue subsides (about 3 to 6 months).

Nursing Care of the Patient with Anemia

Nursing care of patients with anemia requires collaborative interventions to increase red blood cell production, increase available iron if stores are low, and/or decrease blood loss.

- Encourage an iron-rich diet with foods such as liver, lean red meat, egg yolks, raisins, spinach, apricots, beet greens, and whole wheat bread.
- Take supplemental iron (iron sulfate—$FeSO_4$ 325 mg one to three times daily) with food.
- Use a stool softener such as docusate sodium or senna for constipation if this becomes a problem. Warn patient that stools will be black-colored while taking iron.
- Administer intramuscular iron if ordered, using the Z-track method to minimize skin staining and irritation. (See a nursing text for further explanation of this method.)

Two other nutritional deficiencies can result in altered RBC production. Folic acid and vitamin B_{12} are also needed for the synthesis of RBCs. Folic acid deficiency results from inadequate dietary intake, malabsorption syndromes such as celiac sprue, or during times of increased bodily needs, such as during pregnancy and growth. Folic acid is necessary for RBC maturation. It is found in green leafy foods, liver, and yeast. Some drugs, such as phenytoin, phenobarbital (antiseizure drugs), methotrexate (antimetabolite used in chemotherapy), and triamterene (a diuretic), impair absorption of folic acid. Alcoholics frequently have folic acid deficiencies. Because folic acid deficiency is linked to birth defects such as spina bifida, it is important that menstruating and pregnant women have an adequate intake or take a multivitamin supplement.

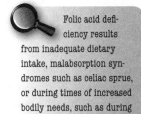

Folic acid deficiency results from inadequate dietary intake, malabsorption syndromes such as celiac sprue, or during times of increased bodily needs, such as during pregnancy and growth.

Vitamin B_{12} (cyancobalamin) deficiency can cause anemia not because of inadequate intake but because the body does not adequately absorb this nutrient. Intrinsic factor produced by the gastric mucosa is needed to absorb B_{12} from food. In cases of atrophy of the gastric mucosa, insufficient intrinsic factor is produced, and B_{12} is not absorbed. Without B_{12}, DNA synthesis of the RBC is impaired and anemia results. Anemia caused by B_{12} deficiency is sometimes referred to as *pernicious anemia*. The RBCs, when examined under the microscope, are abnormally large (macrocytic), oval shaped, and have thin membranes.

Long-term effects of pernicious anemia include neurological manifestations, such as paresthesias of the hands and feet, and spastic ataxia. Treatment involves lifelong injections of B_{12} (100 mcg) to reverse the anemia and try to improve any neurologic manifestations.

Anemias from bone marrow failure are referred to as **aplastic anemias**. Usually the production of all hematopoietic cells (red blood cells, white blood cells, and platelets) is affected and is called **pancytopenia**. The

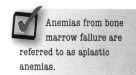
Anemias from bone marrow failure are referred to as aplastic anemias.

anemia results from the failure of the marrow to replace the old RBCs. The cells that are produced are of normal size and color but few in number. The patient presents symptoms of increasing fatigue and dyspnea. Aplastic anemia may develop slowly or acutely and at any age. Possible causes include exposure to toxic chemicals (such as benzene) and high-dose radiation. Half the time the cause is never discovered. Treatment includes removal of the offending substance (if known), immunosuppressive therapy, injections of epoetin, blood transfusions, corticosteroids, and bone marrow transplantation in severe cases.

Anemia of chronic disease is a normocytic, normochromic anemia that is thought to result from uremic toxins destroying the kidney's ability to produce erythropoietin. Causes include diseases such as cancer and chronic infections. The treatments are transfusions and erythropoietin injections (if the bone marrow is functioning).

Transfusion therapy for chronic anemias does have complications. Blood transfusions can result in transfusion reactions and predispose the patient to **iron overload**. Transfusion reactions occur because surface antigens on the blood cells interact with antibodies in the patient's serum. Reactions can be quite serious and blood should always be administered very cautiously. The two most common reactions are hemolytic and febrile reactions. The most serious and feared reaction is a hemolytic reaction from ABO incompatibility. The signs and symptoms are urticaria, flushing of the face, back pain, headache, chills, fever, nausea and vomiting, tachycardia, dyspnea, and hypotension. The transfusion is immediately stopped, and the remaining blood is saved for testing. Intravenous access is maintained for medications. Kidney function must be carefully followed to assess for renal damage from the hemoglobin released from the destroyed RBCs.

 Blood transfusions can result in transfusion reactions and predispose the patient to iron overload.

In a febrile reaction, the patient's blood reacts to the donor's white blood cells, causing fever and chills. Leukocyte-depleted blood is frequently used to avoid this reaction. (Leukocytes are depleted by irradiating the blood.) Antipyretics are used to treat the fever.

Multiple blood transfusions can lead to iron overload. The body metabolizes iron at a fixed rate and recycles it from destroyed RBCs. The iron balance in the body is usually maintained. Each blood transfusion adds another 200 mg of iron to the system, and iron overload can result. Iron can cause cardiac myopathies, liver fibrosis, skin discoloration, as well as endocrine and pancreatic dysfunction. The treatment for iron overload is chelation therapy.

Hemolytic anemia is caused by premature destruction of RBCs, shortened life span of RBCs, or failure of the marrow to replace RBCs.

Causes of hemolytic anemia include immune responses (antigen–antibody reactions, infections, lead poisoning, and chronic diseases such as cancer and lupus). The treatment involves identifying the cause, maintaining renal function, steroids, and possibly splenectomy for refractory cases.

HEMOGLOBINOPATHIES

Defects in the structure of hemoglobin can lead to accelerated RBC destruction and blood vessel occlusion. Two **hemoglobinopathies** will be discussed: sickle-cell anemia and thalassemia.

Sickle cell anemia is a congenital disorder affecting 0.1% to 0.2% of all African-Americans. It is a recessive characteristic that is transmitted either as a trait or as the disease. Almost 9% of all African-Americans carry the gene for the sickle cell trait. In sickle cell anemia, an amino acid is abnormally substituted for a chain in the hemoglobin molecule. The problem with the substitution arises when the hemoglobin deoxygenates and takes on a sickle shape. This deformed RBC can block vessels in the microcirculation, causing tissue ischemia. A crisis occurs when a blood vessel is blocked, causing damage to tissues and organs. **Sickle cell crises** are often very painful for the patient. Common sites are joints, the abdomen, and chest. There is no known cure for sickle cell anemia. Treatment focuses on increasing tissue oxygenation with supplemental oxygen. Patients are taught to avoid situations that could precipitate a crisis, such as infections, cold exposure, excess physical

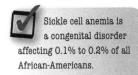

Sickle cell anemia is a congenital disorder affecting 0.1% to 0.2% of all African-Americans.

exertion, dehydration, and acidosis. Bone marrow transplantation, anti-sickling agents, and red cell exchange therapy are also being used to improve outcomes in patients who are unresponsive to other treatments.

Thalassemias are a group of inherited anemias. Occurring mostly in Mediterranean populations, they are sometimes called Cooley's anemia. In thalassemia, one of the two polypeptide chains in the hemoglobin molecule is defective. The anemia results from defective and reduced hemoglobin synthesis. Signs and symptoms are based on the severity of the anemia and include hepatomegaly, splenomegaly, growth retardation in children, bone thinning, and bone marrow expansion with facial changes. The severity of the disease depends on the number of defects in the hemoglobin molecule. The treatment for thalassemias is transfusion therapy and genetic counseling.

ANSWERS TO CASE STUDY QUESTIONS

- What lifestyle patterns would put Miss D at risk for anemia?

Miss D is at risk for anemia because of her diet (low in calories, nutritional value, and probably iron) and her history of heavy periods.

- What is the most common cause of anemia in young women?

The most common cause of anemia in young women is an iron-poor diet.

- What interventions will improve Miss D's energy levels?

Miss D's energy levels will improve over time with rest, increased iron-rich foods in her diet, and iron supplementation.

CHAPTER 8 MULTIPLE-CHOICE QUESTIONS

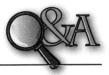

1. A normal hematocrit for women is:
   a. 40–48%
   b. 37–47%
   c. 35–40%
   d. 30–40%

2. The immature form of red blood cells released by the bone marrow is:
   a. Reticulocytes
   b. Erythrocytes
   c. Monocytes
   d. Granulocytes

3. Anemia occurs because of all of the following except:
   a. Renal failure
   b. Chronic blood loss
   c. Increased destruction of erythrocytes
   d. Congestive heart failure

4. Signs and symptoms of iron deficiency anemia are all of the following except:
   a. Fatigue
   b. Dyspnea
   c. Tachycardia
   d. Constipation

5. What portion of the blood's oxygen is dissolved in plasma?
   a. 37–47%
   b. 1–2%
   c. 98%
   d. 50%

CHAPTER 8 ANSWERS AND RATIONALES

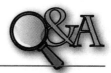

1. **b.**

   Rationale: A normal hematocrit for women is 37–47%.

2. **a.**

   Rationale: Immature red blood cells released by the bone marrow during times of high production are reticulocytes.

3. **d.**

   Rationale: Anemia does not occur during congestive heart failure. Rather, many patients with heart failure have a higher hematocrit in response to chronic hypoxia.

4. **d.**

   Rationale: Constipation is not caused by anemia but may be the result of iron supplementation to treat anemia.

5. **b.**

   Rationale: Only 1% to 2% of oxygen is carried in the plasma; the rest is bound to hemoglobin as oxyhemoglobin.

Bibliography

BIBLIOGRAPHY

Agency for Health Care Policy and Research. *Smoking Cessation: Clinical Guidelines.* No. 18. Rockville, Md: US Department of Health and Human Services; 1996. AHCPR Pub. No. 96-0692.

Ahrens T, Rutherford K. *Essentials of Oxygenation.* Boston, Ma: Jones and Bartlett; 1993.

Baum GL, ed. *Baum's Textbook of Respiratory Diseases.* 7th ed. Philadelphia, Pa: Lippincott, Williams & Wilkins; 2004.

Beers MH, Berkow R. *The Merck Manual.* 18th ed. Rahway, NJ: Merck; 2006.

Bickley LS, Szilagy PG. *Bates Guide to Physical Examination and History Taking,* 9th ed. Philadelphia, Pa: JB Lippincott Co; 2004.

Black J, Matassarin-Jacobs E, Luckmann J. *Medical-Surgical Nursing: Clinical Management for Continuity of Care.* Philadelphia, Pa: WB Saunders Co; 1997.

Burns SM. Working with respiratory waveforms: how to use bedside graphics. *AACN Clin Issues.* 2003;14(2):133-144.

Burrell L, Gerlach M, Pless B. *Nursing Management of Adults with Respiratory Problems.* Stamford, Conn: Appleton & Lange; 1997.

Burrell LO, Gerlach MJ, Pless BS. Nursing management of adults with respiratory problems. In: Burrell LO, Gerlach MJ, Pless BS, eds. *Adult Nursing: Acute and Community Care.* 2nd ed. Stamford, Conn: Appleton & Lange; 1996.

Celli BR. Patient-centered outcomes in COPD. *Clin Rev.* 2006;16(3): 79-93.

Centers for Disease Control and Prevention. *TB Facts for Health Care Workers.* Atlanta, Ga: Centers for Disease Control and Prevention; 1998.

Centers for Disease Control and Prevention. *Core Curriculum on Tuberculosis.* 4th ed. Atlanta, Ga: Centers for Disease Control and Prevention; 2000.

Clinical Laboratory Values Tests: Values and Implications. 3rd ed. Philadelphia, Pa: Lippincott, Williams & Wilkins, Springhouse Division; 2001.

Corbett JV. *Laboratory Tests and Diagnostic Procedures with Nursing Diagnoses.* 4th ed. Stamford, Conn: Appleton & Lange; 1996.

Dubin D. *Rapid Interpretation of EKGs: Dubin's Classic Simplified Methodology for Understanding EKG.* 6th ed. Tampa, Fla: COVER Publishing; 2000.

Fabbri L, Pauwels RA, Hurd SS. Global strategy for the diagnosis, management and prevention of chronic obstructive pulmonary disease: GOLD Executive Summary. *COPD.* 2004;1:105-141.

Fiebach NH, Kern DE, Thomas PA, Ziegelstein RC, Barker LR, Zieve PD. *Barker, Burton & Zieve's Principles of Ambulatory Medicine.* Baltimore, Md: Lippincott, Williams & Wilkins; 2006.

Fischbach F. *A Manuel of Laboratory Diagnostic Tests.* 7th ed. Philadelphia, Pa: Lippincott, Williams & Wilkins; 2004.

Gattinoni L, Tognoni G, Pesenti A, et al. The effect of prone positioning on the survival of patients with acute respiratory failure. *N Engl J Med.* 2001;354(8):568-573.

Guyton AC, Hall JE. *Textbook of Medical Physiology.* Philadelphia, Pa: WB Saunders Co; 1996.

Heart Failure Society of America. The Stages of Heart Failure—NYHA Classification [Web page]. Available at: http://www.abouthf.org/ questions_stages.htm. Accessed September 26, 2006.

Hoffman D. *The Herbal Handbook.* Rochester, VT: Healing Arts Press; 1998.

Ignatavius D, Workman M. *Medical-Surgical Nursing: Critical Thinking for Collaborative Care.* 5th ed. Philadelphia, Pa: WB Saunders; 2006.

Kee JL. *Laboratory and Diagnostic Tests with Nursing Implications.* 4th Ed. Stamford, Conn: Appleton & Lange; 1995.

Kozier B, Glenora E, Berman AJ, Snyder S. *Fundamentals of Nursing: Concepts, Processes, and Practice.* New York, NY: Addison-Wesley; 2003.

Leahy JM, Kizilay PE. *Foundations of Nursing Practice: A Nursing Process Approach.* Philadelphia, PA: WB Saunders; 1998.

Levitsky MG. *Pulmonary Physiology.* 4th ed. New York, NY: McGraw-Hill; 1995.

Lewis SM, Heitkemper MM, Dirksen SR. *Medical-Surgical Nursing: Assessment and Management of Clinical Problems.* St. Louis, MO: Mosby Inc; 2002.

Mahler DA. *Dyspnea.* New York, NY: Marcel Dekker, Inc; 1998.

Martini F. *Fundamentals of Anatomy and Physiology.* Englewood Cliffs, NJ: Prentice Hall; 1992.

Martini F. *Fundamentals of Anatomy and Physiology.* 2nd ed. Engle-wood Cliffs, NJ: Prentice Hall; 1992.

McGowan C. Noninvasive ventilatory support: use of bi-level positive airway pressure in respiratory failure. *Crit Care Nurse.* 1998;18(6):47-53.

Monahan FD, Neighbors M. *Medical-Surgical Nursing: Foundations for Clinical Practice.* Philadelphia, Pa: WB Saunders; 1998.

Corning, HS, Bryant, SL. *Mosby's Respiratory Care PDQ.* St. Louis, MO: Mosby Elsevier; 2006.

National Heart, Lung, and Blood Institute (NHLBI). *National Asthma Education and Prevention Program. Guidelines for the Diagnosis and Management of Asthma: Expert Panel Report II.*). Bethesda, Md: NHLBI; 1997. NIH Pub. No. 97-4051.

Norris J, ed. *Critical Care Skills: A Nurse's Photo Guide.* Philadelphia, Pa: Springhouse Corporation; 1996.

Nursing 2006 Drug Handbook. 26th ed. Springhouse, Pa: Springhouse; 2006.

Pagana KD, Pagana TJ. *Manual of Diagnostic and Laboratory Tests.* St. Louis, MO: Mosby; 1998.

Porth CM, Kunert MP. *Pathophysiology: Concepts of Altered Health States.* 6th ed. Philadelphia, Pa: JB Lippincott, Williams & Wilkins; 2002.

Respiratory Care Made Incredibly Easy. Philadelphia, Pa; Lippincott, Williams & Wilkins, Springhouse Division; 2005.

Roberts N. Selective approach to successful stoma management. *ORL Head and Neck Nurs.* 1995;13(4):12-16.

Shieken LS. Asthma pathophysiology and the scientific rationale for combination therapy. *Allergy and Asthma Proc.* 2002;23(4):247-251.

Swearingen PL, Keen JH. *Manual of Critical Care Nursing.* St. Louis, MO: Mosby; 2001.

Swearingen PL, Keen JH. *Manual of Critical Care Nursing: Nursing Interventions and Collaborative Management.* St. Louis, MO: Mosby; 2001.

Tierney LM, McPhee SJ, Papadakis MA, eds. *Current Medical Diagnosis and Treatment.* 44th ed. Norwalk, Conn: Appleton & Lange; 2005.

Ulrich SP, Canale SW, Wendell SA. *Medical-Surgical Nursing Care Planning Guides.* Philadelphia, Pa: WB Saunders; 1998.

Wilkins RL, Stoller JK. *Egan's Fundamentals of Respiratory Care.* St. Louis, MO: Mosby; 2003.

Wilkinson M, Muzzarelli K. *Tracheostomy Care Practice Survey.* Society of Otolaryngology, Head and Neck Nurses, AACN; 1996.

Zimbler ER. *Fundamentals of Nursing: Review and Study Guide.* Stamford, Conn: Appleton & Lange; 1999.

Zipes D, Libby P, Bonow E, Braunwald E. *Braunwald's Heart Disease: A Textbook of Cardiovascular Medicine.* 7th ed. Philadelphia, Pa: WB Saunders; 2005.

Glossary

GLOSSARY

2,3-diphosphoglycerol (2,3-DPG)—An intermediate product of glyco-lysis.

Accessory muscles—Muscles in the chest, shoulders, and abdomen not normally needed for respiration but which may indicate difficulty moving air through the respiratory passages.

Acidosis—Blood pH is lower than 7.35.

Acute respiratory failure—Condition where the lungs cannot maintain arterial oxygenation and/or eliminate carbon dioxide.

Acute rhinitis—Infection caused by the common cold virus or rhino-virus with runny and stuffy nose (rhinorrhea), malaise, sore throat, coughing, and sneezing.

Adult respiratory distress syndrome (ARDS)—Severe, life-threatening condition manifested by dyspnea, severe hypoxemia, decreased lung compliance, and noncardiac pulmonary edema.

Adventitious lung sounds—Sounds heard in the thorax in addition to normal breath sounds, identified by their pitch, intensity, and dura-tion during the respiratory cycle.

Afterload—Pressure created in the ventricular wall to achieve systolic pressure.

Airway resistance (R_{aw})—Difference between the pressure in the mouth (atmospheric pressure) and the pressure in the alveoli (alveolar pres-sure).

Alkalosis—Blood pH is greater than 7.45.

Allen's test—A test using simple compression of the radial artery to assess circulation to the hand by the ulnar artery.

Allergic rhinitis—Inhaled substances (pollen, animal dander, or dust) cause a type I hypersensitivity reaction producing vasodilation and increased capillary permeability in the mucus membranes of the nose, causing sneezing, watery eyes, and hypersecretion of thin mucus.

Alpha-1-antitrypsin deficiency—Genetic disorder linked to the elastin destruction in the alveoli.

Alveolar air—Air in the alveoli.

Alveolar membrane—Site of gas exchange. Oxygen in the alveoli diffuses across the membrane into the blood, and carbon dioxide in the blood diffuses back into the alveoli.

Alveolar ventilation—Exchange of gases across the alveolar membrane into the circulatory system.

Alveolus (alveoli)—Cup-shaped structures that are grouped like clusters of grapes at the end of the terminal bronchioles and are the site of gas exchange across the alveolar membrane.

Anemia—A reduction in the total hemoglobin concentration in the body.

Angina—Clinical diagnosis and a symptom based on a history of chest pain brought on by exertion and relieved by rest.

Anterior axillary line—An anatomic landmark on the thorax that runs vertically along the anterior aspect of the chest at the anterior fold of the axilla.

Anterior-posterior (A-P) diameter—Measurement of the thorax from front to back.

Aorta—Large vessel that leaves the left ventricle and begins the systemic arterial circulation.

Aortic valve—Valve located between the left ventricle and the aorta.

Apex of the lung—Uppermost portion of the lung located above the clavicle anteriorly.

Aphonia—Lack of sound production when trying to speak.

Aphthous ulcers—Ulcerated and often painful areas in the mucous membranes of the mouth (commonly called canker sores).

Apical pulse—Pulse palpated over the heart, usually at the left fourth or fifth intercostal space at the midclavicular line.

Aplastic anemias—Anemias from bone marrow failure.

Arterial blood gases (ABG)—Laboratory analysis of arterial blood to evaluate respiratory functioning by determining levels of carbon dioxide ($Paco_2$), oxygen (Pao_2), power of hydrogen (pH), oxygen saturation of the hemoglobin (Sao_2), and bicarbonate (HCO_3^-).

Arteriogram—The injection of contrast material or dye into one or more arteries to make them visible on an X-ray.

Arterioles—Smaller arteries that branch off the aorta.

Arteriosclerosis—General term to describe a number of disorders in which the arterial walls thicken and lose elasticity.

Arytenoid cartilage—Cartilage surrounding the vocal cords in the larynx and used in vocal cord movement and sound production.

Asthma—A disease process characterized by increased responsiveness of the tracheobronchial tree to various stimuli with resulting bronchospasm and inflammation of the bronchial mucosa.

Asthma attack—Episode of breathlessness associated with the symptoms of dyspnea, wheezing, paroxysmal cough, and tightness in the chest.

Atelectasis—Collapse of alveoli when the intrapleural pressure exceeds the atmospheric pressure due to accumulation of air or fluid in the pleural space.

Atherosclerosis—Thickening of large and medium-size arteries with the deposition of fatty streaks or plaques that decrease the lumen of the artery.

Atmospheric air—Air in the environment.

Atmospheric pressure—Pressure of air in the environment, measured in millimeters of mercury (mm/Hg).

Atrial gallop—(S4) is sometimes called a presystolic gallop, heard with decreased ventricular compliance (sounds like *Kentucky*).

Atrial kick—Contraction of the atria at the end of diastole, providing a 30% increase in blood return to the ventricles.

Atrioventricular node (AV node)—Area of the heart in the septal wall between the right and left ventricles that receives the electrical impulses from the sinoatrial node and conducts them to the ventricular walls.

Atrioventricular valves—Two valves between the atria and ventricles: tricuspid and mitral valves.

Auscultation—Physical assessment technique of listening for sounds in the body using a stethoscope.

Bachmann's bundle—Bundle of nerve cells traveling from the right atrium to the left atrium.

Barotrauma—Physical injury from exposure to excessive atmospheric air pressure such as occurs from deep sea diving or mechanical ventilation.

Barrel chest—Chest appears round, and the sternum appears pulled out with an increased anterior-posterior (A-P) diameter.

Base—Lower part of the lung that rests upon the diaphragm.

Base of the lung—The lowest portions of the lungs. Anteriorly, the bases of the lungs begin at the sixth intercostal space at the midclavicular line, the eighth space laterally, and the 10th to 12th intercostal spaces posteriorly.

Bicarbonate (HCO_3^-)—Compound measured on arterial blood gases.

Bilevel positive airway pressure (BIPAP)—Pressure-supported ventilation delivered via nasal or facial mask to assist inhalation, increase tidal volume, PEEP, and minute ventilation.

Black lung disease—Lung changes caused by exposure to coal dust.

Blood cultures—Blood obtained by venipuncture at three successive times to identify blood infection.

Bradypnea—Low respiratory rate, less than 12 breaths per minute.

Breath sounds—Sounds in the respiratory tract, classified by their pitch, intensity, and duration in the respiratory cycle.

Bronchi—Two mainstem bronchi, right and left, originate at the bifurcation at the carina and are surrounded by cartilage to maintain their shape.

Bronchial breath sounds—Breath sounds heard over the trachea and main stem bronchi that are high-pitched, hollow sounding, and loud.

Bronchial pneumonia—Infection involving distal airways and alveoli.

Bronchial provocation tests—Used to determine a cause-and-effect relationship between certain inhaled irritants and the reactivity of the airways.

Bronchioles—Smaller tubes without cartilage rings that branch from the bronchi and spread in an inverted treelike formation in both lungs into smaller and smaller bronchioles until they reach the terminal bronchioles.

Bronchitis—Inflammation of the tracheobronchial tree.

Bronchodilators—Quick-relief medications such as short-acting, inhaled $beta_2$-agonists that act to relax bronchial smooth muscle and dilate the airways.

Bronchography—Used to evaluate the structure of the trachea and bronchi, identifying obstruction of the tracheobronchial tree by injecting radioactive iodine through a catheter in the trachea and taking radiographic films.

Bronchophony—An increase in intensity and clarity of vocal sounds through the chest wall. Assessment technique is asking patient to repeat a phrase such as "one-two-three."

Bronchoscopy—Visualization of the trachea and bronchi with fiberoptic or rigid scopes, allowing direct visualization of the anatomy and detection of foreign bodies or tumors.

Bronchospasm—Abnormal contraction of the smooth muscle surrounding the bronchi with resultant narrowing of the airways.

Bronchovesicular breath sounds—Breath sounds heard over large airways such as the bronchi at the first and second intercostal spaces along the sternal border and between the scapulae that are intermediate in pitch and intensity with muted characteristics of both bronchial and vesicular breath sounds.

Bruits—Sounds in large vessels caused by blood turbulence over athero-sclerotic plaques.

Bullae—Air-filled spaces in the lungs following destruction of the alveolar walls.

Candidiasis—Infection of mucous membranes with *Candida albicans*.

Capillaries—Tiny, thin-walled vessels that supply the tissues with oxygenated blood.

Capillary bed—Network of communicating capillaries guarded by a band of smooth muscle called a precapillary sphincter.

Capillary filling—An assessment technique to evaluate peripheral circulation by estimating the time required for capillary refill after compression of tissue.

Capnography—Device to aid in the assessment of proper positioning of an endotracheal tube by measuring expired carbon dioxide.

Carbaminohemoglobin—Molecule with carbon dioxide attached to hemoglobin.

Cardiac catheterization—Invasive procedure using catheter insertion, dye injection, and X-rays to evaluate the coronary arteries and valves.

Cardiac tamponade—Bleeding around the heart caused by damage to the pericardium and pericardial sac with decreased ability of the heart to pump effectively.

Cardiopulmonary bypass—Extracorporeal circulation to allow surgery on the heart when the heart is stopped and the great vessels are cannulated with the circulation and oxygenation facilitated by machinery.

Carina—Location where the trachea branches into the left and right mainstem bronchi.

Cascade coughing—A technique useful in the postoperative period and with patients who have CAL or neuromuscular diseases or those who are bedridden to increase chest expansion during inhalation and more forcefully expel secretions.

Central respiratory center—Respiratory center of the brain located in the medulla oblongata and the pons which detects increased carbon dioxide levels and stimulates respiration.

Central venous pressure—The measurement of blood pressure in the right atrium using hemodynamic monitoring.

Cheilitis—Cracks in the corners of the mouth, possibly indicative of nutritional deficiencies.

Chest physical therapy (CPT)—A method to mobilize secretions and maintain airway patency and alveolar expansion with three techniques: percussion, vibration, and postural drainage.

Chest radiograph (X-ray)—Performed from the posterior-anterior and lateral views to assess pathophysiologic changes in the thorax, such as tumors, inflammation, fluid and air accumulation, integrity of bony structures, and diaphragmatic hernia.

Chronic bronchitis—Chronic condition of the lungs characterized by a hypersecretion of mucus and chronic cough, particularly in smokers.

Chronic endothelial injury theory—Theory of atherosclerosis hypothesizing that lipids deposit over the injury on the intimal wall of the arteries, and a fibrous plaque forms over this fatty core.

Closed chest drainage—Chest drainage that is closed to atmospheric pressure and allows drainage of air and/or fluid from the pleural space.

Clubbing—Increase in the angle between the nail bed and the digit. May be a sign of long-term, impaired oxygenation.

Coarse crackles—Sounds in the thorax that are louder than fine crackles with more intermittent popping sounds.

Columnar epithelial cells—Produce mucous in the respiratory tract.

Compartment syndrome—Compression of tissues and blood vessels from swelling in surrounding tissues.

Compliance—Force required to expand the lungs to a particular volume.

Computerized axial tomography (CAT) scans—Scan using X-rays and a computer to create a cross section of the body through a horizontal plane to provide information about internal structures.

Continuous positive airway pressure (CPAP)—Continuous positive airway pressure (i.e., pressure above atmospheric pressure) throughout a spontaneous breathing cycle.

Cor pulmonale—Enlargement of the heart's right ventricle due to lung disease.

Coronary arteries—Vessels that supply oxygenated blood to the myocardium.

Coronary artery bypass graft surgery (CABG)—Surgical bypass of occluded coronary vessels with blood vessel graft to improve blood flow to the myocardium.

Costochondral cartilage—The cartilage connecting the first seven pairs of ribs to the sternum.

Costochondral pain—Occurs at the connection of the ribs and cartilage and can be elicited with pressure on the area.

Costochondritis—Inflammation at the juncture of the ribs and cartilage.

CPK-MB isoenzyme—Specific component of CPK released into the bloodstream when the cardiac muscle is damaged.

Crackles—Brief, intermittent sounds that indicate the snapping open of collapsed or fluid-filled alveoli.

Creatine phosophokinase (CPK)—A cardiac enzyme when heart muscle tissue has been damaged as in a myocardial infarction.

Crepitus—Crackling feelings under the skin that indicate subcutaneous pockets of air.

Cribriform plate—Area contained in the ethmoid bone and innervated by the first cranial nerve to provide a sense of smell.

Cricoid cartilage—Cartilage that lies below the thyroid cartilage in the larynx and contains the vocal cords.

Cricothyroid membrane—Connects the cricoid and thyroid cartilages and is used for emergency access to the airway.

Critical oxygen (O_2 crit)—Oxygen sufficient for aerobic metabolism.

Cyanosis—Bluish-gray tinge to the skin, nails, or lips.

Dalton's Law—A law stating that each gas in the atmosphere contributes to the total pressure of all the gases in the atmosphere.

Dead air space—Air that remains in the nose, pharynx, trachea, bronchi, and bronchioles that is not involved in gas exchange.

Decannulation—Removal of the tracheotomy tube.

Desensitization—Process of decreasing hypersensitivity reactions and allergic responses to specific substances through repeated, small exposures to the offending substance.

Diaphragm—Principle muscle of respiration, serving as the lower boundary of the thorax and attached to the xiphoid process and the lower ribs.

Diaphragmatic breathing—Slow deliberate breaths using the abdomen and chest muscles, indicated for patients with CAL or anxiety.

Diaphragmatic excursion—The distance that the diaphragm moves with inspiration, normally 5 to 6 cm, but it may increase to as much as 10 cm with maximal inspiration.

Diastole—Resting phase of the heart cycle when the chambers of the heart fill with blood.

Diastolic pressure—Blood pressure when the ventricles are filling.

Diffusion—The random movement of molecules from areas of high concentration to areas of lower concentration; in the respiratory system this occurs across the alveolar membrane.

Diffusion capacities—A test to measure the ability of gases to diffuse across the alveolar membrane.

Directly observed treatment (DOT)—One method to improve adherence through direct observation of patients taking necessary medication.

Doppler ultrasound (DUS)—Apparatus using ultrasound waves, a special stethoscope, and a transducer with an audio unit to detect the movement of red blood cells in the blood vessels.

Dyslipidemia—A disorder of lipoprotein metabolism including lipoprotein overproduction or deficiency. Dyslipidemias may be manifested by elevation of the total cholesterol, the "bad" low-density lipoprotein (LDL) cholesterol and the triglyceride concentrations, and a decrease in the "good" high-density lipoprotein (HDL) cholesterol concentration in the blood.

Dysphagia—Difficulty swallowing.

Dyspnea—Patient perception of difficulty breathing.

Ecchymosis—Bluish discoloration of the skin caused by extravasation of blood into the subcutaneous tissues.

Echocardiograms—Noninvasive test using ultrasound waves to visualize all four chambers of the heart, assess left ventricular and valvular function, evaluate the motion of the left ventricular wall, and calculate the ejection fraction and left ventricular end diastolic pressures (LVEDP).

Egophony (E-to-A change)—Change in voice sounds transmitted through the chest wall, assessed by having the patient say "eee" and hearing "ay" with a stethoscope.

Ejection fractions (EF)—Percentage of blood that filled the left ventricle that is ejected during systole.

Elasticity—The return to the original shape after alteration by outside forces.

Electrocardiogram (EKG)—A graphic representation of the electrical activity in the conduction system of the heart.

Electrolarynx—External electronic device used to produce sounds with patients who have undergone laryngectomy.

Emphysema—Chronic disorder of the lungs characterized by loss of lung elasticity, narrowed bronchioles, and abnormal dilation of the terminal air spaces caused by the destruction of the alveolar walls.

Endarterectomy—Surgically cleaning the plaque from the artery.

Endocardium—The lining of the heart's four chambers.

Endotracheal tubes (ETT)—Polyvinylchloride tube that is passed via either the nares or mouth through the vocal cords into the trachea with the tip positioned approximately 2 to 3 cm above the carina.

End-systolic volume—Amount of blood remaining in the ventricles after systole.

Epicardium—One of three layers of the heart that is part of the serous pericardium.

Epiglottis—A thin, leaf-shaped structure of elastic cartilage that helps to protect the larynx during swallowing.

Epistaxis—Term for bleeding from the nose (nosebleeds).

Erb's point—Anatomical landmark located at the third intercostal space at the left sternal border and used during physical assessment.

Erythroplasia—Premalignant lesions on the mucous membranes or skin resembling red patches.

Erythropoietin—Hormone that stimulates bone marrow to produce red blood cells.

Esophagitis—Inflammation of the lining of the esophagus with pain on swallowing.

Eustachian tubes—A tube that connects each middle ear cavity with the posterior oropharynx.

Exhalation or expiration—Air moving out of the respiratory tract.

Expiratory reserve volume (ERV)—Amount of air that can be forcibly exhaled after normal or tidal expiration (approximately 1100 mL).

Extrinsic asthma—Physiologic change in the lower respiratory tract in response to an allergen or environmental trigger.

Extubation—Removal of a tube, such as an endotracheal tube.

Exudate—Abnormal accumulation of fluid or white blood cells on mucous membranes.

Femoral-popliteal bypass graft—Vein graft used to bypass a femoral artery occlusion from above the occlusion to a point distal to the occlusion.

Fine crackles—Sounds in the thorax similar to hair rolled between the fingers close to the ear.

Flail chest—Result of multiple rib fractures, causing a portion of the chest to "cave in" during inhalation.

Fluoroscopy—Use of a continuous stream of X-rays to assess the motion of thoracic contents.

Forced expiratory flow (FEF)—Rate of air flow during forced expiration on a flow-volume graph.

Forced expiratory volume (FEV)—Amount of air exhaled after full inhalation at various times during the exhalation (e.g., 1 second, 2 seconds, 3 seconds).

Forced vital capacity (FVC)—Amount of air expelled with maximally forced exhalation.

Friction rubs—Harsh sounds made by inflamed and rubbing pericardial or pleural tissue.

Functional residual capacity (FRC)—Amount of air remaining in the lungs at the end of normal exhalation (approximately 1200 mL).

Funnel chest (pectus excavatum)—Congenital depression of the sternum that decreases the A-P diameter.

Gangrene—Necrosis or death of tissue usually as a result of lack of blood supply.

Gingivitis—Inflammation of the gums in the mouth.

Glycolysis—The process of conversion of glycogen in liver stores to produce glucose 2,3-diphosphoglycerol (2,3-DPG), a compound involved in the release of oxygen from hemoglobin.

Goblet cells—Cells in the mucous membrane that produce mucus in the respiratory tract.

Heart failure—Heart's inability to pump sufficient amounts of blood to meet the metabolic needs of the body.

Heart murmurs—Extra heart sounds that signal valvular or other cardiac dysfunction.

Hemodynamic monitoring—System using a catheter, an infusion system, a transducer, and a monitor to directly monitor pressures in the heart and great vessels.

Hemoglobin—A compound of protein and iron in the blood that carries oxygen to the cells and carries carbon dioxide away from the cells.

Hemoglobinopathies—Defects in the structure of hemoglobin.

Hemolytic anemia—Anemia caused by premature destruction of RBCs, shortened life span of RBCs, or failure of the marrow to replace RBCs.

Hemoptysis—Blood tinged sputum arising from the thorax when coughing.

Hemothorax—The accumulation of blood in the pleural space and cavity.

High-density lipoprotein (HDL)—A lipoprotein in blood that is associated with decreased incidence of high blood pressure and heart disease (the "good" cholesterol).

Holter monitor—Ambulatory electrocardiogram.

Hyperbaric oxygen—Use of oxygen at pressures greater than atmospheric pressure to increase the amount of oxygen dissolved in the blood.

Hypercapnia—Arterial carbon dioxide concentration ($Paco_2$) greater than 50 mmHg.

Hypercoaguability—Tendency of the blood to clot more rapidly than normal.

Hyperkalemia—High serum potassium.

Hypertension—Asymptomatic disorder characterized by blood pressure consistently above determined levels.

Hypervolemia—Excessive intravascular volume.

Hypovolemia—Depleted intravascular volume.

Hypoxemia—Arterial oxygen concentration of less than 75 mmHg.

Hypoxia—Inadequate oxygenation of the tissues.

Idiopathic bronchiolitis obliterans with organizing pneumonia (BOOP)—A type of bronchiolitis obliterans, an inflammatory disease of the small airways.

Incentive spirometry—A type of sustained maximal inspiration (SMI) to help visualize inhalation.

Influenza—Infection caused by a viral infection (influenza viruses) of the respiratory tract.

Inhalation or inspiration—Air moving into the respiratory tract.

Inspection—Visual inspection of the chest begins with observing the patient's breathing and watching for chest expansion and the use of accessory muscles.

Inspiratory capacity (IC)—Amount of air that can be inhaled with maximal effort after a normal exhalation (approximately 3000 mL).

Inspiratory reserve volume (IRV)—Amount of air that can be inhaled after a normal or tidal inspiration (approximately 3300 mL).

Intercostal muscles—Muscles between the ribs that pull the ribs upward and forward, increasing the anteroposterior and transverse diameters.

Intercostal pain—Pain between the ribs that is worse during coughing and is often transient in nature.

Intercostal space—Space between the ribs that is numbered by the rib above it; e.g., the fifth intercostal space is just below the fifth rib.

Intermaxillary fixation—Procedures to wire together the upper and lower jawbones by a series of stainless steel wires and elastics.

Intermittent claudication—Pain in the extremities on exertion that is relieved by rest.

Intrapleural pressure—Pressure in the space between the visceral and parietal pleura.

Intrathoracic or intrapulmonary pressure—Pressure within the thoracic cavity, measured in millimeters of mercury (mm/Hg).

Intrinsic asthma—Nonallergic type of asthma where bronchospasm is a reaction to a virus in the upper respiratory tract, to cold air, or to exercise.

Intubation—Passage of a tube into a body opening such as an endotracheal tube inserted through the mouth and into the trachea to ensure a patent airway during the delivery of gases or anesthesia.

Iron overload—Imbalance in the body's metabolism of iron often resulting from too many blood transfusions.

Korotkoff sounds—Sounds made by alternating pressure waves in the vasculature and heard with a stethoscope when auscultating a blood pressure.

Kymograph—Recording device to measure the volume of air inspired or expired during breathing.

Kyphosis—Abnormal curvature of the spine from front to back.

Lactic dehydrogenase (LDH)—Enzyme used as a serum indicator that rises after a myocardial infarction.

Laryngectomy—Removal of the larynx to treat laryngeal cancer.

Laryngitis—Inflammation of the mucus membranes lining the larynx and sometimes the vocal cords.

Laryngopharynx—Most inferior portion of the pharynx, which opens into the larynx anteriorly and the esophagus posteriorly.

Laryngoscopy—Visualization of the larynx with fiber-optic or rigid scopes, allowing direct visualization of the anatomy and detection of foreign bodies or tumors.

Larynx—A structure in the neck commonly called the voice box, including the epiglottis, vocal cords, and glottis, surrounded by nine rings of cartilage to maintain structure, and used for airflow and sound production.

Left atrium—Chamber of the heart that receives blood from the pulmonary veins.

Left ventricle—Thick-walled chamber of the heart that pumps blood into the aorta and systemic circulation.

Left ventricular end diastolic pressures (LVEDP)—Pressure at the end of systole useful in measuring cardiac output.

Left-sided failure—Diminished emptying of the left ventricle with resulting decreased tissue perfusion and backup of blood in the pulmonary vasculature.

Leukocytosis—Increased white blood cell count.

Leukopenia—Low white blood cell count.

Leukoplakia—White patches on the mucous membranes of the mouth and pharynx.

Lobar pneumonia—Infection of entire lobe of the lung.

Lobectomy—Removal of a diseased lobe of the lung.

Lobes—Division of the lungs, two in the left lung and three in the right.

Low-density lipoprotein (LDL)—A lipoprotein in blood that is associated with increased incidence of high blood pressure and heart disease (the "bad" cholesterol).

Lung abscess—Localized inflammation and infection in the lung.

Lung capacities—Measurement of the function of the lungs.

Lung scans—Scans used to assess perfusion of the lungs by the pulmonary arteries using injectable albumin tagged with radioactive technetium and taking radiographic images.

Lung volumes—Measurement of air volumes in the lungs.

Lungs—Spongy, cone-shaped organs that are two functional units of the respiratory system, located within the thoracic cavity on either side of the heart.

Magnetic resonance imaging (MRI)—An X-ray using a powerful magnetic field and computer enhancement to create detailed, cross-sectional pictures of the human anatomy.

Mantoux skin test—Test to detect the presence of the bacillus that causes tuberculosis by injecting a small amount of purified protein (0.1 mL) intradermally on the forearm, and then read the test site 48 to 72 hours later to note any swelling and erythema.

Manubrium—Bony, middle portion of the sternum.

Mean arterial pressure—The arithmetic mean of the blood pressure in the arterial circulation.

Mean capillary pressure—The arithmetic mean of the blood pressure in the capillary circulation.

Mean corpuscular hemoglobin (MCH)—Red blood cell index used to measure the weight of hemoglobin in the RBC.

Mean corpuscular hemoglobin concentration (MCHC)—Average concentration of hemoglobin in the red blood cells.

Mean corpuscular volume (MCV)—The relative size of the red blood cell.

Mechanical ventilation—Machines to assist patient breathing by assisting or controlling ventilations, airway pressures, and percentage of inspired oxygen.

Mediastinal flutter—Movement of internal chest structures back and forth during breathing because of alternating intrathoracic chest pressures.

Mediastinal shift—Shifting the mediastinal contents to one side of the thorax due to injury or accumulation of fluid or air.

Mediastinoscopy—Visualization of the mediastinum using fiber-optic or rigid scopes passed through the suprasternal notch, allowing direct visualization of the anatomy.

Mediastinum—Space in the thoracic cavity containing the heart and great vessels, the esophagus, part of the trachea and bronchi, and the thymus gland.

Metabolic acidosis—A decreased serum bicarbonate level.

Metabolic alkalosis—An increased serum bicarbonate level.

Midclavicular line—Anatomic landmark on the thorax that runs vertically down the anterior chest wall beginning at the center of each clavicle.

Midsternal line—Anatomic landmark that is an imaginary line running vertically through the sternum and is a useful anatomic landmark on the thorax.

Miliary tuberculosis—Spread of the tuberculum bacillus to organs in the body other than the lungs.

Minute ventilation (MV)—Volume of air inspired and expired during 1 minute of normal breathing.

Mitral valve—Valve located between the left atrium and left ventricle of the heart.

Mucociliary blanket—Layer of mucous lining the air passages that protects the respiratory system by entrapping foreign particles and pathogens.

Mucositis (stomatitis)—Breakdown ulceration and/or infection of the lining of the gastrointestinal tract with oral ulcers.

Mucus clearance device (flutter)—Handheld device with a ball valve that vibrates when the patient exhales, causing vibrations to be transmitted in the airways and loosens secretions.

Mucous membrane—Membrane with a rich blood supply that contains columnar epithelial cells and goblet cells and produces mucus for the mucociliary blanket.

Multigated acquisition scanning (MUGA)—Nuclear medicine scan using an injection of technetium pertechnetate to detect ventricular function, detect aneurysms, and evaluate coronary perfusion.

Mycobacterium tuberculi—Bacilli that causes tuberculosis.

Myocardial infarction—Occlusion of a coronary artery with ischemia, hypoxia, and tissue necrosis developing in the myocardium distal to the blockage.

Myocardium—The contractile tissue of the heart.

Nares or nostrils—The two external openings to the nasal cavities lined with skin and hair follicles or vibrissae.

Nasal cannula—Low-flow oxygen delivery system used when patient requires low to medium concentrations of oxygen.

Nasal cavities or passages—The two sides of the nose divided by the nasal septum and composed of bone and cartilage—upper third of the nose, the bridge, is bony and the lower third is cartilaginous.

Nasal polyps—Grapelike masses of swollen nasal mucosa.

Nasal septum—Cartilage and bone that divides the nose into two nasal passages.

Nasal speculum—Tool used to open the nares for inspection of the nasal passages.

Nasal vestibule—Nasal passages in the anterior of the nose.

Nasolacrimal ducts—Ducts from the eyes to the nasal passages that drain tears.

Nasopharyngeal airways—Soft rubber or latex tubes that are placed through one nares into the pharynx to maintain a patent airway.

Nasopharynx—Cavity posterior to the nasal cavities containing the adenoids and the eustachian tubes and utilized for airflow.

Negative pressure ventilators—Air tight devices that enclose either the chest wall cavity or the entire body to enhance ventilatory effort without intubation by creating negative pressure around the thoracic cavity.

Nonrebreathing mask—Oxygen delivery system with a face mask and an attached reservoir bag and a one-way valve between the reservoir bag and the mask to increase the Fio_2 to greater than 60%.

Normal or physiologic splitting—Second heart sound is split on inspiration, but the split disappears on expiration.

Nosocomial pneumonia—Pneumonia that develops after admission to a healthcare facility.

Obturator—Device to block the opening of the tube or cannula during insertion.

Olfactory nerve—First cranial nerve located in the cribriform plate of the nose and used in the sense of smell.

Opening snaps—Early diastolic sound generated by the opening of a stenotic mitral valve and heard best with the diaphragm of the stethoscope.

Oral airways—Rigid plastic devices used to preserve a patent airway by maintaining the normal structure of the oropharynx.

Oropharynx—Cavity posterior to the mouth containing the palatine tonsils and uvula and used for both airflow and food intake.

Orthopnea—Patient perception of difficulty breathing when lying down.

Orthostatic hypotension—A decrease in the systolic blood pressure of more than 20 mmHg when changing from a sitting to a standing position.

Otitis media—Bacterial or viral infection of the middle ear, usually secondary to an upper respiratory tract infection.

Oxygen saturation level (Sao$_2$)—Amount of oxygen bound to hemoglobin as oxyhemoglobin.

Oxyhemoglobin—Oxygen bound to hemoglobin in red blood cells for transport to the cells.

Oxyhemoglobin dissociation curve—Graphic depiction of the relationship between oxyhemoglobin saturation and oxygen tension in the blood.

P wave—Landmark on an EKG that indicates SA node function and atrial depolarization.

Palpation—Use of hands during physical assessment of the thorax to provide information about respiratory excursion, tender areas or masses on the chest, and the presence of tactile fremitus.

Pancytopenia—Lowering of the counts of all blood components as a result of bone marrow suppression.

Papillae—Small pink nubs, often used when assessing the surface of the tongue.

Papilloma—Benign growth in the nose.

Paradoxical blood pressure or pulsus paradoxus—Decrease of greater than 10 mmHg in the systolic pressure during inspiration.

Paranasal sinuses—Mucous-lined cavities in the facial bones that connect with the nasal cavities (sphenoid, ethmoid, and maxillary).

Parietal pleura—Membranes that line the thoracic cavity.

Paroxysmal nocturnal dyspnea—Shortness of breath that awakens the patient at night.

Partial pressure—The portion of pressure contributed by different gases in air.

Partial pressure of carbon dioxide (Pco_2)—The pressure in millimeters of mercury that carbon dioxide contributes to the total atmospheric pressure.

Partial pressure of oxygen (Po_2)—The pressure in millimeters of mercury that oxygen contributes to the total atmospheric pressure.

Partial rebreathing mask—Oxygen delivery system with an attached oxygen reservoir bag to increase the Fio2 to 40–60%.

Peak expiratory flow (PEF)—Amount of air that can be forcibly exhaled after maximal inhalation.

Percussion—Technique to assess lung size, resonance and position, and diaphragmatic excursion using the fingers of both hands in a tapping motion.

Percutaneous transluminal angioplasty (PTCA)—Catheterization of the left side of the heart with fluoroscopic insertion of a balloon-tipped catheter into a blockage in a coronary artery for dilation and/or stent placement.

Perfusion—Process of pumping and circulating oxygenated blood throughout the arterial system and returning deoxygenated blood to the heart and lungs via the venous system.

Pericardium—A fibroserous sac that surrounds the heart and the roots of the great vessels.

Peripheral arterial insufficiency (peripheral arterial disease)—Diminished blood flow to the extremities due to narrowing of the arteries.

Peripheral chemoreceptors—Nubs of tissue in the carotid and aortic bodies that detect decreased oxygen levels and stimulate increased inspiratory effort.

Petechiae—Small red spots from bleeding, often associated with blood dyscrasias.

Pharyngitis—Acute inflammation of the oropharynx.

Pharynx—Cavity and passageway composed of three parts: the oropharynx, nasopharynx, and laryngopharynx.

Phrenic nerve—A nerve that stimulates contraction of the diaphragm and originates from the spinal column at the level of the third cervical vertebrae.

Physiologic dead space—Areas of the lung that are adequately ventilated but underperfused.

Physiologic shunt—Mismatch between ventilation and perfusion with a lack of oxygen to circulating blood.

Pitch—Term used to describe heart murmurs that are detected by the stethoscope; the bell picks up low-pitched sounds and the diaphragm picks up the higher-pitched sounds.

Plasma—Watery straw-colored fluid in blood and lymph that carries erythrocytes, lymphocytes, and platelets.

Platelet aggregation theory—Theory of atherosclerosis hypothesizing that platelets stimulate proliferation of smooth muscle in the vessel wall, blocking the lumen of the artery and leading to atherosclerosis.

Platelets (thrombocytes)—Smallest cells in the blood; they are produced by the bone marrow and essential for clotting.

Pleura or pleural membranes—Thin, serous membranes that encase the lungs and the thoracic cavity.

Pleural effusion—Abnormal accumulation of fluid in the intrapleural space.

Pleural fluid analysis—Fluid obtained by inserting a needle into an area of accumulation in the pleural space.

Pleural friction rub—Harsh, loud, grating sound heard over an area of pleural inflammation in the thorax.

Pleural space or cavity—A potential space between the parietal and visceral pleura in the thoracic cavity.

Pleuritic pain—Pain from inflammation of the pleural membranes that is exacerbated by deep breathing.

Pneumomediastinum—Air in the mediastinum.

Pneumonectomy—Removal of the lung.

Pneumonia—An acute inflammation of the lung tissue usually caused by inhaled bacteria with exudates and plugging of the airways.

Pneumothorax—An accumulation of air in the pleural space.

Polycythemia—An abnormally high percentage of red blood cells.

Porphyrin—The red pigment contained in hemoglobin.

Positive end-expiratory pressure (PEEP)—Positive pressure at the end of the expiratory cycle of a mechanical ventilator to maintain the inflation of the smaller airways and alveoli.

Positive pressure ventilators—Mechanical ventilation by forcing gas into the lungs under positive pressure via an artificial airway (endotracheal tube or tracheostomy tube) during inspiration.

Posterior axillary line—An anatomic landmark that is a line starting at the axilla and extending vertically down the posterior chest.

Postural hypotension—A drop in blood pressure when changing position from lying to sitting or standing.

P-R interval—Landmark on an EKG that indicates AV node conduction time (normal time 0.12 to 0.2 seconds).

Precapillary sphincters—Sphincters that regulate blood flow through the capillaries.

Preload—Pressure on the wall of the ventricles at the end of diastole just prior to contraction.

Pressure gradient—Pressure difference between the aorta, where the arterial system begins, and the right atrium, where the venous system ends.

Pressure support ventilation (PSV)—Mechanical ventilation mode where the patient's spontaneous inspiratory effort is augmented by the delivery of a preset level of positive inspiratory pressure.

Pressure-cycled ventilators—Mechanical ventilator that delivers gas until a preset pressure in the airway is attained, terminating inspiration and allowing passive expiration.

Primary pulmonary hypertension—Higher than normal pulmonary artery pressure (PAP) and increased pulmonary vascular resistance without an obvious cause.

Pulmonary angiograph—X-rays of the lungs using an injectable radiopaque material to assess perfusion of the lungs.

Pulmonary artery catheters—Triple or quadruple lumen catheters that are inserted into a large vein, such as the jugular vein, to measure pressures in the great vessels and the heart.

Pulmonary artery pressure—Pressure required to pump blood from the right side of the heart.

Pulmonary artery wedge pressure (PAWP)—The measurement of arterial pressure in the pulmonary circulation.

Pulmonary contusion—Injury to the lung.

Pulmonary edema—The accumulation of fluid in the extravascular spaces of the lung.

Pulmonary embolus—Blockage in a pulmonary artery resulting in impaired circulation to lung tissue distal to the blockage.

Pulmonary function tests (PFT)—Tests to measure airflow rates and calculate lung volumes and capacities.

Pulmonary hypertension—Condition of chronically elevated pulmonary artery pressure (PAP) and pulmonary vascular resistance.

Pulmonary mechanics—Measurements of airflow in the respiratory tract, calculated by examining airflow versus volume.

Pulmonary ventilation—Flow of gases into and out of the respiratory tract.

Pulmonic circuit—Blood vessels providing blood to the lungs with arterial and venous systems independent from the systemic circulation.

Pulmonic valve—The valve between the right ventricle and the pulmonary artery.

Pulmonic vascular resistance (PVR)—Clinical measure of the right ventricular afterload.

Pulse oximetry—Use of a spectrophotometer to determine the amount of light absorbed by hemoglobin in arterial blood as percentage of oxygenated hemoglobin as compared to the total capacity of hemoglobin available for binding, normally 96–100%.

Pulse pressure—Difference between the systolic and diastolic blood pressures.

Purkinje fibers—Myocardial fibers that carry the impulses to the myocardial cells of the ventricles.

Pursed-lip breathing—A breathing technique to increase pressure in the respiratory tract by forcibly exhaling through pursed lips.

QRS complex—Landmark on an EKG that indicates ventricular depolarization (normal time 0.06 to 0.10 seconds).

Red blood cell (erythrocyte)—Element in blood that carries hemoglobin, the molecule that binds to oxygen during transport.

Regurgitant flow—Backward blood flow through stenotic or incompetent valves in the heart.

Residual volume (RV)—Amount of air remaining in the lungs after forced, maximal expiration (approximately 1000 mL).

Resistance—Force that opposes movement that has an inverse relationship with flow: the greater the resistance, the lower the blood or air flow.

Respiratory excursion—The span that the chest expands on deep inspiration, usually 5–8 cm.

Rest pain—Pain in an extremity at rest as the result of arterial occlusion.

Reticulocytes—Immature red blood cells released by the bone marrow during times of high production or need.

Reye's syndrome—A rare complication of influenza and aspirin therapy that causes liver failure and encephalitis, particularly in children.

Rhinitis—Inflammation of the mucous membranes lining the nasal passages.

Rhinitis medicamentosa—Rebound nasal congestion after prolonged antihistamine use.

Rhinotracheitis—Inflammation of the mucous membranes of the nose and throat from viral exposure.

Rhonchi—Low-pitched snoring sounds, heard on exhalation, that change or disappear with coughing.

Right atrium—Chamber of the heart that receives blood from the vena cavae and the venous systemic circulation.

Right ventricle—Chamber of the heart that pumps blood to the pulmonary artery and pulmonic circulation.

Right-sided failure (cor pulmonale)—Reduced emptying of the right ventricle with right ventricular hypertrophy, systemic venous congestion, and major organ engorgement.

Rubor—Bright red coloration in an extremity—sometimes associated with arterial insufficiency.

Scalene—Muscle involved in thoracic expansion.

Scoliosis—Abnormal curvature of the spine from side to side.

Secondary pulmonary hypertension—Higher than normal pulmonary artery pressure (PAP) and increased pulmonary vascular resistance resulting from cardiac and/or pulmonary diseases.

Severe acute respiratory syndrome (SARS)—A new deadly form of pneumonia that emerged in 2003.

Sickle cell crises—Episodes when a blood vessel is blocked by sickled red blood cells, causing damage to tissues and organs.

Sickle cell anemia—Congenital disorder where hemoglobin deoxygenates and takes on a sickle shape, occluding small vessels.

Sinoatrial node (SA node)—A cluster of cells in the right atrium of the heart that generates electrical impulses to contract the muscle cells of the heart.

Sinusitis—Infection and/or inflammation of the mucous membranes lining the sinuses.

Sonorous wheezes—Low-pitched snoring sounds heard in the respiratory tract, usually produced by secretions in large airways and may clear with coughing.

Sphygmomanometer—A tool for measuring blood pressure with an inflatable cuff exerting pressure over a muscular artery to the point that blood flow can be obstructed and then the pressure lowered so that the pressure at which blood flow returns can be heard by a stethoscope.

Spirometry—Measurement of lung capacities and volumes with a spirometer.

Sputum cultures—Laboratory test of sputum to identify infectious bacteria, check for malignancy, and detect the tubercle bacillus, the organism that causes tuberculosis.

Sputum—Mucous arising from the lower respiratory tract.

ST segment—Landmark on an EKG that indicates time between complete depolarization of the ventricles and complete repolarization.

Starling's law of the heart—The energy of the contraction of the cardiac muscle is related to the stretch of the fibers prior to contraction.

Status asthmaticus—Severe, prolonged asthma attack that does not respond to conventional treatment.

Sternocleidomastoid muscles—Muscles in the shoulder and upper back involved in thoracic expansion.

Sternum—Bony structure at the center of the anterior thorax to which seven pair of ribs are attached.

Stethoscope—Tool to assess and auscultate sounds in the body.

Stress tests (exercise EKGs)—Noninvasive tests used to evaluate cardiac function and perfusion with increasing levels of activity.

Stridor—Coarse loud sounds when breathing, often indicative of airway obstruction.

Stroke volume—Amount of blood ejected from the ventricle during systole.

Subcutaneous emphysema—Air in the tissues around the tracheostomy.

Supraglottic swallowing—Technique to protect lower airways by taking a deep breath and holding it prior to swallowing.

Suprasternal notch—Depression just above the sternum between the two clavicles.

Surfactant—A phospholipid protein secreted by cells called type II pneumocytes within the alveoli that reduces the surface tension in the alveoli, increasing the surface area for gas exchange.

Systemic circuit—Blood vessels that supply all of the body's tissues, except the lungs, with blood.

Systemic vascular resistance (SVR)—Resistance of the entire circulatory system to blood flow.

Systole—Contraction of the heart muscle, expelling blood from the heart.

Systolic pressure—Blood pressure when both ventricles are contracting.

T wave—Landmark on an EKG that represents ventricular repolarization.

Tachypnea—High respiratory rate—rate greater than 20 breaths per minute.

Tactile fremitus—Palpable vibrations of the voice that are transmitted down the tracheobronchial tree and through the chest wall.

Tension pneumothorax—Increased pressure in the pleural space caused by damaged visceral pleura that allows air to escape into the pleural space during inspiration while trapping air in the pleural space during expiration.

Thalassemia—Congenital disorder of defective and reduced hemoglobin synthesis.

Thoracentesis—Insertion of a needle into the pleural space to drain the fluid or air or to obtain samples for pathological analysis.

Thoracic cage—Bony outer shell of the thorax is comprised of the sternum, thoracic vertebrae, and 12 pairs of ribs that are connected to the thoracic vertebrae of the posterior spine.

Thoracoabdominal pump—Pressure changes in the chest and abdomen that facilitate blood return to the heart.

Thoracotomy—Surgical opening into the thoracic cavity.

Thorax—Contains the lungs, heart, and great vessels.

Thrills—Palpable vibrations that may accompany loud, rumbling heart murmurs.

Throat culture—Swab is brushed along the back of the oropharynx and then sent to the laboratory to culture the growth and identify antibiotic sensitivity.

Thrombocytopenia—Low platelet count.

Thrombolytic agents—Medications used to dissolve thrombi that are occluding coronary arteries (streptokinase, tissue plasminogen activator [tPA], and anisoylated plasminogen-streptokinase activator complex [APSAC]).

Thyroid cartilage—Cartilage surrounding the larynx, commonly called the Adam's apple.

Tidal volume (TV)—Amount of air inspired or exhaled during normal, quiet breathing; approximately 500 mL in a 70 kg person but can range from 400 to 700 mL and reach 4500 mL during maximal exercise.

Time-cycled ventilators—Mechanical ventilator that delivers gas for a preset amount of time.

Tonsils—Nubs of lymphatic tissue in the pharynx: lingual, palatine, and pharyngeal tonsils.

Total lung capacity (TLC)—Amount of air in the lungs at the end of maximal inspiration (approximately 6000 mL). It is also the total of the four lung volumes (TV + IRV + ERV + RV = TLC).

Total peripheral resistance (TPR)—Resistance of the entire circulatory system to blood flow.

Trachea—A flexible tube that connects the larynx with the major bronchi of the lungs.

Tracheal breath sounds—Sounds heard over the trachea, normally high-pitched and loud.

Tracheoesophageal fistula—Abnormal opening between the trachea and esophagus due to congenital abnormality or erosion of the trachea from the cuff of an endotracheal tube.

Tracheomalacia—Erosion of the trachea from excessive pressure from the cuff of an endotracheal tube.

Tracheostomy—Surgically created opening in the trachea between the third or fourth ring of the trachea.

Tracheostomy tubes—Type of artificial airway placed into a surgically created opening in the trachea for ventilation, removal of secretions, or after laryngectomy.

Tracheotomy—A surgical incision into the trachea to create an airway in the area of the second, third, and fourth tracheal rings.

Transesophageal echocardiography—Placement of a transducer into the esophagus to evaluate the anatomy and motion of the cardiac chambers.

Transillumination—A technique for examining the sinuses using an external light source to shine through the hollow chamber of the sinuses in the facial bones.

Transmural myocardial infarction—Tissue necrosis developing after blockage of coronary artery, extending through all three layers of cardiac tissue and affecting ventricular wall motion and cardiac output.

Transtracheal catheter—Small catheter percutaneously inserted between the second and third tracheal cartilage for patients who require home oxygen therapy.

Tricuspid valve—The valve between the right atrium and right ventricle.

Troponin (I and T)—Serum indicator of myocardial damage.

Tuberculosis—Infection of lung and other tissues by the *Mycobacterium tuberculi*.

Tunica externa—Connective tissue sheath that protects and supports a blood vessel.

Tunica intima—Innermost layer lining the inside of a blood vessel.

Tunica media—Concentric layers of smooth muscle within a matrix of collagen and elastic fibers in a blood vessel.

Turbinates—Bony projections in the nasal passages that are covered with mucous membrane.

Urticaria—Local wheals or raised, red circular lesions that may be itchy and are associated with allergic responses.

Uvula—Fleshy protrusion from the soft palate in the posterior oropharynx.

Vascular resistance—Friction caused by blood moving along the vessel wall.

Venous reserve—Reservoir of blood for the body in the venous blood system.

Ventilation—Entire process of airflow between the human body and the atmosphere.

Ventilation/perfusion ratio (V/Q)—The ratio of perfusion of the pulmonary capillaries (Q) on alveolar ventilation (V).

Ventilation-perfusion scans (V/Q)—Scan used to assess lung perfusion and ventilation, particularly to detect pulmonary emboli.

Ventricular gallop—(S3) heart sound that is a low-frequency sound and best heard with the bell of the stethoscope, and is one of the first signs of congestive heart failure (sounds like *Tennessee*)

Venturi (Venti) mask—Oxygen delivery under pressure is forced through various-sized orifices in a mask.

Venules—Small vessels in the venous circulation.

Vesicular breath sounds—Breath sounds heard over the majority of the lung fields that are soft, low-pitched sounds heard longer during inspiration than expiration.

Vibration—Technique involving the placement of both hands on the thorax and pressing and vibrating the rib cage over an area of affected lung to loosen secretions.

Vibrissae—Hair follicles lining the nasal passages that are the first line of defense for filtering out foreign objects and preventing them from being inhaled into the respiratory tract.

Visceral pleura—Membranes that cover the lungs and the fissures between the lobes.

Viscosity—Resistance to flow caused by the friction of molecules in a liquid (i.e., thinner liquids, such as water, have a lower viscosity than thicker liquids).

Vital capacity (VC)—Maximal amount of air that can be exhaled after maximal inspiration (approximately 5000 mL).

Vocal cords—Two folds of mucous membrane that when tightened allow phonation to occur.

Volume-cycled ventilators—Mechanical ventilator that delivers gas to a patient at a preset volume.

Wheezes—High-pitched, shrill, whistling sounds with a musical quality heard in the thorax and created by air moving through narrowed tracheobronchial airways.

Whispered petroliloquy—An assessment technique using the transmission of sound through the chest wall when the patient is asked to repeatedly whisper a phrase such as "ninety-nine." It is louder over an area of consolidated lung tissue.

White blood cells (leukocytes)—Component of blood useful in fighting infection.

Xerostomia—Diminished saliva production (dry mouth).

Zone of injury—Myocardium that suffers damage due to hypoxia from the infarction.

Zone of ischemia—Myocardium that is ischemic due to the infarction but is viable.

Zone of necrosis—Myocardium that dies due to the infarction.